CHASING SUMMITS

In Pursuit of High Places and an Unconventional Life

GARRY HARRINGTON

Appalachian Mountain Club Books
Boston, Massachusetts

AMC is a nonprofit organization, and sales of AMC Books fund our mission of protecting the Northeast outdoors. If you appreciate our efforts and would like to become a member or make a donation to AMC, visit outdoors.org, call 800-372-1758, or contact us at Appalachian Mountain Club, 5 Joy Street, Boston, MA 02108.

outdoors.org/publications/books

Distributed by National Book Network

Front cover photograph © Garry Harrington
Interior photographs © Garry Harrington, unless otherwise noted
Maps by Rebecca M. Fullerton and Abigail Coyle © Appalachian Mountain Club
Cover design by Matthew Simmons, myselfincluded.com
Interior design by Abigail Coyle

Library of Congress Cataloging-in-Publication Data
Names: Harrington, Garry, author.
Title: Chasing summits : in pursuit of high places and an unconventional life / Garry Harrington.
Description: Boston, Massachusetts : Appalachian Mountain Club Books, [2016]
 | Includes bibliographical references.
Identifiers: LCCN 2016014913| ISBN 9781628420456 (pbk.) | ISBN 9781628420463
 (epub) | ISBN 9781628420470 (mobi)
Subjects: LCSH: Harrington, Garry. | Harrington, Garry--Travel. |
 Mountaineering. | Mountaineers--United States--Biography.
Classification: LCC GV199.92.H354 A3 2016 | DDC 796.522092 [B] --dc23 LC record available at https://lccn.loc.gov/2016014913

The paper used in this publication meets the minimum requirements of the American National Standard for Information Sciences-Permanence of Paper for Printed Library Materials, ANSI Z39.48-1984. ∞

Interior pages contain 30% post-consumer recycled fiber.
Cover contains 10% post-consumer recycled fiber.
Printed in the United States of America,
using vegetable-based inks.

10 9 8 7 6 5 4 3 2 1   16 17 18 19 20 21 22

FSC
www.fsc.org
MIX
Paper from
responsible sources
FSC® C005010

CONTENTS

CHASING SUMMITS

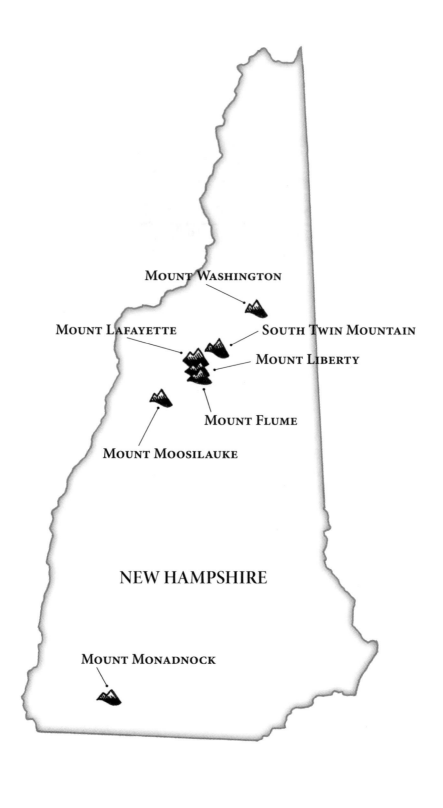

MOUNT WASHINGTON

MOUNT LAFAYETTE

SOUTH TWIN MOUNTAIN

MOUNT LIBERTY

MOUNT FLUME

MOUNT MOOSILAUKE

NEW HAMPSHIRE

MOUNT MONADNOCK

Chapter 1
2000-2004

A PASSION IGNITED

TOO MANY PEOPLE TODAY FAIL TO LIVE MEANINGFUL, FULFILLING LIVES. OH, everyone starts out with good intentions. As children, we all had dreams and aspirations and made bold declarations that we were going to grow up to become astronauts or firemen or even the president.

But eventually most of us forget our dreams and slip silently and willingly into a scripted life marked by a mundane, nine-to-five existence. On the endless, corporate treadmill, we compromise our souls for a weekly paycheck. The grind is punctuated only by vacations—or worse, "*stay*-cations," in which we accomplish little more than catching up on sleep or yard work. And then it's back to the grind the following Monday. Our precious short-term security too often leads to a lifelong emptiness, a soul left catatonic as the body is overtaken by old age and death without ever having really lived.

I know. I too was on that path for much of my adult life. But fortunately, I discovered it didn't have to be that way. I shook off the bonds of an uninspiring existence by rediscovering what I had loved as a youth: the freedom of nature, of climbing to the mountaintops and looking beyond at all the possibilities. Of the crispness of the alpine air in my lungs, the fury of the untethered wind in my face, and the limitless boundaries of my soul being filled with unfettered joy. But it didn't start easily. Or quickly. Or auspiciously. It took more than one hard look at myself and my choices, and the first one may have been the hardest of all.

By sheer coincidence, January 1, 2000—the first day of the new millennium— was the day my life changed forever. My second wife, Debbie, sat on the couch looking at photo albums with some of the kids—one of hers and two of mine. I walked past, glancing at the upside-down album and noticed a picture of her and an overweight man standing on the deck of a ship.

"Who's that fat guy you're with?" I remarked half jokingly.

She raised her eyebrows, tilted her head, and gave me that look that said I should have already known the answer. She slowly spun the album around and my eyes bulged as I recognized the picture from our recent cruise to the Bahamas. The face I was staring at was my own.

What had happened to me? In five years of marriage, I had transformed from an active, fit, everyday competitive runner into a puffy-cheeked doughboy. The scales—and that photo—did not lie.

"My God," I thought, "I look like the Michelin Man!"

In my college days, I ran every day and, blessed with high metabolism, I ate anything I wanted. I never gained an ounce. While attending college close to Burlington, Vermont, I climbed nearby Mount Mansfield often, watching the sun shimmering on Lake Champlain, flanked by the Adirondacks behind. But nearly twenty years had passed since those carefree days.

Upon graduation in the spring of 1982, my life changed in record time. That same year I got married, became a father, and began my career as a sportswriter. Hiking and climbing took a backseat, and those memories were put away as completely as the old external-frame backpack that I found in storage at my dad's house many years later. I had forgotten I ever owned it.

Ten years, three kids, and one divorce later, I was a single dad raising my children by myself in the small town of Hinsdale, New Hampshire, still working as the sports editor of the newspaper in nearby Brattleboro, Vermont. In 1995, though, I met Debbie. She was also a single parent, raising two teenagers. After several months of dating, we decided to blend our families.

But life never stopped. I lost my job as sports editor at the Brattleboro paper after an ownership change, and for the first time in my life I struggled with depression, second-guessing my competence as a journalist. My faith in myself was restored soon after when I landed the same job at the *Keene Sentinel* and we made the 20-mile move to a new town for a fresh start.

At some point during all the tumult, running no longer was a daily priority. In my 20s and early 30s, this hadn't been a problem. Playing softball kept me from being entirely sedentary, but hadn't prevented me from packing on 40 unwanted pounds, and I was putting on weight faster than a sumo wrestler eating *chankonabe* stew. The weight stuck to my 6-foot-1 frame as if I were wearing Velcro. It took seeing myself in that photo to realize that something had to change.

"The streak's over" came the words on the other end of the phone one morning on deadline at the *Sentinel,* where I'd been sports editor for the previous two years.

"Who *is* this?" I asked the caller.

"This is Larry Davis from Jaffrey," the voice said. "My streak of climbing Mount Monadnock every day is over. I got pneumonia last week and it put me in the hospital. My streak ended at 2,850 consecutive days."

Now I remembered. Larry Davis was sort of a local legend, by his own account having climbed the 3,165-foot sentinel that stands over Cheshire County in southwestern New Hampshire every day for nearly the past eight years. Larry had pretty much become synonymous with Monadnock—the most regular climber on what is recognized by many as the most-climbed mountain in the United States.

I quickly wrote the story, located a file photo of Larry, and ran the article on the front page of the Sports section under the headline, "Climber's Streak Ends."

After we went to press, one of my co-workers, who had been at the paper much long than I, pulled me aside. "You know, this Larry Davis guy is not considered very credible," he said. "No one knows if he's really up there every day and a lot

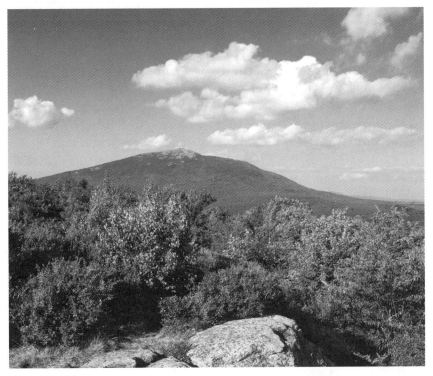

Mount Monadnock as seen from Gap Mountain in Troy, New Hampshire. Photo by Jerry Monkman.

of people don't believe him. I wouldn't have trusted him like that."

"Have you ever met him?" I asked.

"No," he replied.

Well, I thought, maybe I should go meet this guy and find out for myself.

The next day—coincidentally just a few days shy of my fortieth birthday—I packed a lunch and drove the 20 miles to Monadnock State Park. I climbed the White Dot Trail, which ascends about 1,800 feet in less than 2 miles over rocky granite slabs. Monadnock was far from my first mountain—I had climbed it a handful of times previously—but it was the first one I had hiked in quite some time. I'd forgotten how much I had enjoyed hiking and climbing in my younger days. I had forgotten the anticipation of a day above treeline that you get when you pull into the parking lot at the trailhead, your heart racing as you lace up your boots to begin a climb.

Out of breath on the mountain's open, barren summit, I could see snowcapped Mount Washington—the highest peak in the Northeast—far to the north, as well as the entire Boston skyline silhouetted against the eastern horizon. Though it hasn't been possible for decades because of air pollution and haze, hikers could once see all six New England states and the Atlantic Ocean from this perch. But it wasn't always that way.

Legend has it that, in the early 1800s, local ranchers set fire to Monadnock's upper flanks, hoping to drive out the wolves preying on their flocks. The wolves never returned, but neither did the summit's trees. The resulting view has attracted millions of climbers ever since, including the likes of Henry David Thoreau and Ralph Waldo Emerson, both of whom were inspired by the solitude they found on the craggy slopes of what Thoreau called his "temple."

I had barely recovered when Larry appeared out of nowhere, almost like the gray ghosts of the mountain's lost wolves. I recognized him instantly, not from the picture we'd run in the paper, but from the description I had gotten: "He looks like Willie Nelson's *grand*father," I'd been told. Well, not quite. Larry *was* a bit ragged, with his red gym shorts over his sweatpants, crusty T-shirt, and trademark bandanna holding back his long, graying hair. Maybe Willie Nelson's *brother*. Though he was in outstanding physical shape from climbing every day, his face certainly looked well beyond his 39 years.

Introducing myself, I was immediately convinced of Larry's sincerity. He had a firm, matter-of-fact handshake and a straight-shooting demeanor. As I would soon learn, Larry had what many would call "faults." He smoked too much pot, had a considerable drinking problem, was usually in need of a shower, and was always in need of social graces. But I found his word to be as solid as the granite on which we stood. I had no doubt his streak was legitimate.

Larry and I quickly became hiking buddies, and I soon established myself as the newest "regular" on Monadnock.

The mountain was my salvation. I gained its lofty summit often enough that my extra pounds began to melt away as fast as the snow on its precipitous slopes during spring thaw. I reached Monadnock's summit an estimated sixty times in 2000—before I started keeping track. I started looking—and feeling—like my old self again.

Though my life was now firmly implanted on the rocks of Monadnock, my marriage was on the rocks as well. Our chaotic family life resembled *The Brady Bunch* in theory only. Of the five kids, three had grown up and moved out and my youngest would soon be living with his mother during his final year of high school. Debbie and I were on divergent paths. Hers led to South Carolina, where her daughter had moved a couple of years before. Mine led up and down the steep slopes of Monadnock, and I was there almost every day. It became my second home, my sanctuary. On the summit, I was immune to the everyday troubles that lay below. I didn't look back.

The more I climbed Monadnock, the more I wanted to tackle more serious peaks. In May 2001, I traveled to the Canary Islands, intending to climb a 12,000-foot volcano. I decided to take Larry with me, even though he had been outside his native Northeast only once before, when he spent a couple of his high school years in Florida. The highest either of us had climbed before was the 6,288-foot summit of Mount Washington, and my only experience on that famed Rockpile had been a run on the auto road; its trails still scared me. Out of his comfort zone, Larry might as well have been "Crocodile" Dundee.

In fact, that's exactly what the other guests at our condo called Larry during our weeklong stay. With his gray sweatpants, red shorts, and blue bandanna, Larry stuck out like a proverbial sore thumb among the better-groomed guests. But that didn't bother him any.

We spent the first half of the week exploring Gran Canaria, the third largest of the Canaries' seven main islands. A couple of days later, we boarded a hydrofoil to Tenerife, the biggest island in the Canaries. We had been able to see Pico de Teide from the upper reaches of Gran Canaria days before, but now the volcano loomed above us as we approached the port of Santa Cruz. The mountain dominated the landscape, as it had in 1492 when the erupting Teide was the last thing Columbus saw of the Old World as he headed across the Atlantic into the unknown. For us, Teide was more than a landmark: its 12,200-foot summit was the reason we'd come to the Canaries.

The drive from Santa Cruz was scintillating. We climbed through several microclimates and biomes before topping out above 7,000 feet to discover otherwordly views that made us think we had suddenly landed on another planet. In fact, Tenerife's barren, lifeless landscape has hosted tests for NASA's prototype Mars rovers and movie sets including *One Million Years B.C.* and the original *Planet of the Apes.*

We left the car at an abandoned trailhead—wondering whether it would still be there when we returned—then started climbing to the Refugio Altavista, located at about 10,700 feet, where we would spend the night before summiting in the morning. Before long, Larry was laboring in the thin air of an altitude he had never before experienced. Several times he sat down for long stretches, complaining of a violent headache. I eased his burden by taking his backpack—as well as my own—and headed for the hut, still a couple of hours' hike above us.

I was one of only a handful of people at the refuge at first. After a seeming eternity, Larry finally arrived late in the afternoon—long after a gondola had brought the rest of the evening's guests. We were the only ones who had hiked up.

The next morning, Larry was feeling considerably better and we headed for the summit, still about 1,500 feet above us. It was such a cold and windy day—even though it was May—that when we arrived at the summit we stayed only long enough to take some pictures, which is one of Larry's hobbies. But we did exchange a couple of high-fives for achieving new heights for both of us.

We were back at the car by early afternoon, much relieved to see it still there. We headed for the south side of the island, and were back at sea level little more than 2 hours after we had stood on the summit. Where else, we thought, could someone be on a 12,200-foot summit in the morning and swimming in the ocean in the afternoon? Maybe Hawaii is the only other place on Earth where this is possible.

I returned from the Canaries a more confident hiker and looked forward to my next adventure. It came later that fall, soon after 9/11, when I traveled to the tiny Caribbean island of Tobago for a weeklong stay that included some trekking in the rain forest. But, for the most part, I was content to simply continue my nearly daily ritual on Monadnock.

Life was still chaotic over the next few years. Debbie and I had divorced. I entered into a new relationship that ended in late 2003, just weeks before I also lost my job at the *Keene Sentinel.* The mountain was a centering constant amid the variables. I even found a house-sitting gig right at the base just a short walk from a trailhead, enabling me to climb Monadnock every day that winter. And by then, I was looking to up the ante once again.

My opportunity came during a chance encounter on Monadnock on Christmas Day 2003, when I ran into another hiker on the trail, a competitive mountain biker from Shrewsbury, Massachusetts, named Karen Potter, who was hiking alone that morning. In early January, Karen informed me that she and a friend had plans for the following weekend to climb 4,802-foot Mount Moosilauke, and she invited me to join them.

Living in New England, the White Mountains of northern New Hampshire were a logical starting place for more rugged, challenging hikes. My fellow Monadnock climbers were always talking about their weekend trips to the Whites to climb in places I had only read about, such as the rugged trails of Mount Washington and the "Prezzies," the "Pemis," and Franconia Notch. Across the nearly 800,000 acres of the White Mountain National Forest, the forty-eight tallest peaks all stand above 4,000 feet—almost 1,000 feet higher than Monadnock. The Appalachian Mountain Club's Four Thousand Footer Club recognizes those who have climbed them all. Karen was working on this list, and she needed to bag Mount Moosilauke, the westernmost and tenth highest of these Four Thousand Footers.

But for all of my excitement to start a new adventure, there certainly was some trepidation to make my first venture to the Whites. I had read the stories about how dangerous those mountains can be for the uninitiated. At least 150 people have died on Mount Washington alone since 1849, not to mention on peaks elsewhere in the White Mountain National Forest. Many of the victims were skilled, prepared hikers. Many of the deaths occurred on beautiful summer days that turned deadly above treeline, when wintry conditions swept in unexpectedly. These stories confirmed for me that the home to the "worst weather in the world" was no place to fool around.

It was a calm, clear, and cold January day as we began our climb up the Gorge Brook Trail to the summit. When we emerged above treeline, we were greeted by a world I had never before encountered. The wind raged in a tumultuous fury at almost 70 MPH, driving us backward and nearly knocking us off our feet several times. Wind-blown ice crystals stung like tiny shards of glass on our exposed cheeks. We made the summit and then staggered back to the safety of the trees. Once there, we finally caught our breath and could talk to each other.

It was exhilarating.

I was hooked.

Excitedly, I returned to the Whites the next weekend with Karen, climbing Mounts Flume and Liberty with her and some of her cycling friends. We summited despite temperatures that were well below freezing, remnants of an arctic blast that had come through earlier in the week. It had been another exhilarating day.

But on the drive home, I got a jarring phone call from my friend Jay Bradford, who frequently climbed with Larry and me, that left me shaking by the side of the highway.

In the summer of 2003, on the slopes of Monadnock, I had met Ken Holmes, a seasonal Monadnock State Park Ranger who lived in nearby Athol, Massachusetts. Ken, a 37-year-old father of five, often ran up and down the White Dot Trail with no shirt on, carrying a cassette player and wearing headphones. Larry, Jay, and I had thought Ken was a bit standoffish, because he didn't stop to talk to anyone. One day when he darted past us on his way down, I decided to chase him down. Two years of training on Monadnock had turned me into a top downhill runner on technical terrain, and I soon caught and passed Ken, who was so surprised that he almost dropped his cassette player.

At the bottom, we finally talked for the first time, and he asked me to teach him how to descend with such reckless abandon. I agreed, hoping that training with him would help make me faster on the climbs. We quickly became friends, but it was now late in the year and his seasonal position at Monadnock—a job he had gotten after he was laid off from his previous job as a gravedigger—was ending. Our training time was put on hold until the following spring.

In the meantime, Ken's runs up and down Monadnock had been preparing him for a solo winter "Pemi Traverse," a 32-mile loop over eight or more 4,000-footers in the Pemigewasset Wilderness. This was the kind of hike that most people attempt only during the summer, as it is ranked the second-hardest day hike in the United States by *Backpacker* magazine. This type of trek was nothing new to him. He loved being alone, up high, in the harsh winter conditions.

I didn't know that Ken had set out on his traverse in the days between my trips up Moosilauke and the Franconia Ridge. He was out for a few days when that arctic blast started to move in, but had phoned a friend to tell him that while he was pretty cold, he was snug in his tent and looking forward to better weather in the morning.

But better weather didn't come. It turned sharply worse, and the coldest conditions in nearly fifty years descended south from Canada like cruel, icy fingers. Unbeknownst to Ken, he was firmly in its grasp. Nearby Mount Washington recorded temperatures of 44 degrees below zero Fahrenheit, and winds of 92 MPH that created a windchill that neared 100 degrees below; the conditions could have been only marginally better in the Pemis, which are more than a thousand feet lower. Rather than turn back, Ken—never one to quit—

plodded on into the teeth of this wind until he was apparently pinned down near the summit of South Twin, about as far from help as he could be in the remote White Mountain National Forest.

The exhilaration I had felt during my hike on Flume and Liberty that day was still etched in my mind when Jay's phone call jarred me back to reality as I cruised along I-93 toward Tilton. His news of Ken's tragic death stunned me. Ken's frozen body had been found face down in the middle of the Appalachian Trail just below the summit of South Twin, a foreboding 4,900-foot peak in the middle of the remote Pemigewasset Wilderness, just a few miles as the crow flies from where I had been hiking earlier in the day. My heart sank.

Kenny left a wife and five kids—and a lot of questions unanswered. I tried to answer some of them when I researched his final climb and wrote a story that was published in the *Boston Globe Magazine*. Some of the others back at Monadnock wondered if I was wired a little too similarly to Ken and might tempt the same fate someday.

I could understand their concern, but as tragic as Ken's death was, it has always reminded me to make safety my first priority in the mountains, and it never deterred me from my newfound passion. I was determined to methodically check off peaks from lists, one by one.

After just two weekends in the Whites, the peakbagging bug had already bitten me, despite Ken's death. With three of the forty-eight New Hampshire Four Thousand Footers completed, I began looking at the list and planning more trips to the Whites. I dived in with purpose and commitment. I became a peakbagger.

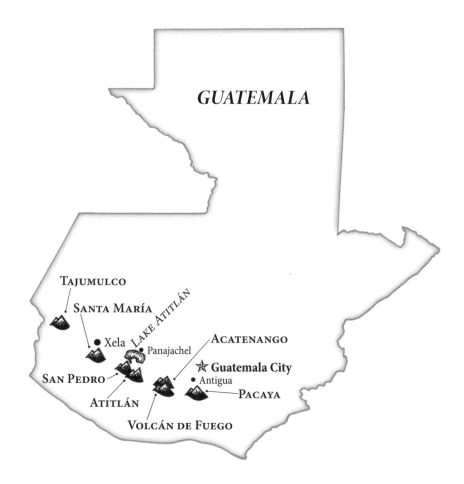

GUATEMALA

TAJUMULCO

SANTA MARÍA

Xela

LAKE ATITLÁN

Panajachel

ACATENANGO

☆ Guatemala City

SAN PEDRO

Antigua

ATITLÁN

PACAYA

VOLCÁN DE FUEGO

Chapter 2
2004–2005

SPREADING MY WINGS

IN EARLY 2004, ABOUT THIS SAME TIME AS I STARTED HIKING THE WHITES IN earnest, my job at the *Keene Sentinel* suddenly ended. And, for the first time in a long time, I considered taking some time off. I began to question why I was working so hard for so little return, in an industry I could clearly see was in a downward spiral because of the Internet. Now, don't get me wrong: I loved being a sportswriter. It had been the only thing I wanted to be from the age of 13, when I was first published in a local weekly newspaper. While still in high school, I had gotten a part-time job covering sports for the local daily, and pursued a journalism degree in college. I had spent the next twenty years in the business, a notebook in my hand and a camera strapped around my neck.

I had covered everything from Little League baseball to the Red Sox and the Patriots, local road races to the Boston Marathon, from cycling in the summer to skiing in the winter. I had interviewed athletes such as Tour de France champion Lance Armstrong; Olympic skiers Phil and Steve Mahre and Bill Koch; tennis players Andre Agassi, Michael Chang, and Jimmy Connors; Red Sox stars Bill Lee and Carlton Fisk; the Celtics' Paul Pierce; and many others. But I will never forget the time I was the victim of one of John McEnroe's famous tirades or the time I made Cal Ripken cry.

In 1985, the Volvo International tennis tournament moved from Bretton Woods in northern New Hampshire to Stratton Mountain, a ski resort within my coverage area as sports editor of the *Brattleboro Reformer*. That first year, John McEnroe—as famous among fans and journalists for his temper as he was for his world-class skill—played Ivan Lendl for the title, and I was fortunate enough to be courtside, taking pictures from the photographers' area during the weeklong event. During one match, McEnroe was serving when the photographer next to me loaded a roll of film. The *click, click, click* of the auto film advance—this was well before the digital days—seemed to echo from the hillsides; the crowd of 10,000 had been completely silent, lest McEnroe berate them, as he was known to do. Distracted by the loud noise, McEnroe stopped. The ball, left untouched in midair, bounced to the hard surface of the court. He erupted into one of his patented tirades.

"Unbelievable!" I remember him screaming.

He turned to the bank of photographers and settled upon me as the probable culprit, since I was on the end closest to him.

"How many times do I have to tell you [jerks] not to do that in the middle of my serve!" he bellowed as he rushed toward me.

He continued screaming, banging his racket on the top of the curtained railing that was only inches in front of my face. All the while, he looked straight at me with those crazed, menacing eyes, ignoring the photographer to my right, who was conveniently "busy" pretending to search for something in his camera bag. I wished I had had the courage to point him out as the real offender, taking the target off my forehead. Instead, I sat there and weathered the beating with 10,000 pairs of eyes piercing the back of my head. It was embarrassing, but how many people can claim to have absorbed one of McEnroe's famous rants?

In 1982, I was at Fenway Park for a game against the Baltimore Orioles, wandering around by the batting cages during team workouts thanks to a pregame field pass. I snapped a picture of Orioles rookie Cal Ripken Jr. standing next to the batting cage talking with his dad, Cal Ripken Sr., who would later become the team's manager, but who, at this time, was still the third base coach. Aesthetically, it may have been one of the best photos I had ever taken—the lighting and contrast were perfect—and the black-and-white photo became one of my prized possessions, sitting framed on my desk at the office for many years.

Nineteen years later, I acquired another Fenway Park field pass before Cal Junior's last game there on his final road trip. This time, I brought the photo with me and when he came onto the field to warm up, I approached him with it. His dad had died of cancer two years before after having spent thirty-six years in the Orioles organization. Cal looked at the photo with keen interest.

"Would you like me to sign it for you?" he asked.

"No," I said, "I want to give this to you. I feel it would mean far more to you than it ever could to me."

Instantly, the bluest eyes I have ever seen started to tear up. Cal Ripken Jr.

was about to cry.

He quickly regained his composure and thanked me profusely, handing the photo to his traveling secretary, telling him not to let it get damaged. Then he asked what he could do for me. I said I would like a photo of the two of us together, which we took with the famed Green Monster in the background, Cal's arm around my shoulder. I had it framed and it immediately became the new prized possession on my desk. Cal Junior retired that year after setting a major league record of 2,632 consecutive games played.

A few years later, a friend who had once worked for the Orioles helped me mail the photo to the club for Cal to sign. It took nearly a year for the photo to be returned to me, but now it sits in my home office adorned by the words, "Garry. Just hanging out at Fenway. Cal Ripken, Jr."

But the career highs were always tempered with lows. By the late '90s, it had been apparent that the Internet would soon make the newspaper obsolete. Dwindling resources and staff cutbacks across the industry made the vocation less and less attractive, to the point that it was no longer fun. The dream had become a job and it was time to get out.

I was suddenly free to go climbing anytime I wanted. A friend on Monadnock tried to console me by telling me he was sorry the newspaper had given me my walking papers, but I replied, "No, they gave me my *hiking* papers!"

That winter, I climbed a couple of more times with Karen and her friends; found a new climbing partner in Lisa Pettipaw, a violin instructor from West Roxbury, Massachusetts, whom I had also met on Monadnock; and even ventured into the Whites alone a few times that winter. Every weekend, I headed north to bag more peaks, eager to check them off my list.

But while I was making quick work of this list, my avoidance of Mount Washington was conspicuous. I was still not sure I was ready to tackle "the beast," which I had summited before only by way of a summer run up the auto road in 1993. After having read all those harrowing accounts of disasters on its upper flanks, I wasn't sure I was up to conquering Washington, and approached the Presidentials cautiously, like a swimmer daring to stick only his toe in the water.

One day that February, Lisa and I met up to tackle Mounts Madison, Adams, and Jefferson—a long day even in summer conditions—and were forced to beat a hasty retreat after the final summit when a typically ferocious storm descended upon the Presidentials. A couple of weeks later, we attacked the Prezzies from the south, turning back on the summit of Monroe, with Mount

Washington looming beyond. I now had only one of the Presidentials left to check off my list: that infamous Rockpile. But I was still not ready to tackle the beast; the peak remained, at least in my mind, beyond my reach.

But before I attempted to conquer Washington, my wanderlust set in again. Without a job to distract me, I began to look for more mountains to climb and more cultures to explore. Since many of the peaks that intrigued me were in Central and South America, I decided that learning some fledgling Spanish would be essential to my journeys. I looked at Spanish-language schools in Mexico, but I found that they were all too expensive for my now limited budget. So I looked farther south, starting with neighboring Guatemala.

I quickly found the Jabel Tinamit Spanish School, in the town of Panajachel, and signed up for a weeklong immersion, which would include the culture shock of staying with a host family. Then I traded a week from the timeshare I owned on Miami Beach to book a second week at a swank-looking resort on the shores of nearby Lake Atitlán, which guidebooks heralded as "the most beautiful lake in the world."

The day after Lisa and I hiked down Mount Monroe in New Hampshire— my forty-fourth birthday—I flew to Guatemala for what was supposed to be two weeks of self-discovery. Other than that week spent in Tobago in 2001, it would be my first time alone outside the comfort zone of my native New England.

Gregorio, the school's owner, arranged for a minivan to pick me up at the airport in Guatemala City. I stepped off the plane into another world and was quickly overwhelmed by what appeared to be pandemonium all around me. I didn't know that it was, in fact, just business as usual in this capital city. I was relieved to find my driver, Carlos, waiting for me with a sign on which my name was comically misspelled. I settled in for the 3-hour ride to Panajachel, a bustling tourist destination today and a favorite haven on the fabled "Gringo Trail."

Looking out the window from the backseat of the minivan, I saw a country-side that was a kaleidoscope for the senses. Everything was brightly colored, especially the "chicken buses," the antiquated yellow jalopies that belched black, noxious fumes and honked continuously as they dueled their way up and down the Pan-American Highway. They were packed well beyond capacity, mostly with native Maya going to and from market. The sights, sounds, and smells were all-consuming.

After a short layover in the former colonial capital of Antigua, a UNESCO World Heritage Site steeped in history, I was 10 minutes late returning to the van after a stroll to the Parque Central, and Carlos almost left without me. Given the frenetic pace, ramshackle feel, and apparent rule of chaos, I was amazed that anything actually ran on time in Guatemala.

Carlos, perhaps a bit miffed by my tardiness, paid me back by driving like a madman the rest of the trip, though compared with the other drivers on the road, he was hardly distinguishable. When he wasn't honking while passing a chicken bus on a blind corner, he was swinging his visor back and forth to block the sun, which glared from a different direction every time we went around another hairpin curve.

Arriving at the school in Panajachel a bit carsick, I got a quick indoctrination from Gregorio and met my host, Maria, a short, rounded Maya with jet-black hair pulled back in a ponytail. She lived just a couple of blocks up the street, which was teeming with activity. Cars, bicycles, and *tuk-tuks*—those three-wheeled, canopied taxis common in many developing countries— were buzzing in every direction.

My room for the week was more like a coffin. It contained a narrow bed with a threadbare sheet and a single blanket, undoubtedly handwoven by the local Maya who sold their wares from almost every inch of sidewalk up and down Calle Santander, the town's main street. A single lightbulb hung by a wire from the ceiling. The room had a pair of shelves next to the bed; the one with a candle on it made me wonder if the power might go out without notice. The walls were bare except for three things: a small, square mirror, a pegboard of hooks, and the requisite picture of Jesus. But at least the window opened, so I could let in the cool, moist spring air carrying in the scent of the colorful flowers blooming in every window box in town.

Following my daily morning class—taught by a young man named Eladio, who was himself a mountain climber—I explored my new world. Panajachel, located at nearly a mile high, lies on the eastern shore of Lake Atitlán in the rugged Western Highlands of Guatemala. The 95-square-mile lake formed in the caldera of a supervolcano that last erupted about 85,000 years ago and sent ash as far away as Panama and Florida. Atitlán was as beautiful as the guidebooks had promised. After traveling through the region on the back of a mule in the 1930s, Aldous Huxley wrote in his book *Beyond the Mexique Bay* that "Lake Como, in Italy, it seems to me, touches the limit of the permissibly picturesque, but Atitlán is Como with the additional embellishment of several immense volcanoes. It is really too much of a good thing." That quote graced every guidebook I picked up.

And the three volcanoes ringing the far shore of the lake were indeed immense. I immediately wanted to climb them and to explore this miraculous world, an area so rugged and remote that the Spanish pretty much bypassed it during their conquest of Mesoamerica in the sixteenth century, leaving the local Maya culture relatively unchanged.

Not long after I arrived, I called my airline and extended my return flight by two additional weeks. I could not possibly adequately explore this incredibly rich, diverse, and beautiful landscape in the two weeks I had initially planned.

Nowhere in Guatemala are the Maya traditions, customs, and languages more intact today than in the Western Highlands. The Maya consider the Lake Atitlán basin the navel of the world, and the lake itself—the deepest in Central America at more than a thousand feet—is reputed to have magical powers. (According to one person I met, there is even a UFO base under the surface.) In recent years, spiritual healers have flocked to Atitlán's shores, setting up meditation retreats in outlying villages. Before that, hippies trying to escape the crackdown by American society in the 1960s and '70s brought their counterculture to Panajachel, where freedom abounded and money was virtually unnecessary. Many of them never left, reinventing themselves as entrepreneurs in a town fondly known as *Gringotenango*, or "place of the foreigners."

And a large number of expats from the United States, Canada, and abroad have since taken up residence in this Shangri-la, finding the climate and the economy too good to pass up. English, I soon discovered, was practically the first language on the streets of Panajachel. So much for practicing my Spanish.

One of the first expats I met was Richard Morgan, a retired U.S. Army colonel who had been wounded in Vietnam in 1972. A New Jersey native, Richard had moved to Panajachel from Tucson, Arizona, in 1998 with his then-wife, Sharon, and son, Luke, and opened Posada los Encuentros, a small hotel, on the out-skirts of town. From there, he ran a business called Adventures in Education, which led guided trips focusing on Maya culture and artwork, and on the three towering volcanoes on the opposite side of the lake.

"Tourism is something this country needs," Richard told me one day while sitting in the enclosed, backyard garden at Posada los Encuentros. "I've been trying to get the Guatemalan government to see the volcanoes as a resource." But in a country that had been locked in a protracted civil war for nearly forty years prior to the 1996 peace accords, self-preservation had been the officials' priority.

I made plans with Richard to conclude my trip with a guided climb up Vol-cán Atitlán, at 11,598 feet the tallest of the three volcanoes that ringed the lake. But he suggested that I first climb the smallest of the three peaks, 9,908-foot San Pedro, which I could do on my own. The biggest obstacle, I soon learned, was not the climbing. Yes, the trail that led from the village of San Pedro la La-guna was steep, muddy, root-infested, and relentless, but what kept many from braving the ascent were concerns about safety.

Guatemala, to be honest, was not a destination for the intrepid. Crime was a legitimate concern, and most tourists—especially women—are warned not to travel anywhere alone. I have been nowhere else where the Coca-Cola delivery trucks have armed guards and the local restaurants have to unscrew the light bulbs out front every night to keep them from disappearing.

Tourists, by their very nature, are targets of the pickpockets and thieves who mainly frequent the crowded markets, but robberies had been reported on the volcanoes, as well. Two French climbers, I was told, had disappeared a few years before on Tolimán—the third volcano on the lake—never to be found. Robberies used to be especially common on the popular Vulcán Pacaya due to its proximity to Guatemala City and the gangs there, and I heard stories that tour guides on the volcano were often in cahoots with the bandits and would lead their unsuspecting charges into prearranged ambushes, deserting them to the robbers.

Fortunately, I was not the only person in my class with an interest in climbing volcanoes. Wendy, a fellow Vermonter in her early 20s, had also wanted to climb San Pedro, but similar concerns about safety had kept her from going. We decided to team up and head across the lake to the village of San Pedro la Laguna and the volcano's trailhead.

Travel on Lake Atitlán is mainly by one of the many *lanchas*—small, motorized boats that comfortably seat up to twenty people, but which are usually overloaded with ten or fifteen more, just like the chicken buses. I heard a joke on my trip that goes like this: "What is the capacity of a Guatemalan chicken bus?" Answer: "Four more." Same thing went for the lanchas. The captains would stop at any dock along the shore to pick up more passengers, no matter how overloaded they already were. On our trip, my eyes were glued to the solitary life jacket in the bow of the boat.

San Pedro la Laguna is considered the new Panajachel in that modern-day hippie backpackers who still follow the Gringo Trail to Lake Atitlán now usually find their way there. Dreadlocks were the main sight, marijuana the predominant smell, and loud music the constant sound. The steep street to the trailhead passed cafés full of patrons idling away their hours, a stark contrast with our day ahead.

From the trailhead, our route tackled a grueling 3-hour climb to Volcán San Pedro's small, rocky summit tucked among trees with staggering views of the other two volcanoes and the immense, shimmering lake below. Wendy and I were overwhelmed by the beauty that unfolded before us. And the ascent had been completely safe; the only others we saw were fellow climbers.

Today, Volcán San Pedro is a national park, with an entry fee and guides, and safety is no longer a primary concern.

But that was not the case on Volcán Atitlán in 2004. When Richard and I finally set out to climb it toward the end of my trip, there was definitely some concern on his part over safety. I met him in the village of San Lucas Tolimán on the southwestern corner of the lake, where we would begin the climb from the home of his own guide, a local man named Carlos.

It was the morning of Good Friday, during the weeklong celebration of Semana Santa leading up to Easter Sunday, when the entire country shuts down for continuous festivals, parades, and revelry. I had gone to bed the night before in my lakeside hotel room—the rate for which had tripled to $9 a night because of the holidays—with a huge celebration going on outside. I had been assured that the party would end around 2 A.M., but when I awoke at 4:30 A.M., the reverberating boom, boom, boom of Latin rock instantly greeted me. The partygoers, many of whom appeared to be little older than 14, were still going strong despite the coming onset of dawn.

I met Richard in the town square, which was decked out for a Semana Santa parade set for later that day. But at this hour of the morning, no one was around except for a handful of locals setting up their craft booths and a few mangy dogs begging for food. We headed to Carlos's house a few blocks away and began the trek in earnest from there. We hiked through alleyways and dirt streets to the outskirts of town and started climbing steadily through coffee *fincas* and fields. A couple of hours later, we reached the saddle between Volcán Atitlán and its shorter neighbor, the double-peaked Tolimán.

Richard carried a .12-gauge shotgun and had given a 9-millimeter pistol to Carlos, "just in case." Carlos, an electrician by trade and the father of six despite his young age of 32 said he had heard about some suspicious activity on Volcán Atitlán in recent weeks, but on this day we saw no one except fellow climbers.

Trash and graffiti polluted what would otherwise have been a pristine landscape. But the views from the summit were absolutely incredible. In every direction, waves of white, puffy clouds bounced along the spine of Central America like a chorus line of Stay Puft Marshmallow Men, each framed by an impossibly brilliant blue background.

To the north, a line of volcanoes popped out of the clouds—literal islands in the sky—stretching hundreds of miles to the Mexican border. To the west, somewhere, was the Pacific Ocean, but on that day it was hidden from view by a band of low-level clouds that resembled stuffing removed from an over-sized pillow.

"This view is magnificent," Richard said, putting away the shotgun in his backpack. "It's one of the toughest climbs in Guatemala; I haven't seen anything as impressive." I agreed. We completed the 10-hour round-trip without incident and my mind was made up: I would come back to Guatemala again soon.

I returned to New Hampshire without a job and without a home. But within days, I had rented a room that I had found in the want ads and was looking for work.

I was a more confident person than when I had left. I put all of the New England Four Thousand Footers on my list. I'd once attempted climbing the highpoints of all six New England states in two days—it'd been 1993, after my first divorce and before I met Debbie. After having run up the Mount Wash-

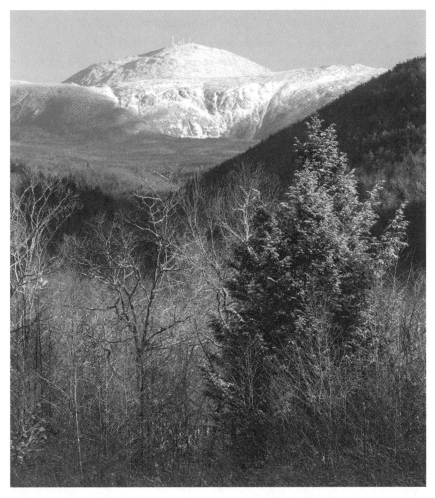

Mount Washington in winter as seen from New Hampshire's Crawford State Park. Photo by Jerry Monkman.

ington Auto Road the second morning, I drove the 7 hours to Baxter State Park where I had to schmooze my way past the ranger at the tollbooth, who had said it was too late in the day to start a summit bid. But a half-mile shy of the summit of Katahdin, Maine's highpoint, I'd turned back, exhausted. After Guatemala, I knew I was better prepared to take on New England's big peaks, including the monster that had me worried: Mount Washington itself.

I set my sights on taking down the beast. Lisa joined me on what was a typical day atop Mount Washington—high winds, blowing snow, and visibility of less than 50 feet. Though the calendar said April 24, winter conditions were still in full force, as they often are even at the height of summer. Yet the day proved uneventful despite my apprehensions, save for one foolhardy decision. We attempted to hike along the lip of Tuckerman Ravine on the descent. We worked our way partially across the top of the steep, 1,850-foot deep, rock-filled bowl below, but without ice axes, continuing would have risked a potentially deadly fall. We abandoned the traverse and retreated the way we had come, via the Lion's Head route.

That summer, I continued knocking off the remaining New Hampshire Four Thousand Footers with expedience, as well as the five in Vermont—including Mansfield again, for good measure. On August 1, I dragged Lisa along on a 19-mile traverse of the Wildcat and Carter ranges. Though she was always eager to join me no matter what the conditions, the weather quickly deteriorated that day, as it always seemed to when Lisa was along. She'd been on twenty-two of the peaks with me, and clear days always seemed to elude us; I called her my jinx. We reached the summit of 4,049-foot Mount Moriah, the last of my Four Thousand Footers in the state, without a view, getting caught in one last thunderstorm and taking several breaks to pick wild blueberries before reaching the parking lot in Gorham just before dusk.

Lisa returned to Boston the next morning, and I headed to Maine. Over the next seven days, I camped in remote locations and made my way over thirteen peaks, getting closer and closer to 5,167-foot Katahdin, the highest point in Maine and the end of the Appalachian Trail.

Arriving in Baxter State Park in remote northern Maine, I climbed North Brother, a 4,000-footer north of Katahdin, spent the night, then tackled the highpoint itself.

Katahdin means "Greatest Mountain" in Penobscot, and it lives up to that billing. The Hunt Trail—the Appalachian Trail's route to the summit—is steep, rugged, unrelenting, and even has *via ferrata*, or metal rungs, hammered into the rock in a couple of treacherous places. Huge boulders often block the path, necessitating a scramble over them. Once, I met a middle-aged couple from Indiana on the summit of Katahdin who were near delirium after climbing the Hunt Trail to meet their two college-age sons, who were completing the entire 2,179-mile Appalachian Trail that day. Apparently, they had previously climbed Mount Elbert, at 14,433 feet the highest point in Colorado. Completely exhausted, the father exclaimed to me, "Elbert was a walk-up compared to this!"

And this is the standard route.

Many people underestimate how tough a mountain Katahdin really is. There have been nineteen recorded deaths on the peak since 1963. I was afraid of adding to that number during a summer day a few years later on a trip with my then-teenage son, Evan. We were crossing the Knife's Edge—a narrow, 3-foot-wide ridge with sharp dropoffs on both sides that connects Katahdin's main summit to neighboring Pamola Peak—when a thunderstorm rolled in. We could see lightning *below* us on both sides, and the air was so electrically charged that the hair on my arm was standing straight up. My ex-wife had made me promise to bring our son home safely, and I wondered how I was going to explain it to her if something went wrong. Fortunately, the storm quickly passed and we escaped an untimely demise. The same conditions in the same location have made for more than one tragedy.

But on that first summit of Katahdin in 2004, I felt a great sense of accomplishment. I'd joined the ranks of peakbaggers to have completed two of the region's most prominent lists. As of 2014, the AMC Four Thousand Footer Club had certified more than 11,000 hikers finishing the New Hampshire Four Thousand Footers; by comparison, only 2,845 have finished the sixty-seven New England Four Thousand Footers.

In hindsight, I should have studied my map a little more closely. In 2007, I decided to finish off the New England Hundred Highest list, which includes all sixty-seven 4,000-footers and the next thirty-three highest peaks in the region. One of them is Mount Fort, which stands just a quarter-mile from the summit of North Brother. At the time, I paid it no attention because it wasn't a Four Thousand Footer. Had I known it was on the Hundred Highest list, I would have gotten both peaks that day, along with South Brother and Coe, which I had also collected on the way out. As it is, I have checked off only ninety-nine of the Hundred Highest, and someday I will have to make the trip back to Maine to bag Mount Fort and finish the list.

In the fall, I got hired as a seasonal driver by UPS and soon discovered I was well suited for the job. The pace was hectic, similar to the deadline pressure I used to encounter daily working for newspapers, but there was so much more freedom. I would be outside all day, and as long as I got my work done, no one was looking over my shoulder.

By the end of the year, I'd climbed Mount Monadnock 210 times.

After completing my first "Christmas rush," I was offered a full-time job, but turned it down. I told them I would be back the following June to begin a new "season," which would take me through the following Christmas, a regimen I would follow for the next five years. That gave me the first five months of 2005 to explore, and I headed back to Guatemala.

My second trip to Guatemala began on a sour note that made me wonder if I would reach any of the peaks I had hoped to climb on the trip, which included Guatemala's three then-active volcanoes and the highest point in Central America.

My first scheduled climb—a guided overnighter on conjoined peaks Acatenango and Volcán de Fuego—was canceled at the last minute because of dangerous activity in the hulking, steaming crater atop Fuego, which was venting almost daily. Sometimes, the volcanoes were the only things running on schedule. I quickly changed itineraries, which I learned was an almost daily necessity. I called Patrick Vercoutere of Adrenalina Tours in the northern city of Quetzaltenango, hoping to climb the active Santa María Volcano. Its shoulder cone of Santiaguito was erupting with a huge plume of ash every 40 minutes or so, reminiscent of Old Faithful, and I wanted a look.

"Sure," Patrick said, quickly switching from Spanish to English, both of which he spoke with a native Belgian accent. "We're climbing tonight at midnight under a full moon. We'll be on the summit for sunrise."

Perfect, I thought. But I had a problem. I was in Antigua, a good 5 hours by chicken bus from Quetzaltenango—or Xela, as the country's second-largest city is commonly known—and it was Good Friday. I had once again arrived during Semana Santa, when virtually the entire country of 13 million people shuts down to celebrate Easter. I bought some apples and bread at the market and stepped on a northbound chicken bus with fingers crossed.

Riding the chicken bus is an experience every visitor to Guatemala should share. I boarded the gaudily painted former school bus that had been shipped down from the States along with its equally eye-popping cousins, each decorated with beads and baubles hanging from the mirror and with a picture of Jesus above the driver's head, for obvious reasons I would soon discern.

Traveling in a country like Guatemala, I gave no thought to putting my life in the hands of a complete stranger. If you want to get around, you just get on a bus and go, and I did.

Although spring is generally much drier than the fall, which is the traditional rainy season, on this day it was raining hard and the windshield wipers on the bus apparently weren't working. This had probably been the case for some time, since the defroster didn't work either, and the driver was constantly wiping fog

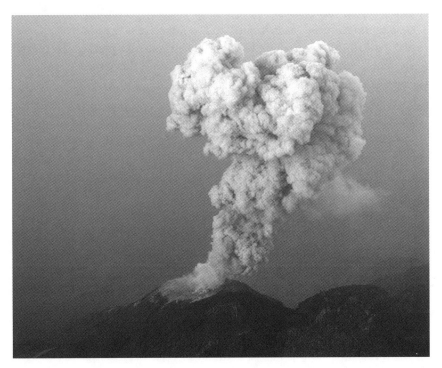

Santiaguito, the small volcano born in 1922 on the shoulder of much-larger Santa María, erupts just before dawn as I summit Santa María.

off the windshield so he could see. The other half of the windshield sported a massive spiderweb crack, which made seeing out of it impossible even if the wipers *had* been functional. But heaven forbid the horn didn't work; the bus probably would have been impounded immediately. Our driver constantly yanked on a chain tied to the air horn to let people know to get out of the way.

While one may actually see a chicken poking its head out of a basket on the lap of one of the Maya passengers, I decided they were more aptly called chicken buses because the drivers all had a morbid fascination—no, make that an ordained obligation—to drive recklessly and pass at every opportunity. They were like matadors, but instead of sidestepping bulls with a wave of a cape and an *"¡Olé!"* they played chicken with oncoming traffic. On one blind curve, our driver gunned it as he passed two cars and a pickup that had two cows in the back—an experience even more terrifying considering the state of the windshield and the fact that guardrails were a rarity. While the locals sat there stone-faced as the bus careened around corners on the wrong side of the road, all parties narrowly missing a plunge into a thousand-foot ravine, gringos new to the experience had their fingernails dug deeply into the top of the seat in front of them. More than a few, I reckoned, soiled themselves on occasion.

Despite the odds, we made it safely to Los Encuentros, a nondescript cross-roads of a town that was about halfway to Xela and also marked the turnoff to the much-closer Panajachel to the south. Suddenly, the bus pulled over and stopped. Everyone got off, including the driver.

No more buses today, I was informed. Time to party.

"Great," I thought, "what do I do now?"

I was left to deal with the *collectivos*, owners of pickup trucks and minivans who ferry stranded travelers (i.e., gringos) up and down the Pan-American Highway that runs north–south along the spine of the Western Highlands. And gringos started piling up like lemmings on a ledge. A pickup came along, and five stranded travelers paid Q10 (about $2.50) each to ride in the back, crammed in like cattle. A Seattle native named Matt, whom I'd met while we all waited, rode away on the back bumper, clinging to the metal cage welded to the back of the truck. I held out and got lucky. Someone convinced the driver of a minivan to abandon plans to go to Panajachel and instead take a full load to Xela for Q20 each.

I was glad I waited. A couple of hours later, when we caught and passed that first pickup truck, Matt and the others looked pretty cold. Someone asked our driver to pull closer to the pickup and I handed my fleece out the window to someone in the back, since we were all going to the same place.

Matt's friends had passed on the truck but caught a ride in the van with me. Andrew and Galen Huckins, brothers from Northborough, Massachusetts, now lived in Xela, where they were learning Spanish, teaching English, and playing in their own little jazz band. Andrew, who was 20, had been in Guatemala for about fifteen months after having hitched a ride as a deckhand on a sailboat from the Canary Islands; Galen, 18, had joined him after graduating from high school the previous June.

Everyone was crashing at their apartment for the weekend, and I was invited to join them—a miraculous stroke of luck, considering I had been to Xela only once before and had set out with no idea where I was going. I was not one to turn down hospitality while traveling alone, even if it came in the form of a couple of kids half my age. And meant sleeping outside on their patio. In a hammock, in March, at 8,000 feet. In a part of the country that even the Guatemalans affectionately refer to as "Alaska."

I certainly couldn't beat the "rent": three one-liter bottles of Gallo, the rather acrid national beer of Guatemala.

One guidebook described 12,375-foot Santa María as a moderate hike, but I can guarantee those authors never made the climb. It was a relentless 4-hour death march to the summit—switchbacks are unheard of in Guatemala—but the instant our tour group topped out under the shimmering light of the setting full moon, we were treated to an eruption from Santiaguito's crater several hundred feet below on Santa María's western flank. A huge rumble was followed by a big belch as Santiaguito let out a puff of gas and ash that billowed into the predawn sky and roiled like a mushroom cloud. It was amazing.

The Santiaguito crater was formed by a huge explosion in 1902, the third-largest eruption in the Western Hemisphere in the twentieth century. Ash traveled as far as San Francisco, but in Guatemala, the government was busy denying that the eruption had even occurred, despite the fact that peasants working the many coffee fincas on the Pacific slope were standing chest-deep in ash. Turned out, Santiaguito had erupted at the worst possible moment—right in the middle of President Manuel Estrada Cabrera's Feast of the Goddess Minerva, whom he had just made the patron saint of the country's so-called progress.

In the face of plummeting coffee prices, Estrada Cabrera had invited diplomats from all over the globe to attend the festival as a ruse for eliciting investment capital from abroad. He couldn't afford to have something as uncontrollable as a volcanic eruption discouraging foreign investment, so he simply denied its existence. Ultimately, the gambit failed, and the investors went home, taking their money with them.

Sunrise on Santa María was spectacular, except it unmasked all the graffiti and trash so common on Guatemalan summits. Like many of the country's volcanoes, Santa María is also considered sacred by the Maya, who use the volcanoes as ritual sites. As the sun rose, so did a dozen or so chanting Mayans, who had slept on the summit. Daylight revealed evidence of a ritual that had involved a live goat, or so indicated the horns on the charred carcass still smoldering in one of the fire pits. Alas, all our group had to eat were ham sandwiches and some cookies.

Among the volcanoes that stood out against the pink sky was Tajumulco to the north, at 13,845 feet the highest point in Central America. It looked perfectly inviting.

When I got back to the apartment, I announced my intention to climb Tajumulco on Sunday and I asked if anyone wanted to go with me. Tyler—who lived in Brattleboro, Vermont, just 20 minutes from where I lived in New Hampshire— and Matt, immediately wanted in, but the others all laughed. Sunday was Easter, they reminded us, and there likely would be no way to get there or back with the intermittent bus service.

"See you Tuesday!" we heard the others say with a laugh as we left early Sunday morning; we took their derision as a challenge.

As it turned out, the buses *were* running, at least in the morning, and we had little trouble getting to the trailhead, needing to change buses only a couple of times. The climb began through farmers' fields and among tall pines and met a high ridge that led west toward the conical summit cone, likely formed during Tajumulco's last eruption in 1863. Along the way, the only people we saw were two young boys riding a sway-backed old mare.

Beyond the ridge, we faced a breath-stealing climb of at least a thousand vertical feet up the summit cone. Matt and Tyler struggled a bit in the thin air and steep terrain—certainly more than I did—but we reached the top in midafternoon, by which time we could see a storm rolling in from the Pacific. We quickly started back down, but hiking along the ridge, we got lost, unable to differentiate among all the trails that led off to our left, the direction we knew we needed to go. Rain started to fall and the approaching thunderstorm looked like it would soon overtake us, so we hurried to get off the ridge. But soon we came to the top of a deep ravine. We had to try to go around it, either to the right or to the left. As we stood there discussing our options with rain pelting down, we suddenly heard young voices yelling.

"¡El camino! ¡El camino!" It was the same two boys we had seen in the morning. "This way," they yelled, motioning us to go left.

We had gone only a short way when I happened to glance across the ravine at the precise moment that a huge bolt of lightning struck the ground—the exact spot where we would have been standing had we gone to the right. The strike left a glowing, purple orb of energy floating in the air like I had never seen before, and a millisecond later it exploded with such intense fury that a nearby tree was blown into a million toothpicks.

I later learned that it had been something called ball lightning, considered the most unexplained atmospheric electrical phenomenon known to scientists. Ball lightning is exactly what it sounds like; it's typically the size of a grapefruit, but this one was as big as a beach ball.

Matt, Tyler, and I were thankful for the boys' help; they had probably saved our lives. We frantically ran ahead of them as the heavy rain turned into a deluge. I turned back to yell to the others, when, zap, another bolt of lightning streaked horizontally across the sky, just feet above our heads. Instantly, the thunder followed, not in a classic boom, but in a frenzied crack giving chase to its source, as if it were tearing a hole through the sky as it went. It was the first time I had ever heard thunder in stereo.

"Wow! Wasn't that cool?" I yelled over the din, but Matt and Tyler weren't really listening as they picked up the pace and ran ahead.

The rain soon let up and we slowed to a walk as we finally passed a house. We asked a man standing at the front door for directions to the main road, where we hoped to catch a bus. He introduced himself as Pedro—we assumed he was the father of the two boys—and offered to drive us there instead. So we piled into the back of his Toyota pickup and rode a short way down to a gravel road, where he dropped us off in front of a church. We immediately took refuge in its doorway, as the heavy rain had returned. Pedro drove off around a bend, stopped, and backed all the way up the road until he was parked in front of us again. He motioned for us to get into the back; apparently he had taken pity on us and had returned to drive us to the next town.

The back of his truck, however, now had about 2 inches of rain in it, and we got even more drenched, if that were possible. As he sped around sharp curves, the water sloshed up in waves, all while the large raindrops pelted us like hail stones. We could only laugh at our miserable plight as we held on tight.

From our seats we could see the intersection with the main road to San Marcos in the far distance and, to our collective dismay, we also saw what we knew in our hearts to be the last bus of the day pulling out of the village of San Sebastián. Suddenly, Pedro sped up even more and barely slowed down as he rounded the corner and chased the departing bus. He quickly overtook it and cut it off, forcing it to a stop. He gave us a cheerful smile as we climbed out of his truck and onto the bus. We were soaked to the skin, but laughing giddily about our incredible good fortune.

When we arrived in San Marcos, however, our mood quickly soured again. The next bus to Xela was *mañana*. Tomorrow. Dashed again. Matt, who spoke a modicum of Spanish, tried to negotiate a ride in a minivan, but the collectivo, who appeared to be quite drunk, refused to make the trip for less than Q200—about $25. We might have considered the offer despite his inebriated condition had we had that much money on us.

Finally, a taxi driver who had been eavesdropping said he thought there was still one last bus to Xela leaving from the next town, and he would take us there for Q15. The race was on again, even though we had our doubts. Most of the streets were closed for an Easter parade, so the taxi turned down side streets and alleys. We turned the corner onto the town square just as what indeed was the last bus of the day was pulling out. The taxi driver honked his horn, flagged it down, and once again a miracle of hospitality and luck had delivered us.

We were laughing heartily as we walked from the bus station in Xela back to Andrew and Galen's apartment knowing how close we had come to spending a long, cold night somewhere in wet clothes. Tuesday indeed. We had even made it back before nightfall.

We stopped at the neighborhood *tienda* again to celebrate our good fortune with three more Gallos. Suddenly, they didn't taste so bad.

By the following weekend, Fuego had calmed down enough to be climbed. I returned to Antigua to meet my guide, Rafael, for our two-day ascent of Acatenango and its rambunctious and aptly named neighbor, Fuego.

We were driven up a washboard dirt road to the trailhead, only to find the chicken bus already there. It seems there's no place too remote for the chicken bus. Rafael and I hiked up through cornfields and then climbed steeply up the northern slope of Acatenango, at 13,044 feet the taller of the two conjoined peaks. The climb continued through ever-changing ecosystems, through a dense stand of massive, moss-covered canac trees, then a forest of stately ponderosa pines, before reaching treeline. Here, we labored through the conical dust and scree. We slid back a half step for every one we took on the loose stones. After 3 hours of climbing, we emerged on the placid crater rim, and Rafael, without uttering a word, took off his pack, sat down beside it, leaned back, and…went to sleep.

A *siesta*? Now?

Deciding there wasn't much choice, I took a nap myself. Twenty minutes later, I was awake, but Rafael was still as dormant as the volcano beneath us. When he soon awakened, we crossed the barren moonscape of the caldera to the higher summit on the other side of the crater. The black volcanic dirt looked genuinely cobalt in the glint of the midday sun.

Starting down the other side, we quickly picked up speed as we started to ski down the slope, which was like walking on little ball bearings. I immediately wished I had brought my gaiters, because within seconds my boots were full of tiny pebbles as I glissaded amid a small avalanche of my own creation. Soon, we stopped for lunch on a rocky outcropping and I dumped a large handful of stones out of each ash-covered boot.

A loud explosion, followed by a rumbling and what sounded like a rock slide, stopped me midbite. Fuego was awake, somewhere in the clouds in front of us. The volcano repeated this ominous sound several times throughout the afternoon. After lunch—and another nap—it was time for the day's second run, and we boot-skied down to a beautiful, pine-forested glade in the saddle between the two peaks, where we camped for the night at about 11,000 feet.

While it was entirely possible to climb Acatenango and Fuego in one day, it was better to wait until the clear sky of morning to witness the awesome summit of Fuego. Usually, by early afternoon, water vapor coming off the Pacific makes its way into the Western Highlands, obliterating any significant views for the rest of the day, just as it had for us the day before.

In the morning, it took us little more than a half hour of steady climbing to reach the broad shoulder of Fuego, giving us our first view of the heavy plume of smoke that had been pouring out of the caldera almost continuously since

1999. We dropped our packs and continued a few hundred yards closer to a spot where Rafael normally turned his clients around. But things seemed quiet, and I wanted to get closer. Much closer.

We crept higher than Rafael had ever taken a client before and he was understandably nervous. But I could see footprints in the volcanic dirt leading up to the crater rim, so I told him to wait while I cautiously sneaked forward despite the warnings the mountain had given us the day before.

Suddenly, a *golondrina*, or swallow, whizzed past my head. I felt instantly transformed into the brave little hobbit Bilbo Baggins, watching a thrush reveal the secret entrance into Smaug's lair. I didn't need a hidden door, just hidden nerves as I inched higher, the crater rim now just a few yards above me. I felt like I was on Tolkien's Lonely Mountain, sneaking up on the sleeping dragon. But I had no magic ring to make myself invisible, and I would be easy prey if the dragon—er, the mountain itself—suddenly awakened, as it had so many times the day before.

Now I could see fire, like the dragon's breath, coming out of the gaping crater in front of me. I smelled its foul, sulfuric stench emanating from the cracks in the earth beneath my feet. And then I felt the heat of its breath on my face as well. I was much too close. I slowly backed away, but not before I picked up a small volcanic rock and slid it into my pocket as proof of my courage, or foolhardiness, just as Bilbo had grabbed a spoil from Smaug's treasure trove.

Fortunately, the rock was not missed by the dragon, which slept through it all, unaware of my presence. I collected a relieved Rafael, and as we retrieved our packs, a faint murmur rumbled from the mountain, probably just Smaug dreaming about a nice meal of dwarves. We completed the difficult descent in record time and the beast above never awakened.

Perhaps I was wearing a magic ring after all.

The minivan to Volcán Pacaya pulled up in front of my hotel at 6 A.M. on Wednesday, much too early, I reasoned, considering I had been out quite late the night before enjoying Antigua's rigorous night life. The weekend seemed to begin on Tuesday in Antigua, with free salsa lessons at La Sin Ventura, a bustling nightclub just down the street from the Parque Central. But I had been next door at the Monoloco. The bar had quickly become my favorite, not just because it served an enormous nachos *grandes* that could feed three grown men, but because it was a Red Sox bar. Honest. The entire back wall was a shrine to my Boston heroes—the *Medias Rojas*, as they are known in Spanish. The décor and devotion had stolen me away from the brighter parts of the city and kept up my supply of Brahva—which tasted a lot better than Gallo and did not, as I later learned, contain formaldehyde, like its popular competitor did.

Even as I ran out the door and into the van, I was still not sure this was going to be a worthwhile adventure. The brochure I had seen in Antigua made unflattering references to Pacaya and the manliness (or lack thereof) of those who climbed it.

Because it was one of the smaller volcanoes in Guatemala at only 8,373 feet, and because of its proximity to Antigua and Guatemala City, Pacaya was a destination popular with the average tourist, something I did not consider myself to be. I imagined camera-toting, sun-blocked pseudo tourists being carted around in air-conditioned buses and "interacting" with nature by looking at it mostly through tinted glass. "That was nice," I imagined them saying as they returned to their gated four-star resorts to sip margaritas by the pool. *Yanquis*, the locals call them. I know them, unfortunately, as fellow Americans.

But Pacaya was the final active volcano on my list for that trip, and being one of the most-visited tourist sites in Guatemala, it made no sense for me not to go there, despite my reservations about how adventurous this guided tour would be.

Soon, we were on a rattletrap dirt road that led to the visitor center at Pacaya National Park. In the distance, smoke spewed from the summit. We pulled up to the park entrance, where cows blocked the road and no tour buses were to be seen. As I got out of the van, my legs still ached from the Fuego climb of two days before, reminding me why I had passed on the previous night's free salsa lessons.

After paying the Q25 entry fee and meeting our guide, we started hiking on a well-groomed path that was as easy as advertised. I had envisioned a relatively unexciting hike, like a day at the zoo, but when I got to the summit and saw the two smokestacks raining down fiery new earth at our feet while we could feel the heat of the volcano on our faces, I discovered that Pacaya was no mere zoo. It was a safari that brought you so close to the lions you could almost pet them.

We were close enough to the active cone that it would certainly be possible for a large belch to come down on our heads. In fact, our guides later told us that that is exactly what had happened one day a few years earlier, when a molten blob landed on the head of one of the *guias*, or guides. They said it was a slow, painful death as they tried to get him to emergency care.

Standing within spitting distance from where these potentially deadly grenades were landing, there was nothing other than my own fear—and suggestions from our guias—to keep me from inching closer, tempting the volcano to unleash an especially large belch that might turn me into tomorrow's headline. No ropes, no fences, no warning signs, and no lawyers handing out business cards. Talk about your shock and awe. I couldn't have done this at Yellowstone. This was the raw, visceral freedom I had come to Guatemala to experience.

A tour with so real a risk would never be allowed in the litigious United States. At Kīlauea in Hawaii, for example, no one is allowed closer than one-third of a mile from the flowing lava. And despite precautions such as warning signs and roped barricades, there have been more than forty deaths there since Kīlauea began erupting almost continuously in 1983. When I was there in 1995 on my honeymoon with Debbie, a newspaper clipping at the visitor center warned of two Japanese tourists who had ventured beyond the ropes a couple of years before and fallen through the thin crust into the 2,000-degree-Celsius lava flowing below.

But on Pacaya, we ate our lunch, mesmerized and numbed into a jaw-dropping trance by the raw beauty unfolding at our feet. A loud "boom, boom" filled the air as two more chunks of molten lava were hurled hundreds of feet into the sky—a sound much like that of fireworks being launched on the Fourth of July. They quickly transformed from a searing, orange glow at their apex to a blackened, obsidian blob as they cooled slightly before landing with a thud at the base of the summit cone. Shattering upon impact, they skittered across the hardened crust like tinkling shards of broken glass.

This was followed immediately by a chorus of oohs and ahs from a group of mesmerized tourists standing barely a dozen yards from where this brand-new earth was being pumped out of a pair of smokestacks on the summit of Pacaya.

Only when the second cone joined its brother by coughing up some particularly dangerous fireballs did the guides yell, "¡Vámanos!" With hesitation, our group began to head back down. On the way, we passed another group of tourists who, as yet, had no idea what awaited them above.

As we neared the parking lot, the ground shook as Pacaya let out a loud roar that could be heard for miles. I looked back at the rim expecting to see people scurrying for cover. But there they were, still standing side by side, cameras snapping away.

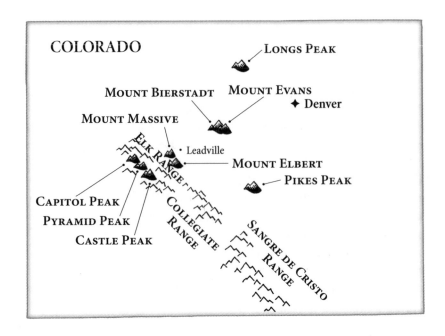

COLORADO

LONGS PEAK

MOUNT BIERSTADT   MOUNT EVANS

✦ Denver

MOUNT MASSIVE

ELK RANGE

• Leadville

CAPITOL PEAK   MOUNT ELBERT

PYRAMID PEAK   PIKES PEAK

CASTLE PEAK

COLLEGIATE RANGE

SANGRE DE CRISTO RANGE

Chapter 3
2006-2007

COLORADO CALLS

AFTER RETURNING FROM GUATEMALA IN 2005, MANY OF MY PEAKBAGGING LISTS in the Northeast were complete. I had completed the New Hampshire 48 in late winter before my trip, and when I got back, I began to tackle the New England Hundred Highest, though I didn't make it back to Baxter State Park to bag Mount Fort, the last peak on my list. Mount Washington had long since lost its luster as a scary monster, as I'd climbed it a handful of times by now, but I had yet to conquer it in winter, a situation I rectified on what turned out to be a particularly nasty day in January 2006, in the company of Karen and Vannak Pol, a new climbing partner I had met on Monadnock the previous year.

The three of us summited via the same Lion's Head route I'd taken on my first ascent in 2004. But this was January, not April, and Washington was in its full winter fury. It was a bitterly cold and blustery day, with wind chills, we guessed, of about 80 degrees below zero Fahrenheit on the summit, not unusual for that time of year. Unlike that first winter summit of Moosilauke two years before, however, I knew what to expect in such conditions. We were prepared accordingly.

As we neared the top, Van stepped on a rock and his crampon broke in half. We pushed on and took shelter in the lee of one of the summit buildings to get out of the raging wind and made a plan. It would have been too dangerous to attempt the descent on the icy trail without crampons, so we used duct tape from our pack and taped the heel plate of his crampon onto his boot. Even with some protection from the building, it was so brutally cold that I lost all feeling in my exposed hands within seconds. By the time I finished the tape job, my hands were so numb I needed help getting my gloves back on. Fortunately, I had not been exposed long enough to invite frostbite. We immediately started down. Fortunately for Van, my hasty tape job held.

With my lists in my native New England dwindling, I started thinking bigger, and to me that meant Colorado and the Rocky Mountains.

*I had been to Colorado only once before, when I was 16 during a family cross-*country trip to visit relatives in Arizona. We visited places along the way such as Bourbon Street in New Orleans, the Houston Astrodome, Carlsbad Caverns, and the Grand Canyon, all of which I remember vividly. But I have little memory of our drive through Colorado, which included a couple of days at a dude ranch outside the ghost town of Tincup, where gold had first been discovered in Colorado in 1859.

So, I had little knowledge of the Centennial State to go on when I started planning my first trip to take on the fifty-four 14ers in 2006, all peaks above 14,000 feet. At least I wouldn't be going alone: Van took time off from his job in a manufacturing plant, where he was a part-owner despite his young age, and decided to join me. It would be the first trip of this nature for Van, a young Cambodian refugee who was nearly half my age and who shared my peakbagging lust.

We flew into Denver on September 12, with plans to climb as many 14ers as we could in the next two weeks. Maybe we'd spot a mountain goat or two on the way; I'd never seen one and made it a goal to spy one before the trip was over. We piled our gear into a rented Jeep Liberty and headed west on I-70 toward Georgetown and Guanella Pass, sleeping under the stars on our first night before arriving the next morning at the trailhead for Mounts Bierstadt and Evans, which were to be our first 14ers.

We began our climb of Bierstadt up the straightforward West Slopes Trail. With us was what we thought was our most essential piece of gear: Gerry Roach's *Colorado Fourteeners*, which would get us into trouble before the day was over.

Bierstadt was uneventful, but we also planned to traverse underneath a dramatic cliff face called the Sawtooth and bag Mount Evans while we were there. Summiting two 14ers on our first day in Colorado was a lofty goal, but we had decided not to waste any precious climbing days on acclimatization.

Roach called the Sawtooth a "classic" route. Though at Class 3—requiring challenging scrambles and presenting the risk of potentially fatal falls—it was relatively mild hiking, yet wonderfully airy for us neophytes. We crossed a broad plateau between the peaks and I arrived at the summit of Mount Evans well ahead of Van, who lingered behind, as he often did.

On the summit, I met two climbers who had bicycled up the Mount Evans

Auto Road—the highest paved road in North America. Learning that I had just bagged my first two 14ers, one of them mentioned that he had previously held the speed record for climbing all of Colorado's 14ers.

I didn't learn his name until years later, but turned out it was Andrew Hamilton of Boulder, who had climbed the 14ers in 13 days 22 hours 48 minutes in 1999. His record, however, was broken just one year later when Ted "Cave Dog" Keizer of Oregon crushed the mark by climbing them all in 10 days 20 hours 26 minutes. A few had tried to break that record since, including Hamilton, but no one came close until Hamilton reclaimed his own crown in 2015 by taking nearly 24 hours off Cave Dog's record.

(Keizer is a hiking and climbing phenom, also having once held the speed records for both the forty-eight New Hampshire Four Thousand Footers and the forty-six in the Adirondacks of New York. Records, though, don't often stand long. Both of Keizer's eastern-mountain records have since fallen, with Tim Seaver of Vermont taking more than 2 hours off Cave Dog's White Mountains record in 2003 and my friend Jan Wellford of upstate New York slicing exactly 1 hour off the Adirondacks mark in 2008. Another acquaintance, Andrew Thompson, would go on to shave nearly an hour off Seaver's time in 2014.)

On Evans that day, I chatted with Hamilton and his friend until Van showed up complaining of a vicious headache, presumably from the altitude. There was nothing we could do but descend, which we had planned to do by reversing course back over the summit of Bierstadt. Once again, I quickly found myself alone as Van struggled to keep up. With the extra time, I spotted a shorter route in the guidebook that would enable us to skip crossing the Sawtooth. Again I waited for Van in the saddle between the two peaks, and when he finally caught up, we set out on the supposed shortcut back to the car.

But Roach's guidebook failed to mention one important element: This trail followed a creek bed that was overrun by willow trees. I soon discovered there is nothing as maddening as having to work your way through a stand of willows, an impenetrable mass of gnarled roots and water-soaked ground. It seemingly took us hours to navigate through this minefield of twisted, scrubby trees, and I made a mental note to avoid willows like the plague in the future.

Once at the car, we decided we had earned a celebration—as much for surviving the willows as for climbing two 14ers on our first day. Heading back to Georgetown, we stopped at the Red Ram Restaurant and Saloon—an iconic Old West tavern in the historic district—and got a table.

Van, who grew up in a refugee camp in Southeast Asia and will eat almost anything, promptly ordered the Rocky Mountain oysters, unconcerned that this supposed delicacy was in reality bighorn sheep testicles. When I told him what he had ordered, he was undeterred, but when the waitress informed him they were out of sheep balls, he ended up with a fat, juicy burger, just like me.

Interestingly, the slim, pretty, heavily tattooed waitress kept coming back to the table asking me if I needed anything, acting as if Van wasn't even there. At one point, Van asked for another fork or napkin or something, and she ignored him. Later, the young woman, who was probably only half my age, came over to the table, stroked my arm and, speaking only to me, asked, "Are you sure you don't need anything else?"

"Uh, no, I think I'm good," I managed.

When she left, Van, unable to control his laughter, said, "I think you have a new girlfriend."

It was all a bit too weird, and we soon got out of there so we could reach our next campsite before dark.

The next day, we climbed Grays and Torreys peaks under beautiful, clear skies. Two young guys from Michigan hitched a ride from us near the bottom of the road leading up to the Grizzly Gulch trailhead, as they did not dare to drive their Honda Civic up the rough track. While we were gearing up in the parking lot, two college-age girls from Boulder bounded suddenly into the parking lot, also driving a Honda Civic. The two Michigan guys looked a little sheepish when they saw this.

The six of us climbed together that day, and we dropped the two Michiganders back at their car without too much teasing.

The following day, Van and I planned to climb Quandary Peak near Breckenridge, one of the easiest 14ers. The peak's standard route is a Class 1 path from the Monte Cristo trailhead to the east, but I desired a little more excitement. I had Van drive me to Blue Lake so I could summit via the Class 3 West Ridge route, another of Roach's "classic" climbs. This route provided "a scenic approach and a sporty scramble," while Van opted to take the comparatively leisurely standard track. Despite having to traverse some snowy, north-facing chutes, I beat Van to the summit by a considerable margin, as he was now fully beset by altitude sickness.

From there, we drove over Hoosier Pass to the town of Alma—the highest town in North America, at 10,361 feet above sea level—and headed even higher toward the trailhead for our next day's climb at Kite Lake.

In the face of bitter cold and wind, we abandoned hope of putting up a tent that evening at Kite Lake. We spent an uncomfortable night, instead, in the back of the Jeep, on top of our climbing gear. In the morning, Van's head was pounding even worse than the wind was howling outside. He waited in the car while I ventured out toward the trail leading up to Mount Democrat along with about a dozen other hardy hikers, all braving the heavy, falling snow. I was the first to summit and return to the saddle, where the trail had come up from Kite Lake. I continued along the ridge toward the summit of Mount Cameron, only to look back and watch all the other climbers bail at the junction and head back to safety. I was the only one to continue on, making my way over Cameron, across a broad plateau to Mount Lincoln, and then into the teeth of the wind as I headed toward Mount Bross, my exposed face being pelted by tiny shards of ice the entire time. I made it back to the car in amazing time, given the wintry conditions—little more than 3.5 hours. The whole route is known as the Decalibron, after the first letters of the four peaks, though Cameron is not considered a full-fledged 14er, as it doesn't rise more than 300 feet from its saddle with Mount Lincoln.

From there, we drove to Leadville—the highest incorporated city in North America, at 10,152 feet—and checked into the Leadville Hostel. We felt as if we had driven up in front of the Ritz-Carlton of hostels. It had a huge living room, with a big-screen TV, a large kitchen and dining area, and plenty of bunkrooms downstairs. And best of all, it had hot showers, something neither of us had enjoyed since we'd arrived in Colorado five days before.

The next day, Van's altitude sickness eased up and we made the short hike to the summit of Mount Sherman, at 14,036 feet probably the easiest of all the 14ers. We were back before noon, in time to watch the Patriots beat the Jets and the Red Sox sweep a doubleheader from the Yankees. What could be better for a couple of New Englanders?

The next day was certainly a contender to best it: We climbed 14,433-foot Mount Elbert, the highest peak in Colorado. The day was unusually clear and calm as we climbed from the South Halfmoon Creek trailhead to the summit. I could have made the entire, gentle ascent with my hands in my pockets; indeed, a Jeep once was driven to the summit in 1949.

It was so calm on the summit that day that when we sat down to eat our lunches, I took my sandwich out of its Baggie and set the bag down on a rock next to my feet. I ate my entire lunch and the bag never moved—not the faintest whisper of a breeze disturbed the summit that day. A couple of locals who showed up about the same time said that Elbert might enjoy only one or two days a year with weather so sublime.

The following day, we climbed Elbert's impressive neighbor, Mount Massive, the third-highest mountain in the continental United States. Massive is only the second highest in the Arkansas Valley, it being 12 feet shorter than Elbert. (Both are outstripped by California's Mount Whitney, at 14,505 feet.) In the 1930s, a rivalry erupted between supporters of the two peaks; climbers built a large cairn atop Massive to make it slightly higher, only to see Elbert enthusiasts climb up and tear it down.

Van was feeling better with each passing day and soon got beyond his altitude sickness, but he was still a ways behind me as I summited Massive. So I killed time by climbing some of the other nubs along the summit ridge, including North Massive, which would count as a ranked 14er itself if it were 20 feet taller. I added South Massive—another unranked 14er—on the way down.

Leaving Leadville the next morning, we headed toward the remote town of Winfield, located at the end of a washboard dirt road that passed the old ghost town of Vicksburg and the Missouri Gulch trailhead, where we expected to be climbing in a couple of days. But first we headed to climb La Plata Peak, the fifth-highest peak in Colorado and one of the most spectacular. The town of Winfield was a bustling metropolis of about 1,500 people in its mining heyday, but now seemed to be abandoned.

At Winfield the road splits, and we took the right fork until the four-wheel track ended just past an old cemetery at a closed gate, and started hiking. This was the easiest route up La Plata, but it also took us past dozens of towers and ramparts that reminded me more of pictures of California's Sierra Mountains than anything I had seen so far in Colorado. Once back to Winfield, we took the left fork and headed into the Clear Creek drainage, one of the prettiest spots I had seen in my life. This high-alpine valley, cut by a deep, clear stream, represented—to me—the quintessential Colorado experience. We went to sleep listening to the rushing stream and to the bugle of a bull elk somewhere beyond the willows. I have camped there several times since, watching shooting stars and satellites streak through the still night sky.

We awoke the next morning with a start, as the roofs of our tents had collapsed onto our faces. About 8 inches of heavy, wet snow had fallen overnight. Being in the backcountry, we had not heard the weather forecast, and were a bit shocked to see so much snow on September 21, the first day of fall.

By about ten o'clock, the weather had cleared, and we decided to proceed with that day's planned summit of Huron Peak, located at the end of this box canyon. It was exhilarating to make first tracks in the fresh snow—something we relished on similar days in the Whites—but we soon came upon something that we likely would not have seen in New Hampshire. Fresh mountain lion tracks suddenly cut in on the trail, and we followed them with trepidation for quite a way before the trail switchbacked to the right and the cat's tracks continued straight into the trees.

Once again I summited well ahead of Van, but did not get the tremendous views the guidebook promised. "The view from Huron's summit is one of the best in the Sawatch," Roach wrote in his guide. But all I could see was another storm descending over the ridge, barreling in on us from the west. I quickly descended, and collected Van on the way—he would have to do without summiting Huron on this day. We got off the mountain, drove back to our campsite, collected our soggy tents, and drove out of there with all of our climbing gear completely soaked from climbing in the snow.

We had not prepared for winter climbing when we planned the trip, and did not have enough dry gear to continue in these conditions. We returned to the Leadville Hostel, spent the night, and decided that because of the change in weather we would have to cut our trip four days short. We returned to Denver and stopped to wash all evidence of our off-road adventures from our vehicle.

Standing in the carwash bay hosing off the Jeep, Van suddenly looked up and said, "I smell Chinese food!"

I looked around, and pointed to the restaurant next to the carwash. "No, it's Mexican," I said.

"No, I definitely smell Chinese food," Van maintained.

Then, looking well down the street, he exclaimed, "There it is!" Sure enough, there was a Chinese restaurant several buildings down. We went in and got the best deal either of us had ever seen—an overflowing plate of everything we could pile on, plus a Coke, for $3.99.

We flew back to New England with both bellies and memories full.

My return to hiking introduced me to a newfound love: trail running. Though I had been a road runner in and after college, I'd trained on pavement and competed in traditional 5K and 10K road races. When I returned to running as an older, slower athlete, the transition to running on trails gave me a renewed sense of accomplishment. My repeated hiking on Monadnock and on other rocky, often more treacherous terrain had transformed me into one of the better trail runners in New England, despite my age. I entered races and consistently finished among the leaders.

In 2006, at the age of 46, I had my pinnacle trail-running season. I competed in the annual Grand Tree Trail Series—trail races held across New England—and finished second in the final standings behind Ben Nephew, one of the nation's top trail runners. Nephew, from Foxboro, Massachusetts, has won the overall title nine times.

Training on Monadnock often took me onto seldom-used trails, and led to some unique experiences. Once, while running down the Smith Summit Trail on the west side of the mountain, I was in midleap between rocks when I heard a loud *crack* below me to my right. I landed and stopped dead in my tracks. The biggest black bear I'd ever seen stepped into a clearing no more than 40 feet below me. Fortunately, the wind was blowing up the ridge and it didn't catch my scent. The bruin, which I guessed must've weighed at least 450 pounds, sat down and started chomping on wild blueberries. I could hear him chewing, and every minute or so he would turn his head to scan the ridgeline above me to search for movement. He was so close I heard him inhale deeply as he sniffed. My heart raced in my chest. Satisfied he was alone, he went back to eating. Several minutes later, he sauntered off. He never knew I was there.

I set a couple of records on Monadnock that year, one of which likely will never be broken, and probably for good reason—it will take someone a bit crazier than me to attempt to break it.

On Memorial Day Weekend in 2006, I climbed Monadnock sixteen times in one 24-hour period, breaking the previous mark of fourteen held by Fran Rautiola, another of the regulars on the mountain. Starting at noon on a Saturday, I climbed repeatedly up and down the White Dot Trail, passing many of the same people four or five times that afternoon, much to their disbelief. It turned into a warm, moonless evening, and the night hikes went very smoothly despite some intestinal issues that sent me to the outhouse more times than I would have liked.

By morning I was still on record pace when Fran showed up to learn I was closing in on his mark. When I returned to the parking lot, finishing my fourteenth trip and tying his total, he was waiting for me. He joined me for the fifteenth climb, timing my 43-minute ascent—a pretty good time for a first ascent, let alone a fifteenth. We returned to the parking lot and, after congratulating me, he informed me that it was only 10 A.M. and I had time to do another one.

"Why not?" I thought, and back up I went.

But the adrenaline that had carried me throughout the whole ordeal had now worn off. I struggled with cramps the entire sixteenth lap. I could barely walk when I finished, and, in fact, had to call for a ride home, as I was unable to drive.

My numbers were staggering: sixteen round-trips amounted to 64 miles, all of it on the mountain's steady grade. I gained nearly 29,000 feet of elevation, roughly the height of Mount Everest.

While I suspect that record will stand the test of time, my second likely will not. Later that same year, I went after the single round-trip speed record for the White Dot Trail. I was informed that Ken Peterson, a now-retired park ranger, had once done the round-trip in 43 minutes flat some years before. For fun, I timed myself during a workout one day to see how close to the record I was. I left my watch at the bottom and started up. I treated it as a training run and did not try to push it too much, given that the rocks were still a bit damp from rain earlier in the day. When I got back to my car I stopped my watch; it read 40:50, more than 2 minutes under the record. I never did attempt to lower that time and I am sure that I could have broken 40 minutes if the rocks had been dry. I have taken too many hard falls over the years to try it now.

Surprisingly, I have never broken any bones on these falls. But my friend Larry was not so fortunate. We were climbing together one winter day, a couple of years before my banner season, just after a storm had coated Monadnock with a thick coating of ice. Just below the summit on the White Dot Trail, we had difficulty getting past one treacherous section of steep, smooth rock leading up from Paradise Valley. At the summit, I pulled my crampons from my pack and strapped them on for the descent, and advised Larry to do the same. Unfortunately, he decided against it.

A few minutes later, when we got back to that spot, Larry slipped and fell forward onto his chest on the icy chute. He rocketed past me in an instant and was catapulted off a small ledge into a stand of short, scrubby pines. It happened so fast I could do nothing but watch in horror.

I quickly climbed down to where he had disappeared into the woods and called his name. Nothing. Again, I called his name, and again, no response. I thought he might be dead. Then I heard a groan and saw movement. Slowly Larry crawled out of his tomb. He was bleeding from a puncture wound to his leg and complained of trouble breathing. But he strapped on his crampons and hiked off the mountain under his own power.

Later, Larry went to the hospital and learned he had broken several ribs. Unable to climb for many months, his physique changed dramatically. Hiking every day as he had in the past had enabled him to stave off the effects of his alcohol intake. But when he could not climb, his excessive drinking quickly began to consume him. Soon, he was very out of shape, had developed a serious beer gut, and really did start to resemble Willie Nelson's grandfather. We thought he was done for.

But, much to our surprise and relief, Larry pulled himself together, quit drinking, and started hiking again. It took a couple of years, but he eventually regained much of his former ability. Now, you can see him on Monadnock almost every day, just as before. He rides his bike from his apartment in the town of Jaffrey, about 4 miles away, and volunteers much of his time, as he always had, doing trail work and picking up all the trash left behind by inconsiderate hikers.

My 2006 trip to Colorado had gone so well that the following year, when I announced plans to continue bagging the state's 14ers, not only did Van want to go back again, but my friend Brian Rusiecki also decided to join us. I had first met Brian in 2004 during one of those first winter hikes in the Whites with Karen Potter. They were both competitive mountain bikers, but Brian was making the transition to trail running. We trained and raced together often in 2007 and '08, when I was still able to keep up with him, and I even beat him a few times. Now Brian is one of the top ultradistance runners in the country.

Brian stated well before agreeing to join us on this trip that he would not be climbing any routes that were exposed, and Van wasn't particularly fond of dizzying heights, either. We planned the vacation over the summer and mapped out an itinerary that would begin with Longs Peak in Rocky Mountain National Park and conclude two weeks later with Pikes Peak in southern Colorado. Then, I would drive them back to the airport in Denver for their return flights, and I would stay on an extra week to continue peakbagging alone.

The three of us were to meet in Denver on September 8, 2007, each flying in from New England out of different airports: Van was leaving from Boston's Logan; Brian booked his ticket from Bradley in Hartford, Connecticut; and I would fly out of Manchester, New Hampshire. I was supposed to arrive first, secure our rental vehicle, and pick them up. But it didn't work out that way.

The night before, I had been out until after 1 A.M. drinking with friends, and then got up 2 hours later when my mom picked me up for the 90-minute drive to Manchester. When we got to the airport, she asked if she should wait for me, but I said not to bother, since I could see the Delta counter through the glass doors. I grabbed my two overstuffed backpacks and trudged inside.

"What do you mean, I don't have a ticket?" I asked incredulously when I tried to check in. "I made this reservation months ago," I exclaimed, my head still pounding from my night on the town.

"Yes, I see you did," the Delta agent said, "but then it was canceled on July 19."

"What?" I shot back. "Who would do that?"

"It appears your credit card company did, sir," she said.

Incredible. I had made the reservation months before using reward points on my credit card, and thought all was set. I had not even bothered to call the airline the day before to confirm, something I usually did before a flight. There was nothing I could do except to buy a new ticket on the spot and deal with the bank when I got home.

"How much is it?" I asked.

The reply: "It's $765."

I bristled as I slid my credit card across the counter.

Because of the mishap, I arrived in Denver late. Brian had been wandering around the airport for nearly an hour looking for me before he spotted me and gave me a start just as I was about to have him paged. I went to get our rental—this time, an all-wheel-drive Toyota Highlander. I wisely agreed to the extra insurance, a decision for which I'd be thankful before the end of the trip. When Van arrived soon after, we piled in and headed to Boulder, intent on climbing Longs Peak the next day without any acclimatization.

Longs Peak is probably the most famous of Colorado's 14ers, perhaps only rivaled in popularity by Pikes Peak, which has both a paved road and a cog railway to the top. Longs Peak stands sentinel over the entire Front Range and is the gateway to Rocky Mountain National Park. It is not an easy climb, and it is not for the faint-hearted, either. Most climbers hit the trail in the wee hours of the morning in order to be off the summit before early afternoon thunderstorms descend on the peak. Given that reputation and Roach's guidebook description of the technical terrain, I was surprised that both Brian and Van agreed to come along, but come 3 A.M., we were off. In the dark of early morning, Brian was unable to see the seriousness of the route until we had put so many miles behind us that it did not make sense for him to turn back.

Daylight came as we approached the Keyhole, a notch on the ridgeline at 13,150 feet that signals the beginning of the serious climbing. The Keyhole Route is the single-most-climbed route on any Colorado 14er; about 25,000 people a year attempt it, and 10,000 of those successfully summit. But it can also be one of the most dangerous; about sixty people have died on Longs Peak since it was first climbed in 1868 by a party led by none other than the famed Grand Canyon explorer John Wesley Powell.

Climbing through the Keyhole onto the other side of the ridge, we then traversed the Trough, which leads to some dramatic cliffs that rise to the summit. From here, the trail skirts these cliffs along a ledge system known as the Narrows, leading to the Homestretch, a 250-foot gully up smooth slabs leading to the broad, flat summit. Only one person—a trail runner—had passed us all day.

We completed the round-trip in just 8.5 hours; not bad for three flat-landers who had just stepped off a plane the day before. Van, fortunately, did not suffer from the altitude this time.

The next day, our route up Mount of the Holy Cross was much less severe, a veritable walk in the park in comparison.

From there, we drove into Aspen and headed for Montezuma Basin, for what we expected to be a relatively simple climb of Castle Peak the next morning. Past the small town of Ashcroft, the road became much rougher, and at one point we came to a halt as the road dropped into a fast-flowing creek. Undaunted, however, I plunged the Toyota Highlander into the torrent and climbed out the other side without bottoming out on any of the massive boulders that threatened to prevent passage.

Ironically, Brian and Van had agreed to climb Castle Peak only because it was considered so benign. At 14,265 feet, Castle is considered the monarch of the Elk Range by virtue of its height, but it is not at all like most of the other 14ers in the range, many of which can be climbed only via treacherous Class 4 ascents. The famed Maroon Bells, for example, are probably the most dramatic and photographed mountains in the state and are also known by many as the "Deadly Bells." They earned their name in 1965 when eight people fell to their deaths in five separate accidents. The main culprit is the so-called "rotten" rock, made of a metamorphic sedimentary mudstone, not the solid granite of other peaks in the range. Not a year seems to go by without at least one recorded death on the Bells.

The trail up Castle Peak, on the other hand, was rated a moderate Class 2, "the easiest route on any Elk Range 14er," according to our guidebook, and we anticipated an easy day.

But I was not able to navigate this diminishing road all the way to 12,800 feet and to Montezuma Basin as I had hoped. A large rock protruding into the road denied passage, and we drove back to a road junction and set up camp. A pair of nearby waterfalls lulled us to sleep. The next morning, we hiked up the road a couple of miles to reach the old Montezuma Mines, where we met a man with a high-clearance vehicle who had been up there to photograph Castle at dawn for a calendar he said he was shooting. We should've pressed him for more information about the route, but he had told us it was a "cinch," and the guidebook had said the same thing. From Montezuma Basin, Roach wrote, "the climb becomes a lark."

With that in mind, we should have been alarmed when we left Montezuma Basin and did not find a well-established trail. No route was readily apparent to us through a thin layer of snow that had fallen overnight. Though it was late summer, the day was chilly. We looked at the map in the book and guessed that the peak we needed to climb was the one to our right. It was a mistake that almost cost Van his life.

We climbed a ways and I lost myself in the exuberance of being in the Rockies. We were so high. I felt so free. And I just kept at the steep scree slope. It angled away from me at 45 degrees, giving me a clear path to push on without worrying about dislodging rocks and sending them flying back toward my friends. But a voice interrupted my progress.

"Don't climb any higher!" Brian yelled some hundred yards below me.

I looked back and realized that I had gotten too far ahead of Brian and Van, a dangerous situation I had known I should avoid. In the moment, I had forgotten the first rule of climbing safety: never put those below you in harm's way. The slope had steepened to a 60-degree pitch and had become a Class 4 scramble.

"Don't move," Brian yelled again.

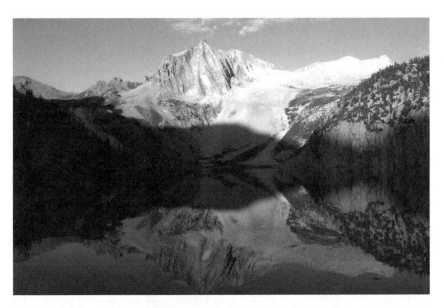
Hagerman Peak, a high 13er in the Elk Range outside of Aspen, reflects off the calm surface of Snowmass Lake on a picture-postcard afternoon.

I had already stopped, finally admitting to myself that this could not possibly be the trail up Castle Peak. The guidebook had said nothing of this.

"Okay," I yelled back. "I won't move."

But the rock under my right foot did not appear as stable as a flatter one a few inches away, so I took my foot off the round stone about the size of a melon to step over to the other one. When I did, the first stone dislodged and tumbled down the slope. At first, I was not concerned. The rock appeared to be heading harmlessly well to Brian and Van's left. But then it hit another rock and I watched—horrified—as it made an abrupt 90-degree turn and rocketed straight for my unsuspecting partners.

"Rock!" I yelled as loudly as I could.

Brian, standing in front of Van, saw it barreling toward them, and quickly dived to the ground, taking cover behind a small rock, only his backpack protruding above it. Van, however, was transfixed like a deer in headlights, not seeing any immediate shelter and not knowing which way to move.

The scene that unfolded felt almost like it had devolved into slow motion. Picking up speed, the rock continued on a direct line toward them, like they were wearing some sort of magnet. The rock took one last bounce and flew airborne, straight at Van's head. Van's eyes bulged. At the last second, he lunged to his left. The rock sped past, missing them both and continuing down the slope to join so many others that had fallen into the basin over millennia.

I had a long climb back down to their position, where I could do little more than apologize profusely. They were understandably upset with me; I had foolishly put their lives in danger. We returned to the basin, where the snow had melted and the real trail to Castle Peak revealed itself. In addition, we could hear voices coming from that direction, meaning other climbers were ahead of us.

But Brian and Van were still visibly shaken. They refused to continue with me up the true trail, and, instead, slowly made their way back to our vehicle. It was probably good that we separated for a while. I was just as upset with myself as they were with me.

Climbing on alone, I followed a trail that traversed up the side of the mountain to a saddle, leading to a short, steep climb to the summit. I arrived just in time to see three people on the summit, one of them whacking golf balls into the ravine thousands of feet below.

Things were understandably quiet when I got back to the vehicle. Brian and Van were waiting to read me the riot act. They said that we could not put ourselves in such a position again. I completely agreed, and spent the remainder of the day apologizing. But it would be several days before either of them would agree to climb with me again.

Fortunately, there were other things to enjoy besides summiting at our next destination. The following day, we planned an 8-mile hike in to camp at Snowmass Lake, which turned out to be one of the most beautiful campsites any of us had ever seen.

We hiked in with heavy packs, yet still covered the 8 miles in less than 4 hours. It had been warm the night before, probably because we were sleeping relatively low at 7,000 feet, and I was glad I had strapped my tent to the outside of my pack after it wouldn't fit inside for the hike in. At 11,000 feet, it was much colder at Snowmass Lake that night, too cold to entertain sleeping under the stars, it turned out. But the lake was magnificent; across the water from our campsite rose 200-foot granite cliffs that glistened white in the afternoon sun, as if covered in snow. It was an idyllic spot.

After lunch, we hiked around the lake to scout out the trail to Snowmass Peak, our goal for the following day. On an unexpectedly steep scree slope, Brian and Van decided the memories of the day before were too fresh, and they headed back to camp. They ended up finding a good hiking trail through a nearby pass with which to occupy themselves.

Continuing up the slope alone, I eventually lost the trail when I could not find any more cairns to follow. So I headed up a basin to my left and found a good chute leading me to the ridgeline, and then followed a narrow ridge over jagged yet solid rock about a half-mile to the summit.

The views from the summit were staggering. I felt I could almost touch near-by Capitol Peak, with perhaps the most impressive ridgeline of any 14er in the state. I would see it soon enough: it was next up on our schedule. In the opposite direction were the deadly Maroon Bells. I dreaded to think that I was planning to climb them in a few days. After signing the register book, I began my descent and arrived back at camp just 5 minutes before Brian and Van.

After hiking out the next morning, we drove to the Capitol Creek trailhead and hiked another 6 miles in to the beautiful, hidden valley underneath the magnificent profile of Capitol Peak, considered by many to be Colorado's hard-est and most majestic 14er. "Singular and stoic, Capitol stands supreme as the northernmost Elk Range 14er," Roach heralded of the granite behemoth.

The campsites beneath Capitol's great north wall were almost as spectacular as the one at Snowmass Lake. There was a grassy depression on top of a small hill with several available sites, one in the process of being vacated by three hikers who had climbed Capitol that day. They said it took them 9 hours round-trip and was harder than the Bells. I found that hard to believe. I feared the Maroon Bells the same way I used to fear Mount Washington.

Capitol Peak's signature feature is its famed Knife's Edge, a 100-foot-long section of smooth rock shaped like the ridgeline of a steeply pitched roof. Crossing it is like walking a tightrope 2,000 feet above the ground. Most people traverse it with their feet below the apex, walking hand over hand across the

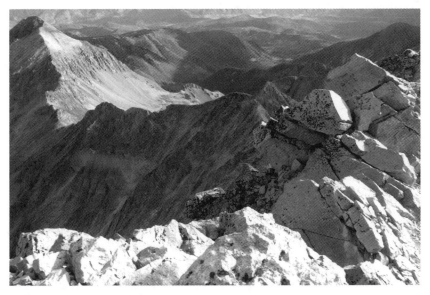

Capitol Peak, one of the most difficult of Colorado's 14ers, features the treacherous, and only non-technical route to the summit, the famously exposed "Knife's Edge."

span; others sit atop the ridge as if riding a horse and scoot their way across on their butt. Some don't cross at all. Incredibly, while Capitol has claimed its share of lives over the years, there have been only two recorded deaths from falls off the Knife's Edge, both in the 1950s.

Needless to say, neither Brian nor Van accompanied me the next morning when I began climbing up to the ridge above. Van, complaining of flu-like conditions, stayed in camp and slept, while Brian continued on the trail that led past the lake for a long run that would include a close-up encounter with an elk.

After reaching the ridgeline, the trail led me onto the far side of the mountain and through a boulder field before leading up the back side of the ridge to a point at an elevation of 13,664 feet known as K2. This was where things got interesting. When I got to K2, I found a local guide with a client on a rope; the guide was lowering him off the knob of K2 down to the ridgeline leading to the Knife's Edge. The client, a man in his late 50s or early 60s, was not liking his predicament, and the guide was having a tough time convincing him to descend to the ridge.

Getting impatient, I simply downclimbed the steeper cliff face next to the other two, and continued on my way. It was amazing how confident I had become on exposed rock since my early days in the mountains just a couple of years before. When I got to the Knife's Edge, there was no hesitation as I simply grabbed the ridge and proceeded across hand over hand as I walked my feet underneath me.

I was quickly beyond the danger and very relieved as I scrambled the final few hundred yards to the summit and its tremendous views in all directions. It was one of the most well-earned summits I had ever stepped onto.

Making my way back to the Knife's Edge, I saw that the guide and client were now hung up on the other side. The client would not budge. In no time, I retraced my steps underneath the razor-thin crown and, moments later, was standing next to them.

"That's some impressive climbing," the guide said. His name was Scott, and he worked for Aspen Expeditions, a local outfitter. "But get yourself a helmet!"

Scott told me I could stop by their shop in town to get one, and asked what else I intended to climb while in Aspen. When I told him I planned on doing Pyramid Peak and the Bells over the next two days, both sporting harrowing Class 4 climbs, he said it would "probably be suicide" to climb either of them without a helmet, as those peaks were notorious for rockfall because of their "rotten rock." I told him I would stop and buy one as soon as we got back to Aspen that afternoon.

When we got to town, I headed for the climbing store, while Brian went in search of a map of other hiking options in the area, and Van wandered over to the town common, where a rugby match was going on. Turned out, it was the annual Aspen Ruggerfest, when more than fifty of the top teams from all over the world descend to scrum. I bought a helmet for $50, successfully negotiating a 10 percent discount that I said Scott had extended to me on the mountain, which was not entirely true.

That night, a violent thunderstorm hammered our campsite, soaking everything and short-circuiting our plans for the next day. In the morning, we drove back into Aspen looking for a laundromat and a place to shower, as none of us had bathed since we'd arrived in Colorado a week before—not counting an ice-cold dip Brian and Van had taken in Snowmass Lake.

Hail the size of quarters pummeled the ground as we drove into Aspen, and, when we drove past the town common, we were amazed to see that the rugby match was still going full tilt despite the deluge. Those rugby players are animals.

We found a laundromat—probably the only one in that ritzy town— but when the weather unexpectedly cleared, we hustled back to our campground without stopping at the Aspen Rec Center to take that $4 shower. Instead, we made afternoon plans: I felt it was still possible to climb Pyramid, despite the late start, while the others planned an overnight hike in to Willow Lake. Brian dropped me off at the Maroon Lakes, one of the most scenic places in all of Colorado. Just about every calendar you will find with mountains in it has a shot taken of the majestic Maroon Bells from this spot. Sure enough, a professional photo shoot was in progress when we arrived.

Pyramid Peak is listed as one of the five toughest 14ers in Colorado, and even the standard route is a Class 4 scramble over loose, crumbly rock all the way to the summit. As I started up the climber's trail, I quickly met a hiker coming off Pyramid who did a double take when he saw me, warning that it was too late in the day to begin a summit bid. While it was after 1 P.M., I figured that if the weather held, I would be fine, and if it didn't, I would bail. Everyone I met coming down advised me to turn around, but I assured them I would be fine and kept climbing.

Following a good trail all the way, I stayed out of the gullies with the loose, dangerous rock that Scott had warned me about the day before. On his advice, I climbed the green band of rock, which was much more solid than the rock around it. Several times, the trail narrowed to a 6-inch-wide ledge and I had to hug the cliff face as I worked my way around a tight corner. Another time, there was a place where I had to leap across a 4-foot-wide gap in the ledge. Four feet is not very far, but with the prospect of a deadly 2,000-foot plummet if I missed, the gap seemed to span eternity.

Pyramid's summit is one of the smallest I would find on any 14er, but with impressive views. The Maroon Bells were directly across the valley, appearing as ominous as ever. Fresh mountain goat scat littered the summit, but although I looked over the edge of the cliff on all four sides, I could not see one of those elusive creatures. Again, I had come up empty in trying to spot one.

Descending by the same route I had taken on the way up, I got back to the main trail at 5:42 P.M., and arrived back at the campground with plenty of daylight left. However, it soon began to rain again, and I ended up having to cook dinner in a downpour, wondering if Brian and Van were also getting soaked.

It was still raining in the morning when I headed back to the trailhead to climb South Maroon, at 14,156 feet the taller of the Bells and, according to most lists, the only one that counts as a ranked 14er. But ranked 14er or not, Roach called the crossing between South and North Maroon "one of the four great traverses" on any of the 14ers. Those who succeed "ring both Bells." I had hoped it would stop raining as it had the day before, affording me a window of opportunity to climb and take both peaks. And by the time I had covered the 3.3 miles on the trail to the turnoff for South Maroon, that's exactly what happened. I hoped it was a good sign.

From there, it was a brutal "forever" climb of nearly 3,000 feet straight up the side of South Maroon to reach the Southeast Ridge. As soon as I got there, a squall of ice pellets driven by 60-MPH winds beat me back. I hunkered down in the only shelter I could find—a small crack between two buttresses—to wait out the storm. Breaks in the swirling clouds teased me with views of the summit, still a long way away across now even-more-dangerous wet rock.

Even though the rain soon abated, I decided my best recourse was to retreat the way I had come and not risk it. I wouldn't be ringing either Bell on this day, but I wouldn't risk becoming a statistic, either.

Just as I got back to the Maroon Creek Trail, it began pouring and hailing again, with lots of thunder and lightning, so I'd certainly made the right choice. Incredibly, just as I got back to the Maroon Lakes, where the car was parked, I spotted Brian and Van on the trail just ahead of me. It was just after noon, and we had earlier agreed not to meet back at the car until three. What good timing for everyone, especially in that miserable weather.

From there, our plan was to drive to the Missouri Gulch trailhead and camp, but when another wild rain-and-hail storm chased us over Independence Pass, we instead beelined it to our favorite hostel in Leadville, where our first showers in more than a week brought us back to civility. It sure beat another long, cold night camping in the rain.

Again, it poured all night and, from the looks of the river running down the street outside the hostel and the fresh snow on Mount Massive in the distance, we were not going to be climbing anything that day. So I went back to bed. Later, we decided to stay a second night at the hostel and discussed changes to our schedule to ensure we could climb something more before I had to bring Brian and Van back to the airport in Denver in six days. We decided we might be able to drive the 5 hours to the San Juans in the southwest corner of the state to find mountains not covered in snow. We set out south, toward Salida, and noticed that the farther south we went, the less snow we saw on the Collegiate Peaks to the west.

In fact, from Poncha Springs, we could plainly see that the two southernmost Collegiates—Mount Shavano and Tabeguache Peak—were free of snow. So we drove to the trailhead and set up camp in a beautiful, open field ringed by some quaking aspens already beginning to change into their shimmering, golden yellow.

It was good to hike with Brian and Van again, as we had not summited anything together since before the rock incident on Castle several days before. But while the trail up Shavano was steep and rocky, it was by no means technical, and the descent over the other side and the traverse up Tabeguache was pretty mellow. If Brian and Van were still wary, they didn't show it. We had a leisurely lunch on Tabeguache's airy summit, returned over the top of Shavano, and completed the 11-mile out-and-back in 6.5 hours.

We resupplied in Salida, then headed for Mount Antero by way of the Baldwin Creek trailhead. Brian didn't like the description of the road in the guidebook and wanted us to hike the 3 miles and 1,400 feet up to the four-wheel-drive parking spot, but Van and I outvoted him. This road was nearly as bad as the one leading into Montezuma Basin, but we made it to its junction with an old mining road without incident and set up camp in a beautiful spot right next to an oxbow in roaring Baldwin Creek.

After a quick breakfast the next morning, we drove across Baldwin Creek at a shallow spot and left our vehicle to begin hiking up the old mining road leading to some of the many still-active mines on Antero. The peak is well known for its aquamarine content, having one of the highest concentrations of that semiprecious gem of any mountain in the world.

We could have driven much farther, but the accepted rules of peakbagging the 14ers call for climbers to ascend at least 3,000 feet under their own power in order for the climb to count. All these crisscrossing roads on the peak made Antero's upper reaches easily accessible to ATVs, dirt bikes, and even regular four-wheel-drive vehicles, and we regrettably met dozens of recreational enthusiasts at a large turnout just below the final climb to the summit. It was probably the least-enjoyable summit day we had yet experienced.

That afternoon, after our descent and a stop at Mount Princeton Hot Springs, we negotiated another steep, rutted road in the Highlander that was so narrow in spots that two cars couldn't have passed without one of them plunging off the cliff into a deep ravine. Fortunately, we were the only ones up there heading to Mount Princeton's trailhead. Our climb to the summit the next morning was uneventful, except that we had to spend most of it on unwelcome talus, making both the ascent and descent tougher than we had expected.

Still, we were back at the car by 11 A.M., and decided we had enough time to drive to the trailhead for Mount Yale and attempt the peak that afternoon, since the weather was holding. By chance, the Delaney Creek Trail out of Cottonwood Pass was by far the best trail we had hiked during our two weeks in Colorado. It was wide, well groomed, and wound its way to treeline through some open, grassy meadows and through some tall stands of aspens. It climbed steeply to the ridgeline at 13,700 feet and presented only a short scramble from there to the summit. We decided that Yale had been the most enjoyable mountain we had climbed so far. We got back to the car in time, we thought, to make it to our trailhead for the next day's ascent of Mounts Harvard and Columbia before darkness overtook us.

We didn't realize, however, what a rough-and-tumble drive Chaffee County Road 365 would turn out to be. Huge rocks and cavernous holes threatened to swallow up the Highlander, which had performed incredibly well so far despite all the scratches we had put into its white paint during our off-road excursions. We made the trailhead just at dusk and had to set up camp and cook dinner by headlamp.

As much as we had enjoyed Mount Yale the day before, the climb up Harvard was even better. The trail was incredibly well manicured; a lot of hard work had gone into maintaining this route up the third-highest peak in Colorado. Rocks had been moved to make steps, especially near the summit. While most trails on the 14ers top out in a saddle between peaks, this one switchbacked from a wide, grassy basin directly to the summit. Harvard had one of the prettiest summits we had seen.

We had planned to traverse over to neighboring Mount Columbia by hiking across the ridge separating the two peaks, but as soon as we descended off Harvard's summit, a large boulder immediately blocked the trail. There was quite a bit of snow in a little gully that we would have to climb down to get around this rock outcropping, and Brian didn't like the looks of it. He decided to skip Columbia and return the way we had come.

Van and I negotiated the turn and continued along the narrow ridgeline, scampering over large boulders with huge dropoffs on either side. We got about a third of the way along this ridge when we came to another large buttress blocking the path completely. Without a rope, it would have been risky working our way over or around this roadblock, so we decided instead to downclimb to some grassy slopes we could see to our left and then reclimb the ridge nearer Columbia's summit.

But it turned out we had underestimated how far we would have to climb down before we could start back up, and must have given up almost 2,000 feet of elevation before we got around the last of the obstacles. It was a quad-burning, lung-busting ascent over dreaded talus blocks to gain the summit, which we did not reach until 3 P.M., very late in the day to be atop a 14er.

Continuing over the summit, we descended a steep scree slope to the valley floor then hustled the 4 miles back to the car, expecting Brian to be waiting impatiently for us because I had forgotten to give him the car keys. Unbeknownst to us, however, he had spent time exploring on his way down, and had been waiting only about 15 minutes. Still, we had a long drive out on that rock-strewn road, followed by a 2-hour drive to get to the base of Pikes Peak for the final climb together.

In our haste, we bottomed out several times, and at one point Brian had to get out and remove a big rock from the path. Van and I could only laugh when he struggled to heave the large stone up an embankment, only to watch it comically roll back into its original resting place. We stopped only once after that—to snap pictures of one of the prettiest sunsets any of us had ever seen.

The most interesting way to climb Pikes Peak is to hike up the Barr Trail from Manitou Springs on the east side of the mountain. This 26-mile round-trip is the same course used by the famed Pikes Peak Marathon, considered the toughest marathon in the world by many and dubbed "America's Ultimate Challenge" by race organizers. It climbs more than 7,000 feet from Manitou Springs to the summit. For hikers, this route is often a two-day ascent, with climbers staying at the fully stocked Barr Camp overnight and summiting the next day. I've enjoyed this route a few times, but in 2007, we didn't have two days, or even one long one. We had to climb Pikes Peak and still have time to drive the two hours to Denver so Brian and Van could fly home the next morning. So we chose the alternate route from Crags Campground, which starts at 10,100 feet and is only 11.4 miles round-trip—less than half the other route.

For all of the upside to its speed, this route also followed the Pikes Peak Auto Road, right from the point where it then turned from pavement to dirt (the road has since been paved all the way to the summit). This meant that in the final 3 miles of our climb, the cars constantly kicked up dust that a ferocious, bone-chilling wind blew into our faces. It was not a joyous ascent.

Once at the summit, the scene was eerily similar to what we had seen many times before in New Hampshire: lots of cars, too many people, ugly buildings, and a cog railway.

"This looks like Mount Washington on crack!" Brian exclaimed of the din surrounding us. Things only got worse when the cog locomotive arrived shortly thereafter with a train full of underdressed tourists, many wearing shorts, while we were bundled against the cold in all our gear. Time for us to leave.

As enjoyable as the climbs on Yale and Harvard had been in the previous two days, Pikes Peak was our least-favorite climb of the whole trip, Antero's crowd of ATVs included. Pikes Peak may be "America's Mountain," inspiring Katharine Lee Bates to pen "America the Beautiful," but that particular route was anything but.

We got to Denver by 4 P.M. and took our second showers of the entire trip. It was appalling how bad we smelled after all those days on the trail. I slept on the floor of their motel room, but when they left for the 4:45 A.M. shuttle to the airport, I climbed into a nice, warm bed for the first time since we had been at the Leadville Hostel, and fell quickly back to sleep.

After helping myself to Brian's and Van's complimentary breakfasts later that morning, I headed south again on I-25 and headed for the town of Westcliffe, the gateway to the Sangre de Cristo Range, one of the prettiest and most challenging ranges in all Colorado. I looked forward to soloing these stunning peaks, though I also knew I would miss the company of my friends.

Once again, one of the roughest roads in the state greeted me as I negotiated rocks and mud and three creek crossings to find the South Colony Lakes trailhead deserted. I thought this strange, it being a Sunday and all, but then it started pouring and sleeting, and it dawned on me why I was the only one there—everyone else had heard the forecast.

I hiked the 1.5 miles to the South Colony Lakes and set up base camp so I could spend the next few days while climbing five 14ers, including the daunting Crestones, two of the most exposed peaks on my list. The South Colony Lakes sit in a high basin under the shadow of the Crestones, and, at nearly 12,000 feet, I anticipated another chilly, late-September night. It rained the entire hike in to the lakes and abated only briefly while I set up my tent and crawled in. The deluge started again and lasted several more hours, and I was glad Brian had left me his tarp. I had laid it down as a footprint under the tent, and it kept the rain from seeping through. Eventually, the rain turned to snow, pinning me inside for the remainder of the day.

A violent wind shook my tent all night long and denied me any real sleep, and I awoke to the coldest morning I had yet experienced. All I could see on any of the peaks surrounding me was a fresh coating of snow and ice. Climbing conditions were clearly unfavorable, but I had to climb something. Humboldt Peak was the only logical choice, it being the easiest of the five 14ers in the basin, but it turned out to be a brutally cold climb, with ferocious winds and a windchill that must have dropped well below zero.

Up top, the mountain was coated in a thick layer of rime ice, and I had worn my running shoes, rather than my boots, which were still wet from the day before. Several times on the descent, I felt myself slipping off the side of the mountain but was able to stop my fall by grabbing onto the rocks. The conditions were too dangerous. I returned to camp and quickly packed up for the hike out, planning to continue the trek south, where I had hoped it would be warmer.

At the road, I had a decision: turn left and go into Westcliffe to get gas, or turn right and chance that I had enough to get me in and out of the trailhead to Mount Lindsey, which was 60 miles away and included a 22-mile drive in off the main road. I turned right.

The road into Lindsey was not as bad as the others I had driven the previous couple of weeks, but I did have to detour around one large aspen tree that some beavers had recently dropped across the road. I passed the town of Gardner and its gas station just before the turnoff to the trailhead, thinking I could make it the 22 miles to the trailhead and back. The hike to the summit the next day was cold, and its only highlight was a close-range sighting of three bighorn sheep on the descent. But I had seen dozens of them; it was a mountain goat that I still longed to lay eyes on.

My only concern when I returned to the car was that I was pretty much out of gas, and I had to make it all the way back to Gardner. It was going to be close. Only 4 miles on my way, another big aspen tree had been dropped across the road during the night. Damn pesky beavers! Unlike the one the day before, however, there was no driving around this one, and I felt hopelessly trapped.

Then, I remembered having seen a large meadow about a half-mile back, and it dawned on me that this field might connect to a road that possibly connected back to the one I was on a short way ahead. So I backed up about a half-mile and found a spot where I could drive out into the field of 6-foot-tall prairie grass.

Elated at my good fortune, I recklessly burst out into this field as if I were speeding across the savannahs of Africa, mowing down large swaths of prairie grass as I went. I had no way of seeing where I was going; if there had been any ditches, rocks, or downed trees in the field, I can only imagine the amount of damage I would have done to the rental vehicle. But, sure enough, the field led me straight to an old farm road and then back onto the road I had driven in on. I was feeling pretty invincible at that point, until I looked at the gas gauge again. There had been one other vehicle at the trailhead when I left, and I wondered whether that person would follow my path through the field and figure out this ingenious escape route or be stranded in there for days, until someone showed up with a chain saw.

I got safely back to Gardner, only to find a big sign outside the gas station: No Gas. I was crestfallen again. I denigrated myself for not having noticed the sign the day before. With the needle well below "E" already, I was convinced there was no way I could make it the additional 25 miles to the town of Walsenburg. But I had to try.

Someone was watching over me, and, as the miles clicked away, the needle held steady and I must've rolled into Walsenburg virtually on fumes. I was never so glad to fill up in my life.

Now that I had gas, I turned west and headed for Lake Como, hoping to reach this high valley before dark so I could attempt the valley's three 14ers the next day. The road into Lake Como, however, is known as the "worst road in America," according to Roach's guidebook. I didn't think it could be any worse than the other roads on which I had already driven. I was wrong. It was by far the worst road I had ever seen, with huge, protruding boulders everywhere, like warts on the back of a giant toad.

After a mere 1.6 miles on this road, I gave up and abandoned the car. I am certain I could have hiked the distance in less time, but I was, as ever, determined to see how far I could get.

It was now late afternoon, and I was unsure how many more miles it was to the lake. Not wanting to lose precious minutes by stopping to take off my 40-pound pack in order to put on a long-sleeve shirt and gloves, I was chilled to the bone just as dusk fell 2 hours later when I finally crested the final rise and spotted Lake Como. To my utter relief, the first thing I saw was a roaring campfire on the far side of the lake.

The camper, John, not only was from New Hampshire, but he lived in Milford, not more than an hour from my home in Keene. After quickly setting up camp, I went over to unthaw my hands at the fire before attempting to cook dinner.

Soon, the rising full moon illuminated the clearing and the light shimmered magically off the surface of Lake Como. It was beautiful. Staggeringly so. As I watched, a shooting star streaked across the sky. But, at 11,900 feet, it was still an exceptionally cold night. Three 14ers rose out of a valley directly behind me: Blanca Peak, Ellingwood Point, and Little Bear Peak, the latter of which I knew was considered one of the five hardest 14ers to climb, right up there with the Maroon Bells. I would attempt to climb Blanca and Ellingwood in the morning and then consider whether Little Bear was a good idea for the afternoon.

As I climbed up through the valley the next morning, Little Bear's massive northwest wall cast an ominous shadow over my progress. The valley itself was spectacular, with several more small lakes, called tarns, dotting the way, all of them an indescribable shade of green. Blanca is Colorado's fourth-highest mountain, and perhaps its most beautiful, rising majestically above the San Luis Valley to the south. I had contemplated climbing Little Bear first and then attempting the perilous mile-long traverse over to Blanca, but Roach termed this the most dangerous traverse on any Colorado 14er—"Simply put, this is Colorado's most astonishing connecting ridge." I had learned my lesson with Roach plenty of times before and I wisely decided against it. My route led me directly below the traverse and all I could see above was ice glistening from all the notches and couloirs. I knew a lot of climbers had died on Little Bear.

The climb up the ridgeline to Blanca's summit was some of the best climbing I had enjoyed in Colorado, and the views to the south were stunning, reaching all the way into New Mexico. Below, I could see the town of Fort Garland, where Zebulon Pike and his men had holed up during the cold winter of 1807—briefly being taken prisoner by the Spanish—and where Kit Carson himself was once the fort commander. Returning to the saddle with Ellingwood, I found the trail up this ridge much harder to follow, because probably the only ones who bother to climb this lesser-known peak are peakbaggers.

Scrambling off Ellingwood down a steep scree slope rather than taking the circuitous route I had come up, I returned to the basin, where I stopped to eat lunch at one of the emerald lakes and sat on a rock contemplating my immediate future. While I certainly could have endured another chilly night on the shores of Lake Como and tackled Little Bear the following morning—and avoided the risk of being caught exposed on the peak by an afternoon storm—I also knew I was running out of days on this trip and did not want to waste any of them.

Little Bear was staring me straight in the face, but I knew that not many people attempt to climb all three peaks in one day, completing what Roach called the "Grand Slam." But there was not a cloud in the sky and it was still morning, so I decided to give it a shot.

Reaching Little Bear's dramatic ridgeline was extremely difficult. I had to climb a near-vertical, 2,000-foot chute that was chock-full of deep, heavy snow. There were fresh boot tracks going up, but none coming down, so I thought there might be a climber above me. But I saw no one all day. Perhaps someone was attempting the traverse, though I hoped not. Once on the ridge, I crossed over to the backside of the mountain and soon was staring up at the crux of the climb, the infamous Hourglass—a steep, water-polished slab of Class 4 granite that ascends 250 feet to Little Bear's summit.

Roach called the Hourglass the most dangerous section of trail on a standard route for any Colorado 14er. Water and ice from snowmelt above cascaded down the center of the Hourglass, adding to the difficulty. There were fixed ropes anchored to the rock, intended for climbers like me, but on this day they were engulfed by the water flowing down the smooth slabs.

Cautiously, I free-climbed the dry rock to the left of the ropes and, despite ascending the wrong gully, which sported some low Class 5 rock, I gained the ridge crest and made my way the final 200 yards to the summit. Exhilarated to have summited all three peaks in one day, I was equally concerned about how I was going to get down. Fortunately, from the summit, I spotted a safer route back to the top of the Hourglass—the route I should have taken on the way up. Still, the climb back was not easy, and, once there, it was apparent that the safest way down was to use the ropes and rappel down the cliff face, even though that meant I would be sprayed by the cascading water and crumbling ice. Now wet and cold, I hightailed it back to camp, pretty much skiing down the snow chute back to the valley floor, kicking up a small avalanche that carried me along.

Then came the long hike back to the car and an even longer, it seemed, drive back to the main road. From there, I headed north, past Great Sand Dunes National Park, which I longed to see, until I reached the tiny village of Crestone and the trailhead for Kit Carson Peak and Challenger Point. The town of Crestone is home mostly to a group of spiritual new-agers, and, in 2011, they petitioned the U.S. Board on Geographic Names to change the name of Kit Carson Peak, since it was named in honor of the frontiersman who made no secret of the fact that he had killed more American Indians than perhaps any other white man. Calling Kit Carson a war criminal, they wanted it renamed Mount Crestone, but with two other 14ers in the same range already named Crestone Peak and Crestone Needle, the petition was denied in order to avoid confusion.

The hike in to Willow Lake was extremely tame, with perhaps thirty or forty switchbacks along its 4-mile length. At the far end of the lake was a 50-foot-high cliff with a narrow waterfall running down the center of it. The whole scene was stunning. The trail led up some granite benches to the top of this waterfall, and then the fun quickly ended in the form of a 2,000-foot scramble up a scree slope to the ridgeline of Challenger Point. This peak was renamed in honor of the space shuttle that exploded a minute after takeoff in 1986, claiming the lives of seven crew members, including New Hampshire's own Christa McAuliffe, looking to become the first teacher in space.

From the summit of Challenger Point, I continued along the ridge and descended to a broad ledge called Kit Carson Avenue that traversed underneath the Prow, a huge protruding rock that looks like the bow of a ship. Eventually, I reached a tiny saddle that seemed to separate Kit Carson from its neighboring peak, and, after some initial confusion, found the trail leading to the summit directly behind me.

I returned to the valley floor and stopped to eat my lunch on top of the waterfall overlooking Willow Lake. The wind had picked up from the south and was carrying the mist from the waterfall back over the lip and drenching me with a cold, enjoyable spray. It was the first shower I had had in a week. On my way out, I stopped to take some stunning pictures of Willow Lake, as the afternoon sun was lighting up the cliffs and the waterfall. It was heavenly.

The next day—a Friday—was the last of the trip, and I contemplated trying to climb both Crestones and then driving all the way back to Denver, but decided against it. I had lots of packing to do, a real shower to take, and the car to clean up. In addition to the myriad scratches and dings I had put into the vehicle, it now also had a starburst crack in the windshield, having caught a rock somewhere along the way, and I was certain I would never be allowed to rent a car again. Fortunately, I had taken out an additional $3,000 in insurance, and the damage probably came close to that amount.

Back home in New Hampshire, I began planning my return to Colorado the following September, when I had hoped to summit the twenty 14ers that remained. Van and I also began talking about a backpacking trip through Central America from January to April, when I would again be on layoff from UPS.

But first I called the bank regarding the matter of my plane ticket. I was polite when I contacted the agent for the rewards program and asked him about their having made the flight reservation for me months before.

"Yes, I see we did that," the man said.

"And, did you see that on July 19 you canceled it on me?" I responded.

After a slight pause, he simply said with chagrin, "How much do we owe you?"

I received a check for $765 within the week.

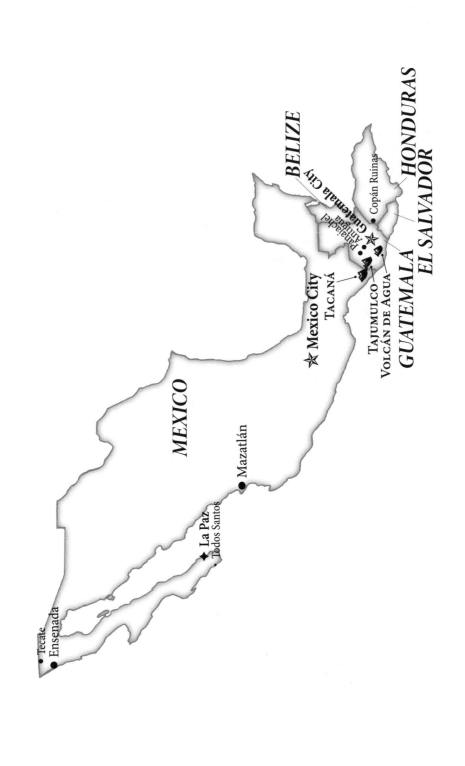

Chapter 4
January 2008

SOUTH OF THE BORDER

VANNAK POL DOES NOT KNOW HOW OLD HE IS. HE DOESN'T EVEN KNOW HIS ACTUAL birth date.

"My driver's license says I'm 33," he told me during a hike on Mount Monadnock on Christmas Day 2013. "But I don't know exactly. My uncle picked my birthday for me. Most Cambodians my age don't know their real age or even their birth date. I'm just lucky to be alive."

Van was born during one of the most unspeakable periods of human history: in the midst of the genocide carried out in Cambodia by Pol Pot and the Khmer Rouge, which was immediately followed by a protracted war with Vietnam that lasted ten years. His parents, who found themselves in Pol Pot's forced labor camps—known as the Killing Fields—could only guess that Van was born sometime in 1980, but even they don't know for sure.

His earliest childhood memories are of death and war. "I remember one day when I was in first grade, a mortar landed in our classroom and a lot of kids were killed right in front of me," Van told me. "Their blood was on my clothes. I ran to my uncle's house crying and crawled into a foxhole. I saw a lot of people get shot and I saw people get their legs blown off by land mines," he said. "That's still my nightmare to this day. I saw a lot of bad things."

Van grew up on the run as first the Khmer Rouge, then the invading Vietnamese chased his family from one refugee camp to the next along the mountainous Thai border. "Our family was running for our lives," he remembered. "We always lived our life on the go."

Ultimately, Van and his family learned they would be allowed to immigrate to the United States, where his uncle already was. "I was ecstatic when I heard we were going to be allowed to go to America," Van said. "We called America 'heaven.' When we referred to heaven in the refugee camps, we meant America."

It was more than a year, however, until they finally were allowed to emigrate, and Van remembers May 26, 1993, as the "most important day of my life."

The family first settled in Cleveland, where Van's uncle then resided. But, not knowing any English, his parents did not get along well there, and they soon moved to Lowell, Massachusetts, which boasts the second-highest concentration of Cambodians in the United States, after Long Beach, California.

"I am one of the lucky ones," Van said, remembering all those he saw die around him as a young child. "I tell myself that every day."

It was in Lowell that Van's passion for hiking and climbing was inadvertently awakened. Van's freshman-year English teacher invited him and some classmates to join her family on a summer hike on Mount Monadnock, located just over the New Hampshire border about an hour's drive from Lowell. At first, he wasn't going to go.

"I didn't think I would like to hike because I was afraid it would bring back all those bad memories," he said. While so many New Englanders fondly remember their childhoods spent outdoors, Van's experiences escaping on foot over the mountains could not have been more different. He went anyway.

"But next thing you know, I was the first one to the top of the mountain," Van recalled. "It was awesome up there. The bug bit me right then."

He began to look forward to joining the teacher on the Monadnock hike every summer. "I would get so excited," he said. "I got into hiking more and more and it built up my confidence as a person. I learned more from hiking than I ever did sitting in a classroom. It changed my life. Now hiking is something I can't live without."

After Van graduated from high school, the same teacher brought him on a trip to the White Mountains.

"They were stunning. Somewhere, I discovered the Four Thousand Footer list, and I remember saying, 'This is crazy.' But in the summer of 2002, I did my first Four Thousand Footer with some friends on the Fourth of July on Mount Liberty. I kept checking off peaks and, by the fall of 2003, I had seventeen off the list. When I completed the list in 2005 on Mount Jefferson, I thought I had seen the whole world. But I was just scratching the surface."

But Van's parents were beginning to worry about their son and his strange hobby. He had three sisters who they thought were "normal," in that they went to clubs every weekend with their friends. Van, however, always went hiking, often by himself.

"I remember hearing my mother telling my uncle on the phone that something was wrong with me and that I needed help," he said, laughing. "She wanted to put me on drugs or into therapy. I told her hiking is my therapist."

Though I had met Van on Monadnock a few times, we had not taken the time to get to know each other. But when we met by chance one winter day in 2004 in the parking lot in Franconia Notch in the White Mountains and spent the day climbing the Kinsmans together, we struck up a friendship despite our twenty-year age difference.

By summer 2006, Van had become a volunteer ranger at Monadnock State Park and had climbed Mount Hood in Oregon with Dave Targan, another park ranger, who had a wealth of big-mountain experience. When I asked him if he wanted to join me to climb 14ers in Colorado that September, he jumped at the opportunity. "Wow," Van said later of the invitation, "that was the first big thing for me. You opened the door to the rest of the world for me."

Just before our second trip to Colorado, in 2007, Van realized another dream. He was informed that he was going to finally become a naturalized U.S. citizen that October. With new rights and responsibilities, he could obtain a passport and explore the world. "To me, that was like an angel getting its wings," he said.

When I started planning a three-month backpacking trip of Central America for early 2008, I invited Van to join me. He immediately said yes, even quitting his job to do so. Van trusted me implicitly—despite that mishap with the rock the year before. But others were not so sure. Many of Van's hiking friends, including Dave Targan, who had become like a father to him, questioned his decision to travel south of the border with me, especially to Guatemala, which had a human rights record nearly as abysmal as Cambodia's.

It took some doing to reassure Van's many adoptive families and friends that he would be safe with me, and I did not take the responsibility lightly.

I'd been back to Guatemala once since my 2005 trip, mostly to finish my book Greetings from Gringotenango, which recounts stories of the characters I'd met on the shores of Lake Atitlán. True to form, I took the chance to summit Volcán Tolimán while I was there. After two years away from the country, I was looking forward to summiting Volcán de Agua alongside Van. But we had plenty of peaks on the itinerary before that. Our plan was to fly to Southern California, walk across the Mexican border, hop a bus, and head south. My brother, Bryon, lives in Alpine, California, in the hills about a half hour east of San Diego, and I arrived there on January 8, one week ahead of Van. Bryon, who is a year younger than me, had headed west not long after graduating from high school in 1979.

My first trip to California was in 2000. That time, after Bryon picked me up at the airport, we had headed straight into the desert for a weeklong camping trip in Anza-Borrego Desert State Park. We had a great time reconnecting; the two of us had never been particularly close, but after that trip we parted as friends for the first time since we were children. Not long after, Bryon moved back to New Hampshire for three years, but by 2008, he had returned to California.

When I arrived that year, Bryon and I again headed for the Anza-Borrego, and eventually worked our way east to Arizona, where the Gaskill Brothers, a team of Wild West reenactors that Bryon was a part of, was competing in an annual event at Yuma Territorial Prison State Historic Park. Both days of the competition, Bryon got "shot and killed," but he recovered in time to drive us home.

Van arrived later that week, and he and I spent that Saturday hiking in the Cuyamaca Mountains near my brother's house. Our climb included 3,838-foot Gaskill Peak, named for the two brothers who successfully warded off a gang of Mexican bandits in the nearby town of Campo, California, in 1875. That battle was also the focus of Bryon's reenactment group and of a book I would later help him write.

Van and I enjoyed a peaceful lunch on the summit looking down at the homes of all the millionaires Van said must live everywhere in California. "But," he exclaimed, looking around at all the natural beauty surrounding us, "we're the ones who are the *real* millionaires."

The next day, we packed and watched as the Patriots beat the hometown Chargers in the AFC Championship Game to improve to 17-0 and advance to the Super Bowl against the New York Giants. Since we did not want to miss the big game, we decided that we needed to be in Panajachel—my "hometown" in Guatemala—in time to watch the Patriots attempt to complete their perfect season. That gave us nearly two weeks to meander our way down the Mexican coast.

The following day—Monday—my brother drove us to the border crossing in Tecate and wished us luck. I knew he secretly wished he were going with us. The immigration officials were somewhat surprised to see Americans crossing the border on foot. Our visas cost us 130 Mexican pesos, or about 22 U.S. dollars at the time. Then we had to pay an additional tax of another Mex$100 on the contents of the boxes of climbing gear we were carrying.

Van and I intended to climb several of the high volcanoes in Mexico at the end of our trip, but we didn't need to carry all our technical climbing gear with us the entire time, so we boxed it up and mailed it directly to our outfitter's office in Tlachichuca, where it would be waiting for us when we arrived sometime in mid-March. It was a great plan, and it cost us each only an additional Mex$90— roughly US$15—to mail the two large boxes from the local post office in Tecate.

After a trip to the ATM to withdraw more pesos, we sat in the town plaza for several hours waiting for the next bus to Ensenada, the gateway to Baja and the Pacific Coast. While the 2-hour bus ride to Ensenada cost only Mex$60, we learned that the next leg from Ensenada to La Paz—more than a thousand miles—would cost almost Mex$800, or about US$130, and would take 20 hours. We were not prepared for the bus to be so expensive, so we had to find another ATM for more pesos.

It was well after dark when we left Ensenada for the overnight ride to La Paz, the capital of Baja California Sur, located on the Sea of Cortez. Our destination, however, was the tiny Pacific Coast town of Todos Santos, and we had to hop on a second bus in La Paz to get there. We arrived after dark. Despite the moon being nearly full that night, it was overcast, and there were few streetlights. We stepped off the bus onto streets that were almost devoid of light just as it started to sprinkle. Knowing no one, and with no clue which direction the ocean was— we had planned to camp on the beach—we were completely lost in the darkness.

Providence then intervened, as it seemingly would so many times on this trip. We turned onto a street lit only by an outdoor café where a young couple was eating dinner and clearly speaking English. We introduced ourselves and told them of our predicament. They quickly invited us to join them. Austin and Joelle Ater were from Washington and, along with their month-old baby, Ocean, were staying in an RV down near the beach on property owned by Austin's uncle.

Before dinner was over they had pretty much adopted us. They gave us a ride to the beach and we pitched our tents in the sand just 30 yards from the pounding surf of the Pacific. Van and I spent three glorious days and nights on what

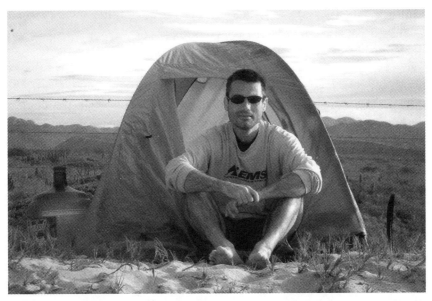

I enjoy an idyllic afternoon watching humpback whales breach offshore while camping on the beach near Todos Santos in Baja Sur, Mexico.

was practically a deserted, endless beach known to the locals as La Pastora. The Aters brought us food and water, and we spent much of the first day watching humpback whales breach the surface about a hundred yards offshore.

On Thursday morning, Austin drove us to the deserted La Burrera trailhead, 11 miles from the main road. We estimated that our packs weighed nearly 60 pounds, including the gallon of water we each had strapped to the sides. This was not a simple day hike: we were starting a two- to three-day hike to climb the highest peak—an unnamed point at 6,857 feet—in the Sierra de la Laguna mountain range that bisects the state of Baja California Sur.

We hiked for nearly 2 hours but gained only about 3,000 feet, according to Van's altimeter, as the terrain was not particularly steep, and decided to set up camp in a small recess off the trail well below ridgeline. Van said the magnificent views reminded him of Cambodia—rugged and remote, but without the land mines, of course.

In the morning, we left our camp intact and climbed on with just our day packs, gaining another 3,500 feet to the rim of a canyon, where the trail leveled a bit as it approached some radio towers. The trail beyond was faint, but we could see our destination in the distance.

The craggy, double-peaked summit was nothing more than a big, granite rock pile that looked like any number of summits in the White Mountains. Another trail continued over to a lower, broader summit, which appeared to have better views to the west and the Pacific. That's when I noticed a teenager sitting there with a "USA" jersey on. And another.

Turned out, they were part of a group of about a dozen teenagers and three instructors from the National Outdoor Leadership School (NOLS) on a seventeen-day camping trip in this remote, barren landscape. And two of them were from New Hampshire and had spent many days training for their trip by hiking Mount Monadnock. They had been out on the trail six days from La Paz, and the first thing they wanted to know was who was playing in the Super Bowl. The two New Hampshire girls were ecstatic when I told them the Patriots had won, but one boy from Wisconsin let out a huge groan when he learned that his beloved Packers had lost to the Giants in the NFC Championship.

We found less to explore in the mountains than we had expected, and in the morning, simply hiked the 2 hours back to the La Burrera trailhead, where we hoped we could hitch a ride back to Todos Santos, as Austin was not supposed to pick us up until the following day. But the only people we saw all day were three men who arrived in a pickup truck with two burros in the back. The two older men quickly unloaded their donkeys, mounted up, and hit the trail, and the teenage boy drove off before we could ascertain his destination.

It was a long, boring day, followed by an equally long night camping behind the locked ranger station, waiting for Austin to pick us up the next afternoon. Sure enough, he arrived right at 2 P.M. as planned, and with a cooler full of ice-cold Pacifico *cervezas,* no less. I drank three of them on the ride back to town, where we stopped at a little streetside café and had fish tacos, which were three for a dollar. We all then drove back to the beach at La Pastora and watched the whales breach until sunset.

We awoke outside their camper in the morning to the smell of Joelle cooking French toast and enjoyed one last meal with our hosts before piling into their pickup for the hour-long drive to La Paz, where Van and I would catch a ferry to Mazatlán on the mainland. We almost missed the boat—literally—as its departure time was 3 P.M., and not 4, as we'd seen posted online. But we got there with 20 minutes to spare and said our goodbyes, and paid US$100 each for the 18-hour crossing of the Sea of Cortez.

The boat, the *Sinoloa Star,* did not dock until 10:30 the next morning. We quickly found a taxi driver who spoke English to bring us to the bus terminal. But first he took us on a side trip to show us the Cerveceria del Pacífico, which brews and bottles the best beer in all of Mexico, he boasted. I could not argue; I told him I'd had three ice-cold ones just two days before.

At the bus terminal, we paid him an extra Mex$10 to come inside with us to help us purchase our tickets. He advised us to abandon our plans to travel down the Mexican coast via Acapulco, as it would be excessively expensive and we would not see much anyway, since most of the journey would be at night. So, instead, we purchased a ticket to Mexico City and hunkered down for a 17-hour bus ride that deposited us in the capital city at 5 A.M. the next day.

Then we had another 5-hour wait for the next bus to Tapachula, Chiapas, on the Guatemalan frontier. That ride took another 18 hours. (Who knew Mexico was so big?) We arrived in Tapachula at 4 A.M. and took a short taxi ride to the border. Our driver had worked for a chicken farm in Delaware before being deported for being in the country illegally, we were told more than once.

Despite the predawn hour, kids as young as 10 jostled with one another begging for tips for carrying our bags, which weighed nearly as much as they did, and for pointing us in the direction of the 'migración office, as if we hadn't seen the sign. The money changers were also there, at first offering only two Guatemalan quetzales on the dollar. From my previous trips to Guatemala, I knew the real exchange rate was closer to seven to one, so I held out until they brought the offer up to Q6 and then only changed US$40, which pissed the man off considerably. But I only wanted enough money to get us to San Marcos, where I knew we could get a better exchange at the bank.

After crossing the border, we took another short taxi ride to the outskirts of Malacatán and then took our first chicken bus ride of the trip. We disembarked the bus just as the sun was coming up. We rented a room at a cheap hotel called The Rabi, located just up the street. We left our big packs there and walked back to the bus terminal with just our day packs. From there, we were headed into the hinterland to climb a remote volcano called Tacaná. Our big packs would stay behind until we returned. Thankfully, I grabbed a business card from the hotel counter on our way out the door, an afterthought that would prove invaluable.

Our chicken bus climbed and climbed and climbed its way out of a steep valley for a couple of hours before we got off at a desolate turnoff for the village of Sibinal. From there, we had a dusty walk of just over an hour to reach the remote village, but at least it was downhill most of the way. It was market day in Sibinal, too, and the place was typically chaotic. What's more, everyone seemed to be thoroughly drunk, and everyone was staring at me, as if I had been the first gringo to step foot in this town in years. Perhaps I was. Van's dark skin, though, helped him go virtually unnoticed. He said the deplorable conditions of this town reminded him of home, except that things in Cambodia, he said, had been ten times better!

We planned to climb Volcán Tacaná the following day. The peak straddles the Mexican border and is the second-highest peak in Central America. But that day we couldn't even see it through the clouds, which hung on the town like a curtain of despair. Though it wasn't that cold despite the 8,200-foot elevation, we could still see our breath in the thinner, alpine air. We found a cheap hotel for the night, but the only place our guidebook said would have Internet access did not, and we were unable to find out anything more about the climb except that we were told that the trailhead was in the next village, a town called La Haciendita.

A loud, constant noise that might have been a bus warming up awoke us from a sound sleep at 3:30 A.M. and made further sleeping impossible, so at first light we began our odyssey. We hiked out of town on the road we'd been told went to La Haciendita, even though there were no signs. We flagged down a ride with the first car that passed, and the driver said we were indeed headed for the *volcán*, which was about the only word we understood, since I don't believe it was Spanish he was speaking, but rather some Mayan dialect.

He dropped us off at a fork in the road and pointed for us to take the turn to the right. We discerned that he would drive us to the trailhead for Q250, which was more than $30, so we politely declined. But perhaps we should have accepted the offer: the badly maintained road climbed many hard miles before descending to a sweeping horseshoe turn, where we finally saw a sign. A straight line to the left was labeled Mexican Frontier; a comically squiggled line to the right said Volcán Tacaná and the town of Vega del Volcán. We never did find La Haciendita.

There were two shacks next to this turn and a couple of women were in the yard talking, so we attempted to ask directions. The younger woman did not know, but the older one pointed and said the trail behind her house went *directo* to the volcano, so we took it. The footpath skirted a ridge that we guessed we had to climb, so we kept on it until we reached a high valley where there were some farms. This, we concluded, had to be the wrong direction; the trail now seemed to be leading us back down the mountain. We soon ran into an old man who told us as much—as best we could comprehend—so, instead, we started bush-whacking straight up the ridge in the direction that he pointed.

Topping out, we came to a barbed-wire fence in the saddle between the ridge we were on and the main peak, and we were much relieved to see our destination. Soon we even found a faint trail that led to the summit, where we were greeted by stones in the ground marking the highest point as well as the Mexican border. We enjoyed views south along the rolling Guatemalan Highlands and north into Chiapas, Mexico. Suddenly, Van realized he was missing the fleece jacket he had tied around his waist when we had started bushwhacking. In it were a $70 pair of sunglasses, his headlamp, and about Q150.

We attempted to head down the same way we had come up, but despite the fact that we came out at the exact spot where we had met the farmer and started bushwhacking, we did not find his jacket. Some lucky stiff likely hit the lottery someday not long after.

Following the trail back to the two shacks, we knew we had a long climb out of the valley ahead of us, followed by a long downhill descent back to Sibinal. We arrived back in town at about 5:30 P.M., or 11 hours after we started. Not bad, considering the guidebook had termed this a "two- to three-day hike." I wouldn't recommend anyone doing what we did without hiring a guide or at least speaking fluent Spanish or Mayan, because we completely winged it, using little more than common sense and good luck. If it had been as cloudy as the day before, we would have been in serious trouble.

Back in town, the owner of the *hospedaje*, or small hostel, where we had stayed the night before was not in and could not be found, so we had to stay at the other hotel nearby. I think we paid the equivalent of $2 each for the night.

The old lady who ran the place would not leave us alone. She just stood in the hallway outside our room as we surveyed our feet—caked in black soot and volcanic dust—and tried to undress for showers. The shower, such as it was, did have hot water—at least to start—but, according to the shrug of the old wom-an's shoulders when we inquired, there were no towels. I located a small hand towel and was at least able to take a pseudo shower and wash my feet. But there was no curtain and the bathroom had no door, and the old lady just stood there watching me the entire time, a toothless grin on her face, much to Van's amusement.

In the morning, we got on the 7 A.M. chicken bus, and it seemed to take forever for the rusted relic to belch its way out of this steep, steep valley up the dirt road that Van and I had walked down the entire length of two days before. A couple of hours later, however, we were dropped off at the same trailhead for Tajumulco from which Matt, Tyler, and I had hiked that Easter Sunday three years before.

Tajumulco being the highest point in Guatemala at 13,845 feet, Van needed to check it off his list, and even though I had already climbed it, I certainly wasn't going to let him go alone. We climbed up the same way I had remembered from 2005, gaining the broad, forested ridge that led to the cinder cone to our west. Reaching the summit, we enjoyed a lunch of cold chicken and fries that we had bought the night before.

This time, I did not get caught in a thunderstorm on the way down. While waiting for a bus after our descent, two men in a pickup truck offered us a ride back to San Marcos, so we hopped into the back. Ten seconds later, however, they pulled into the driveway of a restaurant and asked us if we wanted to get something to eat. I think one of them must've been the owner, and he probably wasn't happy when we ordered only a couple of Cokes. So, they motioned to us and said, *"¡Vámos!"* and we got back into the truck for the promised ride to the bus terminal in San Marcos.

The only thing was, when we got there, we didn't recognize the place. It was not the same bus terminal that we had left from two days before, yet we were assured there was only one bus terminal in San Marcos. Perplexed, I pulled out the business card of *The Rabi*, where we had stashed our packs. An eavesdropping taxi driver said that hotel was in the neighboring town of San Pedro. We had not been in San Marcos at all that first day!

The taxi dropped us off at the front door and, after we banged on the door for what seemed like an interminable time, the same young man who had checked us in two days before let us in. Crisis averted.

The next morning—Super Bowl Sunday—we packed up and left our hotel to the contrived befuddlement of the same 16-year-old who seemed to be running the place. He questioned whether Van had stayed in the room, too, since it had been a room for one. We just pretended we didn't understand. Besides, only our bags had stayed in the room two of the three nights, and Van had slept on the floor anyway.

From San Pedro, it took us four buses and 7 hours to reach Panajachel, my home away from home during my previous visits to Guatemala. The first thing we did was cross the street to Solomon's Porch, a gringo-owned restaurant where I had hoped the Super Bowl would be showing. Indeed, the owners had a huge projection screen TV set up and a big Super Bowl party planned, so we plopped down Q100 each for front-row seats, which would include a huge half-time spread of Buffalo wings and spare ribs.

The Super Bowl didn't go the way we had hoped. Eli Manning, as everyone in New England knows, pulled off a miraculous comeback and the Giants prevailed 17-14 to ruin the Patriots' bid for a perfect season. Van and I were crestfallen as we walked down Calle Santander to the huge villa of Curtis Chapin and his wife, Augusta.

Curtis is a Massachusetts native whom I had befriended during one of my previous visits. I'd interviewed him and several other interesting characters I met in Panajachel for *Greetings from Gringotenango*. And Curtis certainly is interesting; once he had suffered a broken rib at the hands of some rebels he had gotten into an altercation with in El Salvador, and upon returning to Guatemala a few days later, was cured of the ailment overnight by a Maya shaman.

In the morning, I realized I had tilted too many Heinekens the night before. But it wasn't anything to worry about: I didn't have much to do over the next few days except lounge around and reconnect with old friends. I crossed the lake a few times interviewing people for my book and catching up on things. Van, unfortunately, came down with the flu and spent much of the next four days confined to Curtis's house. But he was fine by Friday, when we caught a shuttle to Antigua. We still had peaks to climb.

Van saw it first. Climbing out of the minivan that had brought us from Panajachel— with twenty-one passengers inside, not counting the driver—Van turned as the clouds parted to give him his first view of Volcán de Agua, our next peak. The mountain towered over the city of Antigua, where we would spend the night in a hospedaje. A lot of people had warned us about the danger of climbing Agua— not from another earthquake and landslide, such as the one that had buried the former colonial capital of Ciudad Vieja in 1541, but because of bandits. I wasn't worried, but I could tell Van had a few misgivings.

The Spaniards had built magnificent Ciudad Vieja on the volcano's flanks in the 1530s. But on September 11, 1541, a torrential storm from the Pacific combined with an untimely earthquake to crack the crater wall on the summit of the 12,340-foot volcano. Just after midnight, the resulting earthquake sent the entire contents of a 300-foot-deep crater lake cascading down on the unsuspecting residents of the city, burying thousands under a layer of thick mud.

By sheer coincidence, the calamity had occurred just days after Doña Beatriz de la Cueva had received news that her husband, conquistador Pedro de Alvarado, had died in battle in Mexico. The grief-stricken widow had ordered all the walls in the great castle painted black in mourning and called herself "La Sin Ventura," or "the unfortunate one." The surviving Spanish quickly blamed the disaster on Doña Beatriz; her name went down in infamy.

The Spanish built a new colonial capital a few miles down the road in Antigua, where Van and I were spending the night.

The next morning, we boarded a chicken bus, which took us to the village of Santa María de Jesus, and we began what the guidebook described as a 4-hour hike to the summit. The first half was on a navigable road, then we followed a well-traveled trail that often joined a four-wheel-drive road, which provided access to the many radio antennas that crowded the summit. There was even a little tienda selling snacks and Cokes about halfway up the volcano. We saw no sign of bandits.

When we got to the rim and began our descent into the crater, we found ourselves not on the edge of a 300-foot-deep lake, but rather on the sidelines of a makeshift soccer field. Later, we learned that the Guatemalan national team occasionally practiced on this rock-strewn pitch because of the 12,000-foot altitude.

Climbing above the field to the far rim, which was the highest point, we saw many towers, crumbling cement-block buildings, and plenty of graffiti and trash. It was one of the ugliest summits either of us had ever seen. We ate our lunch of chicken and fries and began the long descent back to town.

That night, we went to the Monoloco—still right next to La Sin Ventura, named for Doña Beatriz, and where I had turned down the salsa lessons on my last visit. We shared the nachos grandes, a plate big enough for four people.

Agua was my tenth Guatemalan volcano, and the last of the major peaks in the country.

The next day, we set out to take the guided tour of Pacaya, the still-active volcano that had mesmerized me years before. But when we got there, things were vastly different than I remembered. The mountain had changed considerably in the three years since I had last climbed it. The top of the volcano had blown off, and we hiked instead to the edge of some large lava flows in a valley to the west of where the summit used to be.

Walking to the edge of the hard, blackened crust, I was surprised to see pockets of orange glowing at several locations out on the charred plains in front of us. There were fresh lava flows all around, and our guide promptly led us out onto the hardened crust right up to the hot spots where new lava was slowly oozing out of the ground. The heat was incredible, like a hundred bonfires roaring at once. I got as close as 3 feet to one of the fissures until the intense heat drove me back. This was almost better than the last time I was here.

Our guia even took his walking stick and poked it into the glowing mass, and when he pulled it out a mere second later, it was on fire. We should have brought some hot dogs or marshmallows to roast.

At precisely four o'clock the next morning, our shuttle arrived to take us to the ancient Maya ruins of Copán, located just over the border in Honduras. I tried to sleep most of the way, having come down with a violent case of Montezuma's revenge at some point during the night. In my five trips to Central America, this was the first time I had been sick, and it came on with a vengeance. When we stopped at a restaurant to eat breakfast, I remained in the van, with my throbbing head buried on my folded arms resting on the back of the seat in front of me. In that seat was a Danish woman, who assumed the same position on the seat in front of her, nursing a colossal hangover, she said.

After crossing the border into Honduras, we reached the town of Copán Ruinas, and I was feeling somewhat better. After dropping our bags at our hostel, we walked a kilometer or so to the ruins. They were quite impressive, but, to me, they paled in comparison to Chichén Itzá, located outside Cancun in the Mayan Riviera, which I had visited twice before. As we exited, we ran into the woman from Denmark, who also appeared to be much better but seemed agitated with the man she was with, some guy from Alaska she had met in Antigua; I would later learn that he had dumped his girlfriend to travel with her, and apparently not at her request.

Later that day, others showed up at the hostel, and one was a guy from Philadelphia named Seth. He told us he was just arriving from El Salvador, where he had climbed El Pital, the country's highpoint, that morning. We quizzed him for information about the climb, since that's where we were headed next. He said the climb was a cinch: there was a road all the way to the summit.

In fact, Seth gave us so much good information about places to see in Central America that Van and I abandoned our plans to go all the way to Panama, and instead set our sights on the Bay Islands of Honduras and, after that, Belize. When I had planned the trip, I had concerned myself primarily with the mountains we would climb, and had overlooked many of the other things we might see or do along the way. Seth helped take my blinders off, and Van and I agreed it was a good thing. A change of plans, we concluded, would free us from turning this vacation into a peakbagging scramble and allow us to slow down and relax.

And that's exactly what I did that afternoon. I climbed into a hammock in the front yard of the hostel and took a much-needed siesta.

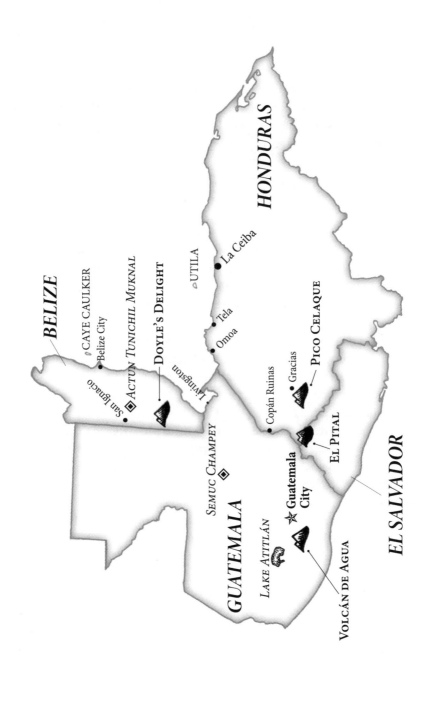

Chapter 5
February 2008

IN THE STEPS OF THE CONQUISTADORS

OUR HOSTEL IN COPÁN RUINAS, HONDURAS—THE MANZANA VERDE, OR GREEN Apple—was quite unusual. Each room had its own name, as did each bed. Our room was the World Famous room, and my bed for the night was named Al Bundy. Van did better: he slept in Madonna's bed. The room's seven beds were occupied on our first night by people from seven different countries; me from the United States, Van from Cambodia, Santiago from Chile (appropriately enough), Oscar from Canada, Erin from Scotland, Teemu from Finland, and Tarso from Brazil.

After breakfast the next morning, we started out for El Salvador's highpoint, El Pital. Van and I climbed into a minivan with twenty other people for a 90-minute ride to the town of La Entrada, where we switched to a bus for a 45-minute ride to Santa Rosa. Here we got lucky and were able to get on a first-class bus—something we hadn't seen since Mexico—for the 2-hour ride to the Honduran border town of Ocotopeque, which cost the equivalent of $3 each. Then we took another *camioneta*, or minivan, to the El Salvador border itself, where we simply walked across without having to do more than flash our passports.

Next came a short bus ride from El Poy to San Ignacio. We felt like we got ripped off when they charged us $1.25 for the 7-kilometer trip. Strangely, the official currency of El Salvador is the U.S. dollar, which we had not used in the five weeks since we had left California.

One last bus brought us to the remote village of Río Choquito. This final leg was only 8.5 kilometers, but it took nearly an hour as the windy road climbed steeply up the side of a mountain. I'm certain the driver never got out of second gear. At least it cut down the elevation we would have to gain in the morning.

Getting off the bus, we saw some cabins for rent nestled in the pines right next to our trailhead; however, the owner was charging $25 a night, which we thought was steeper than the road we had just come up. We negotiated a discount of $40 for two nights, and only after that did we discover that the cabins had no hot water and there was no wood for the fireplace. And, it was cold up there at more than 7,000 feet. The place was beautiful, and safe, too, since two local policemen were staying in the cabin next to ours, but there was nothing to do except go to bed once the sun went down.

The summit of El Pital is not that high at 8,957 feet, so the morning hike up the semipaved road was not long or difficult, just as Seth had told us. As we rounded a corner, we spotted a rickety old shack next to the road that looked like a tollbooth. Van and I laughed out loud at the ridiculous notion that there would be a tollbooth in such a remote location, where they might go weeks without seeing a single climber to charge. We were about to walk right past the decrepit building when we were surprised to see an old man sitting there. We were even more surprised when the man proceeded to charge us $2 to pass. Seth had not mentioned this. Fortunately, we had money with us, or else I am certain he would not have let us through. It reminded me of the tollbooth scene in the movie *Blazing Saddles*. "Go back and get some more dimes!" I could not help but laugh.

The summit, however, may not have been worth the two bucks. There was a large tower on top and a fenced-in building that appeared to be a military installation. Inside the fence, a guard dog signaled our arrival. As we rounded the building, there was a naked man standing in a 55-gallon drum taking a bath. It was all too surreal.

Just like the summit of Tacaná, the top of El Pital stands at the border between two countries, the El Salvador–Honduras border demarcated with a stone pillar in the ground. There was nothing much more to see, so we hiked back to our cabin and I braved an ice-cold shower. That night we hiked what we were told was "2K" to the Miramundo hotel to eat dinner, but it turned out to be at least 5 kilometers. The steak dinner and the tremendous views, however, were worth it, despite the $16 bill and the 3-mile walk back to the cabin.

While we were packing up the next morning to catch the 6 A.M. bus, I looked outside and noticed a shirt with "El Salvador Police" emblazoned upon it drying on the clothesline next to my towel. I desperately wanted to steal it, as the shirt would have made an incredible conversation piece back home. But, I figured, the two cops were still inside their cabin, and they might catch us before we were able to get out of the country. Besides, since they were stationed there with no transportation other than their own two feet, they probably would have had to pay to replace the stolen shirt out of their own paltry paychecks. So I decided against it.

We were back in Honduras in no time, but it took us five buses to get to our destination—the town of Gracias, located at about 2,600 feet in elevation in the mountainous region of western Honduras. Legend has it that the early explorers, tired of trekking through the rugged, mountainous terrain, exclaimed, *"Gracias a Dios hemos llegado a tierra plana,"* or, "Thank God, we have arrived at flat ground," upon first stepping foot in what would become the regional capital from 1544 to 1549, complete with a Spanish-built fort that overlooked the entire town. After that, it was moved to Antigua, which had now been completed following the 1541 disaster in Ciudad Vieja.

However, we were here to climb the country's highpoint: Cerro Las Minas, where the Spaniards must have spent time searching for gold, because the name means "Hill of the Mines." The 9,416-foot peak is also called Pico Celaque, and is the most prominent feature of Celaque National Park, which was (according to our guidebook) reportedly home to jaguars, pumas, and ocelots.

We had contemplated camping in the national park until Van saw the word "jaguars" in the book, and instead we rented a room in Gracias at the Hotel Guancascas, owned by a Dutch woman named Froni, whom our book had said was a good source of information about Cerro Las Minas. The room was expensive, for our budget at least, at $23 a night, but Froni helped arrange for us to be picked up by a taxi at 5:30 the next morning for the 6-mile ride up to the park entrance. We picked up a map at the tourist office that showed the trail to the summit as nothing more than a squiggly line—steep, with lots of switchbacks. The guidebook noted that most of the terrain in the national park exceeded 60 degrees in slope. We envisioned it to be a difficult 10- to 12-hour ordeal.

In the morning, a tuk-tuk driver took us to the park entrance, where we paid a fee of fifty Honduran lempira, which was about $3. From there, we walked about a mile up to the trailhead and then began a grueling hike to the summit that took us 4 hours 15 minutes. The hike was incredible, however. The trail passed through the largest cloud forest in Honduras, with lots of mist in the air and moss hanging from the trees. We thought we had stumbled into a scene from *Jurassic Park.*

Not wanting to run into any velociraptors, or even jaguars, we literally ran off the mountain, needing just 2 hours 25 minutes to get back to the park entrance. The round-trip, which included a half-hour lunch on the summit, had taken just 7 hours 20 minutes, far less than we had expected. Of course, we still had a 6-mile slog back to town, but at least it was all downhill.

After about 2 miles, a dump truck rattled its way down the poorly maintained dirt road and we flagged it down. The driver motioned for us to climb in the back, which was not easy with our heavy backpacks. We must've looked silly riding in the bucket of the truck, but it sure beat walking, even if he did barely ever get out of first gear on the heavily rutted road. After a shower and a shave back in our room, I headed for the hotel bar to get a well-deserved Salva Vida beer—Honduras' national *cerveza*. Froni was surprised to see me back so soon. She questioned whether we had been to the actual summit, but after I showed her pictures as evidence, she was convinced and said we likely had set some sort of speed record.

We ate street food that night, something we always tried to do, since it was cooked right in front of us and was always cheap and tasty. I had three huge chicken *pupusas* and a Coke for only L25, about $1.50. I could live like a king in Gracias forever, thank you very much.

We had originally planned to continue south to climb the highpoint of Nicaragua next. But when Van read that Pico Mogotón, at 6,913 feet, is still riddled with land mines planted by the Sandinistas during the Contra War of the 1980s, he said he was out. After what he had experienced as a child in Cambodia, he wasn't going anywhere near land mines. I was going to explain that there was a local guide who knew the safe path up the mountain, but I knew better than to push Van on this one.

So we put our peakbagging mission on hold and decided to venture in a completely opposite direction for a while: back to the beach. Armed with Seth's recommendations, we headed in the direction of the Caribbean coast and the Bay Islands of Honduras.

It took only three buses to cross Honduras, but the first one, from Gracias to Santa Rosa, had so little legroom that a first-grader would've been cramped.

Our next bus took us to the huge, vibrant city of San Pedro Sula, the second-largest city in Honduras after its capital, Tegucigalpa. San Pedro Sula had a modern, gleaming bus terminal that rivaled anything we had seen in Mexico, and we had little trouble catching another bus to the seaside town of Tela, on the Caribbean coast.

We immediately headed for the water and found the beach crawling with activity. We hadn't realized that it was Saturday, a day when locals overrun the beach. But we found a fleabag hotel directly across the street from the water for just $4 a night, although at that price we had to forego some amenities. For instance, the room had no door, opening directly onto a shared central patio. Likewise, the bathroom had no door, so anyone looking into the room from outside could watch you do your business. What's more, the toilet did not work, so we had to fill a bucket from an outside spigot and pour water into the bowl to get it to flush. Compared to the chilly weather we had experienced in the mountains, it was stifling hot in Tela, and our room also had no ceiling fan, believe it or not. And we had paid for two nights in advance, no less.

But the price was right.

Van soon found a cockroach the size of his thumb in bed with him, but I told him not to worry: there were probably fifty more under it. Welcome to paradise.

Tela, though a bit seedy, was a decent enough town, with national parks flanking it on both sides. We planned to explore both of them over the next couple of days. For Sunday, we booked a snorkeling trip to an offshore coral reef in Jeanette Kawas National Park—known locally as Punta Sal National Park—to the west, and on Monday, we planned to go kayaking through the tidal mangroves of Punta Izopo National Park to the east.

While taking a break from the heat to enjoy a cold beer—well, Van had a coconut shake, since he doesn't drink—we met Howie and Kathy, a couple from Colebrook, New Hampshire, who told us that we should bypass Roatán, the biggest of the three main Bay Islands and a tourist mecca, and instead go to the smaller island of Utila. They said it was less expensive, less crowded, and had all the same activities as Roatán, such as the cheapest scuba diving on the planet. Van said he had always wanted to get certified as a diver, so we put that on the agenda.

That night, we ate dinner at a fish house and I had a delicious red snapper, the first time I had ever eaten a fish with the head still on, its eyeball staring back at me.

Sunday's tour to Punta Sal was disappointing. The reef we snorkeled at had very poor visibility and very few fish, perhaps because the local Garifuna, who were our hosts in the national park, had caught them all to serve for lunch, as once again I ate a fish that winked back at me.

Monday's kayaking tour of Punta Izopo was far superior. Our guide, Melvin, led us up a tidal river through the mangroves that lined both shores. The only others on the trip were Howie and Kathy, and a guy named John, a lawyer from St. Louis. Like me, John had been divorced twice, so we had plenty to commiserate about.

Punta Izopo was much more alive than Punta Sal. We saw white-faced monkeys, poisonous tiger spiders, and more species of tropical birds than we could count. We failed to see any crocodiles, and we fortunately missed the deadly fer-de-lance that the locals told us had slithered by that morning. Melvin took the time to allow us to interact with nature, often pointing out various plants and flowers, rather than hurrying us through as our guias had done the day before.

That afternoon, we took a 2-hour bus ride to the port city of La Ceiba, where we would catch the ferry to Utila the following morning. We checked into our guidebook-recommended hotel, Hotel Caribe, and almost accepted a dorm-style room for L240. At the last minute, we smartly upgraded to a double with its own bathroom for L280, roughly a dollar more each. It's too easy to be cheap on the road.

While Honduras is a Spanish-speaking country, its Bay Islands are nothing like the mainland. English has been the three islands' predominant language since British pirates made them their sanctuary during the mid-1600s. At that time, as many as 5,000 pirates were said to be living on Roatán, by far the largest island, and they often raided the Spanish cargo vessels laden with gold and other valuables headed back to Spain. The famous Welsh pirate Henry Morgan made his base at Port Royal on Roatán during this period.

Not until the mid-1800s did England finally cede control of the Bay Islands to Honduras, but the islands have remained culturally British to this day. Many of the residents are direct descendants of the pirate heyday. The English spoken there is its own, distinctly pirate dialect, and I sometimes had more trouble understanding the locals there than I did those speaking Spanish on the mainland.

Stepping off the ferry after the 18-mile crossing from La Ceiba to Utila, we were immediately besieged by representatives of all the local dive companies. Dave, a Canadian who ran the Underwater Dive Shop, hurried us—somewhat against our wills—from the dock and along the short walk up the main street. A four-day certification course, complete with all meals and lodging, was just $238, a deal too good to pass up. Van and I both signed up.

We spent the early afternoon reading from a diving manual, but I quickly found it too tedious and decided I didn't want to commit to anything that cerebral for four days, no matter how good the price. I backed out of the course and left Van in the room, intensely studying.

Later that night, I wandered down the street to a couple of bars. Jade's caught my eye: the warm sea breeze wafted through the large, open-air tree house and the branches overhead. It was magical, except for the many tiger spiders, which had seemingly spun webs in every corner. I got quite drunk and staggered back up the main street to the dive shop, only to be stopped en route by a guy who tried to sell me drugs and "a really nice woman." I passed. On both.

I much preferred Utila to what awaited on Roatán. The larger island's big hotels, crowded beaches, and international airport with daily direct flights to the United States wasn't the setting I'd wanted for this much-needed break. Utila, in contrast, was a sleepy little island with mostly sandy streets, few cars, and no chain hotels. Everything there was family owned. But as uncluttered as

Utila was, I desired even more solitude. I decided I'd camp out on one of the tiny cays for a few days. It would be the first time on the trip that Van and I had been separated overnight, but he was in good hands in Dave's diving course. I had also watched his confidence grow immensely since we had started the trip six weeks before. At first, Van had never left my sight, but now he was fully willing to venture off on his own, and often did. I would not see him again for several days.

I went down to the docks and hired Captain Hal to taxi me on the 15-minute ride out to a tiny islet called Water Cay for L700—about $35—and pick me up again at noon on Friday, two days later. Captain Hal must've been a descendent of Henry Morgan, because I couldn't understand a single word he muttered in his gravelly voice. It was like listening to Ozzy Osbourne. But, he managed to assure me, he would be back as we arranged, which was all I needed to hear.

There were six others on the tiny cay when I arrived, but they were all day-trippers. A family from Syracuse, New York, lent me some snorkeling gear for a short while, and I went swimming along the reef off the northern tip of the island. After a boat picked them up later that afternoon, I had the entire island to myself.

My kingdom was only about a quarter-mile long by a hundred yards wide, but for the next two days it would pretty much be mine. Except, that is, for the mangy dog that came over from the mainland across a sand bar during low tides. With only about a foot or two of water covering this sand bar at low tide, the dog would wade across and hang out with me. A few hours later, she would go back over before the onset of high tide, when the crossing would become impossible. This dog evidently knew the tidal charts. Some locals later told me her name was Rosie, but since I felt like Robinson Crusoe on my little island, I had already renamed her Friday in my mind. It may not have been the top of a mountain, but the isolation and solitude brought about the same flood of emotions I had felt while on the summits of 14ers in the Rockies. This was my world, and I was king.

Once I was alone, I again explored the reef, which was teeming with life. It was infinitely better than the depleted reef we had visited at Punta Sal. After sunset, I promptly stripped naked and went skinny-dipping off the north end of the island, where a large reef extended just under the surface.

Fixing breakfast the next morning, I was surprised to see none other than John—the lawyer from St. Louis whom I'd met on the kayaking tour—get off the first boat of the day. I had run into him briefly after arriving on Utila, and met the Canadian couple he was with—Greg and Jane from British Columbia— and I had told them I was going to be roughing it out on some small island, but they did not realize it was Water Cay.

I gave them the grand tour of the island, which took all of about 10 minutes, and then John and I sat in the sand at the north end of the island and chatted most of the day. We made plans to go whitewater rafting together when we returned to La Ceiba in a couple days.

Captain Hal was right on time the next day and returned me to the main dock on Utila. I walked up the street to the dive shop to get the rest of my gear; John and I had plans. Van was probably underwater somewhere learning how to read a depth gauge. I left him some money and a note to take the 6:20 A.M. ferry on Sunday and meet me at the Hotel Caribe in La Ceiba.

After disembarking the ferry in La Ceiba, John and I grabbed a taxi for the ride to the Jungle River Lodge to go whitewater rafting. Enormous potholes riddled the dirt road leading inland to the lodge and the driver swerved from side to side to keep the huge craters from swallowing the car whole. The lodge, a stunningly modern-looking log cabin, was located on the banks of the Río Cangrejal opposite the border of Pico Bonito National Park, at a spot in the river where deep pools and huge rocks made for excellent cliff jumping.

We enjoyed a barbecued pork dinner on the open-air patio that evening and listened to two Canadian women talking about marine biology. In the background, croaking elephant frogs sounded strangely like goats and were so loud that they could easily be heard above the thundering roar of the river long into the night.

In the morning, after a huge pancake breakfast, everyone assembled for the day's rafting trips, and John and I were excited to learn that we were the only two who had signed up for the full-day trip. The half-day rafters loaded into the back of a truck and we followed them in a pickup for what seemed like only a couple of miles up the road, where they stopped to begin their adventure. We continued on nearly a half hour more, climbing higher and higher into this valley. John and I agreed that we had made the better choice, even though the Río Cangrejal appeared to be getting smaller and smaller beside us.

We were dropped off underneath a bridge along with our captain, Darwin, and his first mate, Roberto. The put-in looked doubtful: we could practically hop across the river. We wondered how we could possibly navigate this narrow river in such a large raft, but Darwin said he grew up on the Río Cangrejal, and had been guiding it for years, even though he didn't appear to be older than 20.

Once on the water, we came to appreciate his experience. Incredibly competent, Darwin navigated us through small cracks between the rocks, and we zipped through almost continuous sections of whitewater. We got hung up on some rocks a few times and had to climb out to unwedge ourselves, and we did have to portage around one unrunnable section. Three times the boat capsized coming over small waterfalls, but that just added to the adventure. On one of the upendings, I lost my sunglasses in the deep pool under the falls, and Roberto offered to dive down to find them. *"No necessito,"* I told him in my pidgin Spanish, since they were a seven-year-old pair I had purchased in Tobago in 2001, but he put his mask on and jumped in anyway, promptly coming up with them. However, we flipped again moments later and I lost the sunglasses for good. Fortunately, my contact lenses remained intact.

We stopped for lunch on a wide, sandy beach near the only village we passed all day, and about fifteen young kids—none appearing older than 10—commandeered our raft and had a great time paddling it around the calm pool while we ate. They were laughing and screaming and were about as unspoiled as any children we had ever seen. Our full day did not end until we paddled directly into the Jungle River Lodge at 4 P.M. John and I agreed that we couldn't remember having so much fun, and I told him it was the best day of my trip so far.

It soon ended, however; I had to catch a ride back to La Ceiba to meet Van. John and I vowed to stay in touch, since he often came to Vermont, where he owned a second home. But when I got back home weeks later, I could not find the business card he had given me and we lost contact.

Van arrived at the Hotel Caribe early the next morning, beaming from his scuba diving experience. We hopped the first bus to San Pedro Sula, where I bought a new pair of sunglasses for $3. We took the next bus headed toward Puerto Cortés, planning to catch the ferry to Belize to continue our slow tour, but our bus broke down halfway there, leaving a dozen of us on the side of the road. *Pero no problema:* the next bus, not much bigger than a minivan, promptly stopped. We all crammed into the van, along with our two overstuffed backpacks, though a dozen or so people were already in it. Arriving in Puerto Cortés, we extracted ourselves from our sardine can and grabbed another bus headed for the beach resort of Omoa, a few miles to the west.

Omoa was once home to a huge Spanish fort that King Charles I had built as a terminus for all the gold-laden ships sailing back to Spain from the New World and for the shipments' protection against the constantly plundering pirates. Once, legend has it, the king was seen peering through a telescope in his palace in Madrid and was asked what he was looking at. He is said to have responded, "I should think that with all the money it cost to build Omoa, I should be able to see it from here." Now, only a few of the outer walls remain.

It being a Sunday, the beach was crammed with native Hondurans, but they soon started packing to head home, and all was tranquil again as the sun began to go down across the bay. In this place where the Honduran coast juts into the Carribbean's Bahía de Omoa, the views out onto the water are west facing, rather than to the east as you might expect. It was a little disorienting to see the sun setting out over the bay from my location sitting on the porch of the Sueños de Mar bed-and-breakfast, drinking a cold Salva Vida with the Canadian owners, Mark and Karen Hislop. Later, I went next door to the Sunset for dinner, and spent the last of my lempira and had to inform Mark and Karen that I would have to come back in the morning to pay my beer tab, which was about $4. No problem, they said. "See you mañana."

But when I got back to our hotel room, Van informed me he had been reading the guidebook, and the ferry from Puerto Cortés, he had discovered, was leaving the next morning, and not on Tuesday morning, as we had thought. So in the morning we packed up quickly and caught the first bus back to Puerto Cortés. It was the first time I had ever welched on a bar tab, but I sent Mark and Karen an apologetic email a few days later and they told me just to pay up the next time I came through. They are still waiting.

Arriving at the docks in Puerto Cortés, we were immediately approached by the captain of the ferryboat, who led us to the ticket office to purchase our $43 tickets and to the immigration office to get our exit stamps. We returned to the dock and waited. And waited. We were supposed to have departed at 11:30 A.M., but by well past one o'clock, we still hadn't boarded. The captain said it was immigration's fault, but really it was because he kept accepting late-arriving passengers in order to ensure a full boat—and everyone had to go to immigration first.

Once we did depart, the initial part of the crossing was very rough because we were out in open water on the Gulf of Honduras, and one girl got seasick. But soon the many Belizean islands protected us and the water calmed, and we arrived after 3 hours in the port city of Dangriga, in southern Belize. Our plan had been to head to Belize City and then directly to Caye Caulker, an offshore island, but the next bus leaving Dangriga was going to the inland town of San Ignacio, located deep in the jungle near the Guatemalan border, so we went there instead. We had planned to visit San Ignacio anyway, so the itinerary change made little difference.

Following our guidebook's recommendation to talk to Bob at a hotel called Eva's, we rolled into San Ignacio just after dark and headed straight for the hotel. Only Bob didn't work there anymore. But the office for Mayawalk Tours across the street was still open, and we immediately booked two tours for the following two days. They directed us to a hostel around the corner called the Hi-Et—not to be confused with the Hyatt—but, we were told, they too were full. Steve, the owner, made a quick phone call and booked us a room down the street at J&R's Guesthouse for twenty-two Belizean dollars, which was slightly more than US$22, we were told. In

Belize, it appeared, we were dealing with real money again.

The next day Van and I booked a US$60 cave-tubing tour at a place called Cave's Branch, but we began to doubt the wisdom of this decision when our driver left a half hour late for the hour-long drive to get there. But when we got to the entrance to the cave, its beauty changed my opinion in a flash.

We put in at a spot where the river came out of one cave and then slipped silently into another, and we all jumped from a ledge into the crystal-clear water and linked up our tubes as our guide, a local man named Lion, backstroked his way into the cave entrance. We floated gently along what felt more like an amusement park ride, gliding through an immense room with a high roof overhead. Then all went dark as we rounded a corner, blotting out the sunlight. Eventually we came back out into daylight, but the current picked up speed and pulled us back underground.

Stalactites hung from the ceiling like crystal chandeliers, and a roar from an unseen waterfall got louder and louder as we were swept along in the darkness. Soon we came into a huge room where there was an opening to the sky and everything was basked in a brilliant, emerald green where the sun shined in. The cascade we'd heard was from water pouring down from this opening in the roof to join our river. The rocks were otherworldly, all smoothed and sculpted by centuries of running water. They looked more like glass with the rushing water gently tumbling over and around them.

We got out and walked over the rocks, which kind of felt like walking on the lava fields of Pacaya. Lion showed us some faint, ancient carvings on one of the stalactites near the mouth of the cave, where Maya had etched seven faces vertically and one more on each side. He said they represented the levels of the underworld as told in the Popul Vuh, the legendary Maya book that tells of the creation of the world.

We continued floating down the river until it reemerged into the sunlight and, finally, deposited us at our waiting vehicle.

The next morning, a dozen of us boarded a fifteen-passenger van for a long ride over a bumpy dirt road and through several creek crossings as we made our way into the Tapir Mountain Nature Preserve. We then hiked through the subtropical jungle for another 45 minutes, wading across Roaring Creek three times, before reaching our destination. Crystal-clear turquoise water gushed from a cave entrance that looked like an eerily misshapen mouth, with moss and vegetation hanging above the opening like the unkempt bangs of a teenager. The water collected in a deep, calm pool in front of the opening before spilling over rocks and rushing quickly downstream, seemingly in a hurry to leave this foreboding place.

We were at the entrance of Actun Tunichil Muknal, considered the top-rated tourist attraction in Belize and one of the greatest archeological finds in all of Central America. Discovered in 1989, the cave was opened to tourists about ten years later, but this tour was not for the faint of heart. Inside were dozens of human skeletons, all victims of Maya sacrificial rites dating back more than a thousand years, now calcified into the cave floor by centuries of water seepage. Translated from Mayan, its name means "Cave of the Crystal Sepulcher," but it was called the "Cave of Doom" by *National Geographic Adventure* magazine in a 2001 article. Locals simply call it Xibalba—gateway to the underworld.

To get inside, we swam across the deep pool, through the entrance, to a knee-deep section of the subterranean river where we could stand. Our Maya guide, Martin, had us turn around to look back at the inside wall of the cave mouth we had just entered. Sunlight filtered in to illuminate a huge, grotesque image of a face on the wall; I couldn't tell if the visage was human-made or not. Martin said it depicted the sun god Chac, who was responsible for seeing that the sun rose from the underworld each morning.

The cave was narrow enough that we could reach out with our hands and touch the smooth walls on both sides as it wound for several kilometers deep into the mountainside. The fluted, crystalline calcium deposits dripping down the walls were simply spectacular to look at.

Martin had us turn off our headlamps and hold onto the shoulder of the person in front of us. He led us, single file, through the twisting labyrinth for nearly a minute without banging us into the walls. That's how well he knew the cave.

We left the water and climbed up a sidewall into a huge, cavernous room known as the Cathedral. Here, we were instructed to take off our shoes to reduce the impact of foot traffic, and we continued on in stocking feet. Artifacts littered the smooth, rocky floor of the cave. Dozens of nearly intact pottery jars, large and small, were frozen into the floor in the calcite that had accumulated over the centuries. This remains the largest collection of such earthenware ever discovered.

While the pots appeared to be strewn about haphazardly, Martin offered a different theory. He believed each pot was purposely placed where it was found, each used by the priests, or shamans, as part of a sacrifice of food or blood to the fertility and rain goddess Ixchel, whose silhouetted likeness was also part of an immense rock column nearby that indeed appeared to be an intricately carved figure of a woman.

Moving farther into the cave, we came upon the first of the many skeletons encrusted by the mineral deposits, victims of the human sacrifices carried out in this deep underground chamber. The skulls, though, had less sediment built up on them and stared blankly back at us, almost grinning in death. Martin said the skeletons date back to as early as AD 250.

While the skeletons in the cave ranged in age from infant to adult, one in particular stood out above all others: the Crystal Maiden, the nearly intact skeleton of an 18-year-old girl. We reached her upper chamber by climbing a ladder. She lies on her back, calcified into the floor with her head tilted forward, as if trying to rise to greet us.

Her sparkling skeleton is missing two vertebrae from her lower back. Scientists have proposed that this is likely the result of her falling when she died, but Martin said that is incorrect. He suggested that the vertebrae were skillfully cut out by shamans using an ax that was found near her body so that they could reach up inside her while she was alive and rip her still-beating heart from her chest. That way her unmarred frontal features would still be a pleasing sacrifice to Ixchel, an offering of thanks after the sought-after rains finally came.

The next day I spent some time contemplating what we had seen during our veritable Indiana Jones expedition. I had much appreciation for the Belizean government for allowing this site to exist as a tourist attraction. It was fortunate that the cave was discovered undisturbed—it had never been looted—and it was a brave decision to leave most of the artifacts and all of the bones exactly where they were found, trusting tourists to comply with strict, rigid guidelines to ensure that there is no damage to these fragile, irreplaceable relics. The only mishap, Martin said, had been when a tourist accidentally dropped a camera and broke two teeth off one of the skulls (it has happened more than once since my visit). Such an attraction could never happen in the United States; there would be extreme liability issues because of the danger and degree of difficulty in entering and negotiating the cave system, let alone the risk posed to the ancient artifacts.

These revelations seemed to come in regular succession as we continued from one country to another.

The next morning, we headed to the beach yet again. After a brief stop at the famed Belize Zoo, we arrived in Belize City in time to catch the next high-speed water taxi for the half-hour crossing to Caye Caulker. Once there, we learned that the hotel recommended by our guidebook was full, so we ended up staying at a place called Sandy Lane, where we got a clean, basic room for BZ$6.25 a night. While the rooms were inexpensive, the beers were not; I wandered up to the Lazy Lizard, a bar located at the northern tip of the island where a tropical storm had years earlier cut the island in half, and paid US$2.50 for a cold Belikin.

The tiny, idyllic island measured 5 miles long and less than a mile wide. There were no cars on the island—only golf carts—and the streets were not paved. I pretty much went barefoot the entire time we were there. Its peaceful, laid-back atmosphere reminded me a lot of Utila. It was going to be hard to get me to leave this paradise after just five days.

The next day, February 29, was a windy, blustery, and rainy day in paradise. But it was still paradise. I didn't see Van the entire day; he went off exploring on his own. I was increasingly proud of the confidence he had gained since we had left California fifty-three days ago.

The next morning I walked down the street to the Happy Lobster and got an outside table next to a couple of animated women from the States who were enjoying catching up with each other. Kathleen Moore was from Sacramento and Kari Montrose lived in Salida, Colorado; the two had been friends since their high school days in Redding, California, and had flown in the day before. Turned out, we were all the same age—all 1978 high school graduates.

Kari captivated me. She was tall, slender, and athletic, and had a beautiful smile, a great laugh, and wild hair that made it look like she had spent too much time in the wind. But she was married, I discovered, though I could not quite ascertain the dynamics, which seemed somewhat disjointed.

Whatever her status, we hit it off immediately and spent the rest of the day together. After 3 hours chatting at the Happy Lobster before paying our bills, we walked up to the Lazy Lizard for a couple of Belikins. Walking barefoot along the sandy street on our way back, it started to rain again, so we ducked into the Rainbow Café on a dock over the water and stayed for lunch.

It rained off and on the rest of the day and we kept ducking into whatever bar we were near when the next squall came through. After dinner, we bought a couple of bottles of rum and went back to their place and talked some more until we must've run out of things to talk about. The weather cleared by morning, and we all booked a snorkeling trip to the barrier reef for the following day.

Van had made himself scarce since we had arrived on Caye Caulker, having befriended another guest at the hotel, a fisherman named Marv. Van said he had seen Marv one night fishing off the end of a pier down near the main dock, and he had walked out to see how he was doing.

"As soon as I arrived," Van related to me some time later, "he started catching a bunch of fish. He hadn't been having any luck until I arrived, so he called me his good luck charm." When Marv caught a fish, he snaked a chain that he had fastened to the dock through its gills and dropped it back into the water to keep it alive longer. Not long after Van's arrival, Marv had several fish dangling in the water next to the dock.

"All of a sudden, the pier started to shake like an earthquake," Van remembered. "I said, 'What was that?' Then, we saw the chain being pulled tight and heard it snap in two. We shined our light out on the water and we saw a shark swimming off with the chain in its mouth."

It was a scene straight out of *Jaws*.

"The shark must've been 5 or 6 feet long," Van said. "It was pretty exciting."

The Mesoamerican Barrier Reef that lies off the coast of Belize is the world's second-largest barrier reef system after the Great Barrier Reef in Australia. It is one of the most diverse ecosystems in the world, and almost a quarter of a million people a year scuba dive or snorkel there. It has been a World Heritage Site since 1996.

Just off the northern tip of Caye Caulker, in the trough between it and larger Ambergris Caye, is perhaps one of the best snorkeling locations on this Caribbean reef: Shark Ray Alley. The water here is only 8 feet deep, has a sandy bottom, and has countless numbers of nurse sharks and stingrays. This was where Kari, Kathleen, and I were heading for the day.

At our first stop that morning, we had dozens of nurse sharks up to 10 feet in length swimming all around us, almost begging us to feed them. They were quite harmless and almost tame. Later, at another spot, I got quite a start when I came face to face with a barracuda that was bigger than I was. It continuously opened and closed its gaping mouth to show off row after row of razor-sharp teeth. Fortunately, it was just posturing and soon swam off.

The best thing about Shark Ray Alley, however, was the stingrays. They were everywhere. We dived down to touch their very soft and gelatin-like bodies. They seemed to like getting their backs scratched, almost like puppies.

We stopped for lunch at Ambergris Caye, which is far more touristy than tranquil Caye Caulker, and made one more dive before heading back. It had been another great day. Kari and I walked around some more that evening after dinner and I made plans to stop and see her that fall, when I planned to return to Colorado to complete the 14ers. Van and I were up and gone on the 6:30 A.M. water taxi the next morning, heading back to Guatemala once again.

Doyle's Delight, at 3,688 feet, is located in the Cockscomb Range, an extension of the Maya Mountains of western Belize. It is also, perhaps, the newest highpoint in the New World: it was discovered to be higher than the previous accepted highpoint—3,675-foot Victoria Peak—only around the turn of the twenty-first century.

As such, there is no real trail system leading to Doyle's Delight. A group of mountaineers who had attempted the hike in 2007 required eight days to traipse through the virgin jungle to obtain their objective. The peak—named for Sir Arthur Conan Doyle from a line in his book *A Lost World*—also has no discernible summit, just a broad, vegetated hump. Victoria Peak, in contrast, has three dramatic summits, which require ropes to reach. Neither peak, however, fit our agenda. A full-scale jungle expedition to reach either summit would take several days that we did not want to waste.

Instead, we took a bus from Belize City to the southern city of Punta Gorda en route to the outlet of the Río Dulce. We missed the day's ferry over to Livingston but caught another heading to Puerto Barrios. Both Guatemalan cities are located on the Gulf of Honduras, on either side of the outlet from Río Dulce. Upon arrival, we grabbed the last two spots on an already overloaded boat going back to Livingston. This lancha was no bigger than the ones on Lake Atitlán, but this one needed to cross the exposed expanse of the Gulf of Honduras. I was a bit concerned. It was the one time when I actually wore the life vest they handed out.

Livingston may be the most cosmopolitan town of its size in the world. It is probably the only place in Guatemala where English is nearly as prevalent as Spanish, and the town has a large black population—more than 6,000—who are known as the Garifuna, the descendants of slaves who escaped after a revolt on the island of St. Vincent, which was British, in 1795. There are no roads leading to Livingston, and it is accessible only by boat.

Typical border-town characters crowded us as we got off the boat. We shook them all except one, but he turned out to be useful, as he went to retrieve the men from the immigration office, who were at dinner. Also, he talked us out of paying Q150 to stay at the hotel our guidebook recommended (notably, the hotel had purchased an ad on the facing page). We went to the Viajero instead and got an end room right on the water for Q60.

After a tasty dinner at the Happy Fish, I went back to the hotel and sat on the porch watching a pretty good display of heat lightning over the gulf.

The next afternoon, we boarded our ferry for the ride up the Río Dulce, but it turned out we were about thirty years too late.

There was a time when the Río Dulce really was the "sweet river" that its name implies. Centuries ago, the Spanish-built Castillo de San Felipe guarded this once-important port at the outlet from Lake Izabal from pirate attacks. Even decades ago, its idyllic charms were known to only a handful of modern sailors. They had glided their sailboats up the wide, turquoise-blue river and anchored in the town of the same name to sit out hurricane season; no hurricane has hit Río Dulce in recorded history. Most had wintered there, too, as the place was a veritable Garden of Eden.

In 1972, Mark Hassall ended his 40,000-mile, around-the-world trip on his 37-foot SeaRunner on the Río Dulce. With him were his wife, Bonnie, and David, his son from a previous marriage. I met Mark on Lake Atitlán in 2005, and his description had stayed in my mind since: "We came up that river and it was the most gorgeous place I'd ever seen. There were parrots and pelicans, and we were the only foreigners there."

Then the Río Dulce got discovered. Hassall watched helplessly as an invasion of people and their boats overran the place. Soon, he said, Río Dulce became known by many as "the river that swallows gringos."

By the time Van and I navigated the Río Dulce in 2008, the river had long since lost its luster. The water was now brown and murky, no longer the pristine blue that had greeted Hassall decades before. Don't get me wrong: it was still one of the most beautiful rivers I had ever seen, and the 1-hour ride was over way too soon, but imagine how captivating it must have been in years past.

We spent no time in the town of Fronteras, where the Río Dulce emerges from Lake Izabal, Guatemala's largest lake, and where the great Spanish fort still sits. The fort, constantly plundered by pirates and rebuilt several times since it was first constructed in 1595, was restored in the 1950s and is now a major tourist attraction. But we weren't feeling touristy.

We traveled west by bus along the north shore of Lake Izabal and got off at Finca el Paraiso—Paradise Farm—where we expected to camp for the night and enjoy the "hot waterfall" that our guidebook said was a must-see.

After paying Q10 to enter, we hiked down a trail to a spot where a clear-running creek rushed through a little ravine. A large rock jutted out into this creek, and over the top of it rushed a 30-foot-high waterfall that came directly out of a nearby hot spring and cascaded into this deep pool. The water in the main creek was ice cold, but the water coming over the falls was as hot as any hot tub I had been in. It was almost too hot. I would stand on a rock, getting hammered by the force of the hot water coming over the falls until I couldn't stand it anymore, then jump off into the deep, cold water to keep from getting scalded. It was the best shower I had taken in weeks.

After an hour of bliss, we hiked back to the restaurant and inquired about the camping arrangements. Turned out the campground was located more than a kilometer away by the shore of Lake Izabal and we would need to pay Q25 for the campsite and another Q70 for a tractor ride to get there, including the return trip in the morning. It was more than Van or I wanted to pay, so we said we would return to the main road and catch the next bus to El Estor, where we knew we could get cheaper lodging.

"Oh, there are no more buses today, *señor*," said the man at the front desk. But before he had finished his sentence, we watched out the window as a chicken bus raced past.

"What was that, then?" Van and I asked in unison.

"Oh, *that* was the last bus," the man replied.

We decided to take our chances and started walking along the dirt road toward El Estor as darkness began to fall.

Just as we were about to give up and pitch our tents out of sight in the woods, another bus came along, and we flagged it down. It dropped us off in the center of El Estor, and minutes later we had a room in a hospedaje for just Q25 each.

In the morning, we left the edge of the lake and began a long, hot ride through some of the most beautiful mountainous terrain I had yet seen. We kept getting handed from bus to bus all day long, with the *ayudantes*—young boys who ride the bus and collect fares from passengers—tossing our backpacks from the roof of one bus to the next at each transfer. At one point, our bus stopped to pick up a young woman named Anna from the Czech Republic who had been stranded there for 4 hours. She said she had left El Estor at 6 A.M., nearly 6 hours before us.

A short while later, the bus stopped and everyone was directed to get off. We collected our packs and we all walked across an aging, sagging steel-arch bridge over the raging Río Cahabón; it was buckling in the middle and was therefore no longer navigable by vehicles. On the other side, another bus waited to take us the final 3 hours to the town of Cahabón over another twisting, turning, steep mountain road where the driver may never have seen third gear.

From there, we still had another 1.5-hour ride to the town of Lanquin, and the best we could do was to squeeze into a minivan that had twenty-five people in it at one point, including the Czech woman. It was sweltering inside; fortunately, when we got to Lanquin we were able to secure a ride in the back of a pickup truck for the final 10 kilometers to our destination, which was the incredibly beautiful and remote Semuc Champey, perhaps the best-kept secret in all of Central America.

Most of the others in the pickup were staying at the larger Posada Las Marias, but we remained in the truck and got dropped off at a smaller hostel named El Portal. It was a nice-looking place, nestled in a grassy glade, and the food appeared good. Plus, we had a loft in a thatched-roof bungalow to ourselves that night. We immediately walked down to the river to cool off from a long, hot day of travel.

When we walked the short distance to the entrance in the morning, we found no gift shops or tour buses along the way, just a few local women selling trinkets or chocolate and one old man collecting the entrance fee. The trail was a wet, slippery path that at first followed the Río Cahabón, which suddenly disappeared from view, and all became quiet. And incredibly peaceful.

Semuc Champey is as hard to describe as it is to get to. The natural, 300-meter-long limestone bridge stretches over the Río Cahabón, which flows through a cave underneath. Its name means "where the river hides beneath the earth" in the local Mayan dialect.

The seven tranquil sacred pools soon came into view and their stunning beauty instantly mesmerized us. Each pool gently flows into the others via a series of tiny waterfalls before a larger cascade connects to the torrent of the reemerging Río Cahabón below. The pools were shades of blue and green and turquoise that I had never seen before. The water was so placid and serene that you would never have guessed that just a few yards beneath your feet, the Río Cahabón was raging in tumultuous fury through its hidden cave. The colors, as it turned out, depended on each pool's depth and even the time of year. They ranged from 3 to 10 feet deep, and the water was so clear that if a dime sank to the bottom of the deepest one, I would have been able to tell from the surface whether it had landed heads or tails.

We immediately went swimming, joining Anna and two other young women, from Germany, at one of the larger pools. The high concentration of limestone in the natural spring water made one especially buoyant, and floating on the surface was a cinch. Lush, steep mountains rose majestically on both sides. Mist hung in the air. Birds sang, monkeys howled, and butterflies flitted past silently. I had died and gone to heaven.

On our way back to El Portal, which was just a few hundred feet from this paradise, Van and I noticed a group of about twelve tourists near the outlet to the cave, where the Río Cahabón spilled violently back into daylight. Here, their guide, Josue, had lowered a rope ladder from the top of the roof down along the edge of the waterfall created by the water from the pools as it cascaded gently over the lip of the roof and dropped about 65 feet to the river below.

They climbed down, and then Josue led them into the mouth of the cave next to the raging river, where many interesting stalactites and stalagmites could be seen. We climbed down and peered in, but since we were not part of the tour, we were excluded. I did ask Josue if it was safe to jump into the Río Cahabón here, since the water looked plenty deep as it exited the cave, and he said people often did.

So Van and I climbed back up the ladder and contemplated our futures, peering over the edge of the lip, staring down at the frothing Río Cahabón with lumps in our throats. It looked a long way down. In fact, had I been on a mountainside staring over a 65-foot cliff, I would not have dared to venture this close to the edge. But somehow, the unknown depths of the water far below buoyed my courage.

I flung myself into the abyss.

It seemingly took forever for me to fall the height of a six-story building into the water, plenty of time to reconsider my folly. I smacked the water hard, but popped back to the surface and swam around a large boulder into an eddy. Then I climbed back up and did it again. And then Van went too. And so did one of Josue's group, a Brit who had been watching us anxiously.

Then, Josue was next to us, out of breath and appearing very concerned. He had not realized we meant we had intended to jump from the top, pointing to a small outcropping well below us only 10 feet above the water.

"*That's* where people jump from," he said, "not from up here! This is 20 meters up!" The last person who jumped from the top, he said, was a Swiss man who hit an underwater ledge and had to be air-lifted out by helicopter with a shattered leg.

"But you can see the ledge, and we avoided it," I pointed out.

"Yes," he said, "that's because the river is as low as I've ever seen it. I don't know how deep it is there."

Nice to find out all this after the fact. We all survived with nothing worse than sore tailbones.

After a fitful night in paradise—logging trucks clanked across the nearby wooden-slat bridge most of the night—we found out that a large group of rich Guatemalans was arriving that day and had rented our bungalow. We thought we would have to leave El Portal, but they allowed us to set up our tents down by the river instead.

Later that afternoon, back at El Portal after another day swimming in the sacred pools, a group of Europeans arrived by bus. Among them was Natasha, a beautiful Greek woman with flowing auburn hair and the most compelling green eyes I had ever peered into. We spent the rest of the day discussing subjects such as spirituality, Maya mysticism, and the speculation around the then-impending end of the Maya calendar.

She also had a Maya Yucatán calendar and, using my birth date, calculated my Maya sign as "White Cosmic Wind." I liked that. We seemed to have a strong connection and talked well into the night. I decided not to risk certain rejection by inviting her back to my tent. In any case, we had talked until 11 P.M. and Van and I planned to catch a 7 A.M. bus to Cobán.

Getting ready to leave in the morning, I had hoped Natasha might awaken so she could see the White Cosmic Wind one last time before it blew out of town. But, alas, she never stirred, unlike the rich Guatemalans, who were up at the crack of dawn despite having partied late into the night. Several empty tequila bottles sat on a table nearby.

In Cobán, we checked into the Hotel La Paz to find Anna, the Czech woman, already there. Since our bus back to Antigua wasn't leaving until the following morning, we had the rest of the day to laze around, and I spent most of the warm spring afternoon sitting in a local park reading. It was relaxing just to do nothing for a while, since there had been very few rest days on this action-filled vacation. Not that swimming in the tranquil pools of Semuc Champey had been work.

Monday, March 10 dawned bright and beautiful. It was the day before my birthday and our last full day in Guatemala. We had long since decided to fly from Guatemala City to Mexico City to save two days of travel by bus—the cost of the plane ticket was only slightly more—and we had a flight set for the next day. On the way back to Antigua by bus, we worked a side deal with the driver to pick us up the next morning for Q100 to bring us to the airport.

That night Van went to bed early, but I headed back to the Monoloco to celebrate my forty-eighth birthday. I certainly didn't feel or act 48, but that's what my driver's license said. And, unlike Van's, I knew mine was correct.

A woman sat down next to me at the bar, and we stared at each other with that hesitant look of familiarity for a few moments before she introduced herself as Trine from Denmark. We were several minutes into our conversation before we both finally realized that we had met on the shuttle to Copán Ruinas the month before, when we were both sick in the minivan. After enjoying a good laugh, I asked her what had happened to that guy from Alaska we had seen her with at the ruins. She said he had latched onto her after they had met one night here at the Monoloco, and the guy had even dumped his girlfriend to travel with her to Copán. She said it was a couple of days before she was able to ditch the guy. Now, at least, she was out having shots with her friends.

When the clock hit midnight, the bartender, Zach from Minneapolis, gave me a free beer to celebrate my birthday.

In the morning, our shuttle driver, whom we'd paid in advance, failed to show at the pre-arranged hour. As the minutes passed, Van and I began to panic, fearing we would miss our flight and be stuck in Guatemala City, a place I had carefully avoided during my previous visits because of its dangerous reputation.

We were just about to pay another driver about twice that amount to bring us to the airport when our driver pulled up. We got to the airport with only an hour to spare, but it proved to be plenty of time. We boarded the plane and put Guatemala behind us. It was time to get back to the peaks, and we were about to embark on what we anticipated would be the highlight of the entire trip: the high, majestic volcanoes of Central Mexico and the dizzying depths of Copper Canyon. We could hardly wait.

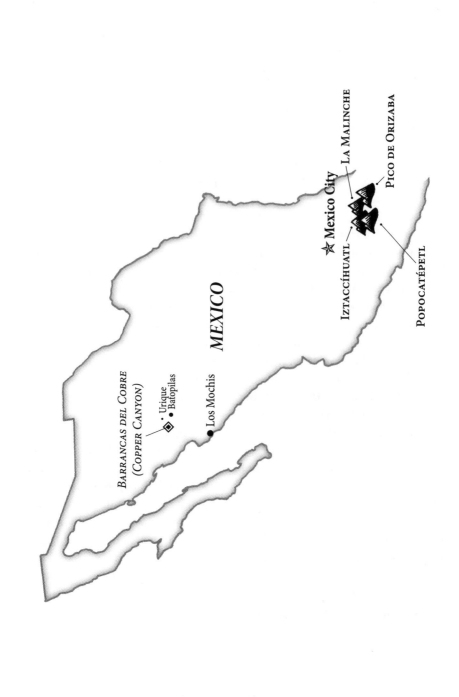

MEXICO

BARRANCAS DEL COBRE
(COPPER CANYON)
· Urique
● Batopilas
● Los Mochis

☆ Mexico City

LA MALINCHE

PICO DE ORIZABA

IZTACCÍHUATL

POPOCATÉPETL

Chapter 6
March 2008

THE MEXICAN VOLCANOES AND COPPER CANYON

IT'S CALLED LA MORDIDA, OR "THE BITE," AND I SHOULD'VE SEEN IT COMING. BUT, when the transit cop stuck his hand into our rental car 5 minutes after leaving the Mexico City airport, in my naïveté I simply reached out and shook it, thinking he was welcoming me to his fine country.

"¡Mucho gusto, amigo!"

Moments later a swarm of white-uniformed officers surrounded our tiny, blue Chevy whatever-it-was. And then it dawned on me: our new friend wasn't the welcome wagon. He was the paddy wagon. Or would have been, he made it clear, if I didn't pay the US$180 "fine" for supposedly running a red light at the Calzada Zaragoza intersection. This was precisely the spot our guidebook, *Mexico's Volcanoes: A Climbing Guide*, had warned us about. The transit cops, who were waving cars through the crowded intersection with disregard to the traffic light overhead, also loitered at this intersection to shake down tourists.

So far on our trip, Van and I had flown totally under the radar, unlike millions of our American compatriots who more visibly relied on Mexico's amenities for tourists. But that all changed as soon as we flew into Mexico City the morning of my birthday and picked up a rental car. It's amazing how quickly one can be transformed from a traveler to a tourist. For us, it only took putting four wheels under our feet.

When I refused to cooperate, the fine was quickly reduced to $100, but I still had no intention of paying.

"Señor," the officer snarled in halted English, "you don't want to go to jail. Just pay the fine and you can be on your way."

As I held my wallet in my hand, trying to explain to him that I had only

$5 on me, he actually reached through the open window and grabbed the billfold, and an honest-to-goodness tug-of-war ensued. When I finally was able to wrest my wallet from him, he reluctantly agreed to the fiver, since he was losing "business" with every passing minute. Opening my wallet, I was surprised to see a US$20 bill staring me in the face, and I'm sure he saw it too. But I reached behind it, grabbed a US$5 bill instead, and quickly handed it through the window.

As the officer begrudgingly snatched the bill from my hand, Van yelled, "Go!" and moments later we were speeding down the road to Puebla and the three high volcanoes on our list for the next five days. Not the best way to start one's birthday.

Our main objective over the next few days was the literal highpoint of the trip: Pico de Orizaba, a massive, conical, dormant volcano 2 hours east of Mexico City. At 18,491 feet, it is the third-highest mountain in North America. It's also relatively easy to climb, making it perfect training ground for any climber looking to do the bigger peaks of Alaska, the Andes, or beyond. Both Van and I had aspirations of climbing even higher someday.

But Orizaba was not going to be our first peak after weeks of relaxing in Guatemala, Honduras, and Belize. Five volcanoes rise from the central plain surrounding Mexico City, which itself is at 7,000 feet, and all five are taller than anything we had climbed in Colorado. We had planned on climbing three of them. Our first destination was La Malinche, at 14,640 feet the shortest of the five, but a perfect acclimatization climb.

La Malinche is named for the woman who is said to have betrayed an entire empire. When the great conquistador Hernán Cortés landed in Mexico in 1519, the Maya he met along the Yucatán coast honored him with the gift of twenty women; one of them, an Aztec slave named Malintzin, he soon discovered, spoke the Nahuatl language of the Aztecs. She promptly became his translator, mistress, and, not long after, the mother of his first-born son. Most historians agree that the Spaniards would not have survived long enough to have reached the Aztec capital of Tenochtitlán, let alone conquer it, if not for the resourcefulness of the woman they would call La Malinche.

Her mountain namesake lies within Malinche National Park, where there is a government-owned resort at the end of the road sitting at just over 10,000 feet. There were cabins, a large restaurant, and also campsites, which—at just US$3.70 a night—were perfect for our backpacker's budget. We pitched our tents in an open grassy area among some hedges and went to bed. We had seen no one else in the campground and expected a quiet night. But at about 10 P.M. we were startled awake by a mob of screaming children running all over the place, shining lights onto our tents, and generally going crazy, until the melee stopped so suddenly that I had to ask Van in the morning if it had all been a dream. He assured me it had not.

But there was no sign of these kids, or anyone else, for that matter, as we hit the trailhead shortly after sunrise. Soon we overtook the first of three climbers from California who were on the same itinerary we were—using La Malinche as a tune-up for Orizaba two days hence. It was perfect timing for Van and me, since one of the three, Doug Nidever, was a guide from the Mammoth Lakes area and had climbed Orizaba a handful of times, including once the previous month, and had always used La Malinche for an acclimatization hike. When we met him, he was guiding two of his friends, Ken and Larry.

It took Van and me only 3.5 hours of straightforward hiking—there were no switchbacks—to gain more than 4,500 feet of elevation and the summit of La Malinche; it was as easy as any 14er we had climbed during two previous trips to Colorado. The trail climbed through scented pine forests and wind-swept grasslands before gaining the summit ridge up a deeply eroded scar. From there it was a short climb to the summit, which afforded incredible views of the towering hulk of Orizaba to the east and of the twin volcanoes of Iztaccíhuatl and Popocatépetl to the west (better known by the diminutives, Izta and Popo). It marked a new high for both of us, as La Malinche stands 207 feet higher than Mount Elbert, which we had climbed in Colorado on a similarly perfect day.

That evening we joined Doug, Ken, and Larry for dinner at a small *comedor* just outside the resort's front gate. Though they were using a different outfitter on Orizaba, we all would be transported to the Piedra Grande hut, located at 14,000 feet on Orizaba's north face, the next day, and we tentatively agreed to climb the glacier-capped volcano together.

The next day, after eating breakfast at the comedor with the other three, Van and I drove to Tlachichuca, which—at 9,000 feet—is base camp for most foreigners climbing Orizaba. We arrived at the headquarters of our outfitter, Servimont, and met owner Gerardo Reyes, who informed us that the boxes containing our high-altitude gear had arrived by mail weeks before, as expected. The century-old building, located a block from the town square, was a former soap-making factory that the Reyes family had converted into a compound, from which they've been serving the climbing community for three generations.

Late that afternoon, the clouds parted long enough to reveal our first up-close view of Orizaba. The perfectly symmetrical, conical volcano glistened white in the afternoon sun, which reflected off the Jamapa Glacier that guards the upper reaches of the peak. Cortés and his men were surprised to see snow at such a southerly parallel when their ships arrived in Veracruz; Orizaba is just 60 miles inland from the coast and visible even today from the Gulf of Mexico.

The next day a pickup drove us the roughly 13 miles up a dusty, deeply rutted road to the Piedra Grande hut. It was barren except for a couple of long tables meant for gear and cooking, and six wooden sleeping platforms stacked three high from floor to ceiling. It looked like the hut could sleep upward of sixty, if necessary.

When we arrived, though, only Doug and Larry were there. Ken was out celebrating his fifty-eighth birthday with an acclimatization hike to about 15,500 feet, and Van and I soon followed, meeting him about a thousand feet above the hut on his way down. Van made it to Ken's turnaround point at a small campsite marked by flapping Tibetan prayer flags, but I climbed higher, making my way up a tricky gully over the headwall to the base of the Jamapa Glacier at about 16,200 feet. This row of parallel gullies represents the crux of the climb, as the marked trail effectively ends at the prayer flags.

Above that, the mountain rose steeply and majestically another 2,500 feet in the classic conical shape of a volcano. Despite its nontechnical slopes, Orizaba was not summited by a European until 1838, though it is surmised that the Aztecs ventured to its upper slopes, since the summit afforded views all the way to the coast.

It was an uncomfortable night at the Piedra Grande hut. As I had only a thin foam pad for a sleeping mat, the hard, wooden planks of the bunks prevented me from getting much sleep. But apparently no one else had that problem. A Frenchman tiptoed in well after dark and no one else noticed. I spoke with him briefly before he turned in too. Doug's alarm rang at 3 A.M., but only the Frenchman and I noticed. The Frenchman had a 2-hour head start by the time everyone else awoke and packed.

Oversleeping a whole hour might have been a major concern on a typical 18,000-foot mountain, but not on Orizaba. We reached the prayer flags and the first unsteady climbing just as the sun made its appearance over the Gulf of Mexico somewhere off to our left. I scampered ahead and watched from atop a boulder at the edge of the glacier as the Frenchman, visible above us, traversed the glacier from left to right and passed underneath a band of exposed rock. He slowly climbed out of sight over the curved edge of the crater rim more than 2,000 feet above.

When the others caught up, I showed Doug the route the Frenchman had taken—and the wands with little red flags on top sticking out of the snow to mark the way—but he ignored me. He said he was taking his charges to the left, which to me seemed ridiculously out of the way, but since he was a professional guide, even Van decided to follow.

Having watched as Van was plagued by acute mountain sickness two years before in Colorado, I could understand why he chose to cautiously hang back with the Californians. I continued on alone. Trudging up the breath-stealing 45-degree slope, I stopped briefly to chat with the descending Frenchman, and reached the gravelly summit after about 2 hours of steady climbing from the edge of the glacier. The wind-sculpted snow proved so hard and sure that crampons were unnecessary.

The summit crater was enormous—more than a quarter-mile across—and the crater walls were so steep that from the rim I could not see the crater's bottom. I decided to lie down near a twisted piece of metal that appeared to be part of an old tower, and took a short nap in the brilliant sunshine. After waiting for what seemed an interminably long time for the others (it was really only about 45 minutes), I arose from my siesta and started down, thinking they may have turned back for some unknown reason.

But I met them a few hundred feet below, still climbing, though Ken was spent and said he could not continue. Doug said he was going to push on with Larry—and with Van in tow—leaving Ken where he currently was, sitting on a rock with his head in his hands and apparently feeling the altitude. Even though they were all friends, I found this considerably unprofessional of Doug, who apparently expected me to watch over Ken, though he never asked. I stayed with Ken until the others returned, even though Van and I ran the risk of missing our ride from the hut. Soon, the sun began to set behind the summit dome, throwing me and Ken into shadows. It was a long, cold 2 hours awaiting the successful return of the conquistadors.

We got back to the hut at 5 P.M. to find that our ride back to the Servimont compound had waited for us, despite our being an hour late. Driving back down, we had to pull over to let pass two vehicles carrying climbers who were having difficulty negotiating a particularly rutted section of road.

While the three Californians were headed back to the States in the morning, Van and I were not done. After a hot shower and a restful night in Tlachichuca, we were awakened at six the next morning, which was Palm Sunday, to the very loud sound of rockets going off all over town, marking the beginning of the weeklong Semana Santa celebration. After breakfast, we set out for Iztaccíhuatl—the striking 17,160-foot volcano in the Paso de Cortés—with handwritten directions from Gerardo Reyes himself.

But even though we could see the twin towers of Izta and Popo rising majestically to the west, we got lost. Had our circuitous course through the cities of Puebla and Cholula been charted on a map, it would have looked like a 4-year-old's Etch a Sketch drawing.

We had to stop and ask directions several times before we eventually found the unmarked dirt road leading up to the Paso de Cortés, the 11,000-foot saddle separating Izta and Popo, from where Cortés had first laid eyes on the great

Valley of Mexico and its gleaming city of Tenochtitlán. Cortés may have had an easier time finding the pass than we did.

We stopped at the visitor center at the national park and paid twenty pesos to stay at the hostel located at a microwave antennae installation facility about a mile from Izta's main La Joya trailhead. From there, we had incredible views of both Iztaccíhuatl and Popocatépetl, the latter of which was still smoking from its giant crater after what we had been told was a sizable eruption just the weekend before. Not surprisingly, the volcanoes are tied together for eternity in Aztec legend.

Izta is known as the "white woman"; viewed from the west, the volcano does appear to take the appearance of a woman lying down. In fact, the various summits on the elongated ridgeline are known by various body parts, such as "the knees," "the head," and "the breasts," which mark the true summit.

According to legend, Popocatépetl was a warrior who was in love with Iztaccíhuatl. As he was returning to claim her after a victory in battle, rivals sent notice of Popo's death instead. Izta immediately died of grief. Popo then built the two facing mountains, placing her lifeless body atop one and standing sentinel over it on the other. Indeed, Popocatépetl means "smoking mountain," and his namesake has been one of the most volatile volcanoes in North America since Cortés's day. It has been almost entirely off-limits to the public since its most recent spate of eruptions began in 1994.

Amazingly, five of Cortés's soldiers scaled the erupting Popo during the siege on Tenochtitlán, and two of them were lowered into the hulking, bubbling crater to retrieve sulfur for gunpowder—an act that would have been unbelievable had it not been recorded in transcripts sent back to the King of Spain. Thousands—Cortés's troops and the native tribes aiding his conquest—turned out to watch as the party ascended the snow-capped volcano; during the climb, Popo erupted, lobbing hot rocks toward the climbers. One of the rocks landed in the snow nearby, and the men huddled around it to get warm.

Reaching the crater rim at 17,880 feet, the soldiers endured another eruption, but after the smoke cleared, they looked into the crater at the pools of molten lava below. Then, one of them, Francisco Montaño, was lowered seven times by a hemp rope about 200 meters into the boiling cauldron, each time coming up with a bagful of sulfur. Exhausted, he was replaced by Juan de Larios, who repeated the descent six more times, all with fumes and eruptions occurring around him. In all, they obtained 140 kilograms of sulfur—more than 300 pounds. Afterward, the two men were carried on the shoulders of the crowd all the way to the town of Coyuhuacan on the outskirts of Tlaxcala. Even Cortés was said to have embraced them upon their triumphant return.

It would be nearly 300 years before another European climbed higher; not until Baron Alexander von Humboldt reached 19,286 feet on Chimborazo in Ecuador in 1803 did anyone surpass the high-altitude mark set on Popo that day.

That night in our bunkhouse—a barren, cement-block building with three rooms that looked more like jail cells—we were awakened at 11:30 P.M. by a late-arriving group of climbers. We did not know it at the time, but it was the same group we had seen in the trucks heading to the Piedra Grande hut on Orizaba the day before. In the morning, I headed to Iztaccíhuatl alone, as Van, satisfied after his successful summit of Orizaba two days before, decided to sleep in and join me later at the trailhead.

Climbing by myself, it didn't take long for me to catch up to and fall in with the late arrivals from the night before, who had hit the trail shortly before me. One of them was a gringo from Washington, D.C., named Zachary Bookman, a 27-year-old University of Maryland graduate on a Fulbright fellowship to study Mexico's recently passed Freedom of Information Act. Zac was climbing Izta with a handful of locals he had met at a climbing gym in Mexico City. In fact, they were completing their self-proclaimed *La Triada*: having summited La Malinche and Orizaba over the previous two days, they were tackling Izta on the third day, as opposed to my five-day plan.

Zac, who was training for what would be a successful summit of Denali later that year, had invited his father, Charles, to join them. Charles had climbed Mexico's big volcanoes fresh out of college in 1970 "on the heels of a solar eclipse." He jumped at the chance to do it again on the cusp of his sixtieth birthday, and had flown in from Seattle, arriving from sea level just in time to jump into a four-by-four and head to La Malinche.

The elder Bookman wasn't able to summit all three mountains, but that was due more to the rigid schedule of their La Triada than his stamina. He said he had reached the summit of La Malinche on the first day to be greeted by a wizened old man offering tequila and hot serrano peppers, telling the group, "You're not done until you drink and take a bite."

On the second day, Charles surpassed 17,000 feet on Orizaba before Zac collected him on the way down. And on Izta, Charles made it another 4,000 feet up to "the knees" before rejoining us at the La Joya trailhead, where some local women were cooking tacos on a grill set up in one of several shacks located in the parking lot. We were all gluttonously washing them down with cold cervezas as quickly as they could prepare them.

Later, Van joined us at the trailhead, and we enjoyed a glorious afternoon swapping stories over endless tacos and beer. Then, to top it off, Popo joined the show, throwing up big plumes of ash three times as we sat at La Joya enjoying the remainder of the day. The ash clouds soared several hundred feet into the atmosphere, roiling into grotesque shapes before dissipating in the wind and floating gently in our direction as Popo paid tribute to his lost love, Izta. This was all capped by an unforgettable sunset of brilliant pinks and purples, probably the result of the volcanic gases and ash.

Then someone suggested we all climb Nevado de Toluca—the 15,500-foot mountain on the west side of Mexico City—the next day to make it four in a row, and I think the beers were talking when we all agreed it was a great idea. Zac said we could follow them back to his apartment and crash on the floor that night. But that meant doing something Van and I had pledged not to do under any circumstance: drive in Mexico City after dark.

Assured it was not dangerous, we packed up and fell in line behind Benito, the driver of the pickup, whom I was convinced drove as if he was trying to lose me at every opportunity. Somehow, I kept our tiny Chevy sardine can glued to his bumper for 60 miles as he raced through stop signs, failed to slow for speed bumps, and once even darted across several lanes of two-way traffic without warning. All, I imagined, while laughing maniacally at the white-knuckled gringo in his rear-view mirror.

Then, on the outskirts of the city, he pulled to the side of the road after hearing what he said was a strange rapping noise in the engine. Comically, we tried to shoehorn Zac and Charles and all their gear into our Matchbox rental, but then, thankfully, Benito announced there was no problem after all. He had called the pickup's owner on his cell phone to learn that the truck was *supposed* to make that noise.

Back at Zac's apartment, more friends stopped by, and we all walked to a taqueria for late-night *chilangos* and more beer. Nevado de Toluca was soon forgotten.

The next day, we said goodbye and drove back to the airport to drop off the car, glad we didn't have to pass Calzada Zaragoza once again. Though I did learn from Zac how to avoid any future run-ins with the transit police: just bring a video camera and point it in the officer's face.

Too bad I hadn't thought of that before. I just might have saved five bucks.

Van and I were very relieved to have gotten rid of the rental car and to have simply become travelers again. From the airport we took a taxi to the Zócalo section of Mexico City, the large main square in the modern part of the city and one of the largest city squares in the world. In pre-Conquest days, the Zócalo was a large open space in the center of Tenochtitlán, and was just one block southwest of the Templo Mayor, a temple considered the center of the universe by the Aztecs. Nowadays, that is pretty much the site of the Hostal Moneda, where we were headed on a gorgeous Tuesday morning.

We got a noisy dorm room right off the lobby for just Mex$50 a night, which included dinner, served nightly on a rooftop patio overlooking the entire Zócalo district. The first thing we did was walk seven blocks to the nearest post office to mail our boxes of climbing gear back home, since we would no longer need any of it. Incredibly, my box cost the equivalent of US$95 to mail, while Van's was a pricey US$75. But what were we going to do? We certainly didn't want to tote that gear with us the rest of the trip.

After some sightseeing to the impressive ruins of Teotihuacan the following day, during which the teetotaling Van surprised me by trying samples of *pulque* and *mescal*, we boarded a bus for a 23-hour ride to the city of Los Mochis on the Sea of Cortez to catch a train to Barrancas del Cobre— Copper Canyon. For the first time, I was getting tired of traveling and was looking forward to the end of our journey. It was March 20—day 73 of our trip. But I was glad we were finishing up with Copper Canyon, one of the deepest, most remote canyons on Earth.

The next morning, the first day of spring, dawned bright on the day after a full moon, but it found us still on the bus. The night before, when we pulled into the city of Tepic at nine o'clock, I had calculated that we would not arrive in Los Mochis in time to catch the 8 A.M. train. Even though I failed to factor in crossing a time zone, which would have worked in our favor, we still missed it by half an hour. At the bus station, we decided to take the next bus to the tiny town of El Fuerte so we wouldn't have to spend the day in such a large city, and catch the train from there the next morning.

The Mexican army ensures that bus travel throughout the country is quite safe. There are military checkpoints every few hundred miles, and at these stops everyone has to get off the bus while soldiers board and search everything. Once, when we stopped at a checkpoint, a soldier boarded the bus and went down the aisle asking for everyone's passport. When he got to Van, his eyes lit up, as he was certain he had discovered an illegal from Guatemala. The look on his face was priceless when Van forked over his brand-new U.S. passport.

When we arrived in Los Mochis, I had only four Mexican pesos to my name— about thirty-eight cents—and that was only because I'd saved three pesos by climbing over the cage to use the restroom instead of paying, which I had no qualms about doing. Arriving in El Fuerte a couple of hours later, we found an overpriced hotel for the equivalent of US$25 and spent the rest of the day sleeping. By then, we were both road-weary. Plus, it was hot out. We were now in the northern, semi-arid part of Mexico, not far from the edges of the Sonoran Desert, where the average daily temperature in March is 89 degrees Fahrenheit. We didn't emerge from our siestas until dinnertime.

Its official name is the Ferrocarril Chihuahua al Pacifico, but everyone knows it simply as "El Chepe," or the Copper Canyon railway. It runs 418 miles from Los Mochis to the city of Chihuahua, and is one of the most scenic and gravity-defying railroads in the world. Begun in 1898 by a group of Americans looking to set up a socialist society in Mexico, construction was abandoned for more than fifty years because the technology did not exist to complete the arduous route. When finished in 1961, the track passed over thirty-seven bridges and through eighty-six tunnels, climbing to the Continental Divide at 7,900 feet above sea level near Divisadero.

The entire journey would have taken about 16 hours, but we were not going all the way to Chihuahua, located on the other side of the rugged Sierra Madre Occidental. We were headed for Creel, a small town high in the mountains that is considered by many to be the adventure capital of Mexico. We booked passage on the first-class train, which had a restaurant car and ran express to the major towns along the route. The second-class train would have been cheaper, but it would stop anywhere along the route to let passengers on and off, sort of like the chicken bus.

Rolling out of El Fuerte, the train picked up speed through the desert lowlands, but that soon changed as we began climbing up the side of a canyon with a precipitous drop appearing beside us. The first major bridge we crossed was more than 1,600 feet long. We plunged into darkness when we entered a tunnel that was well over a mile in length. Before we had reached the tiny village of Témoris about 2 hours into the trip, we had already passed through twenty tunnels totaling almost 2 miles.

After a brief stop at Témoris, the train crossed the Santa Barbara Bridge high above the Septentrion River and turned back to the west along the wall of the steep canyon. Then all went dark again as we entered the La Pera Tunnel, perhaps one of the most remarkable engineering feats in the history of railroading. This horseshoe-shaped tunnel—more than 3,000 feet long—not only made a sweeping 180-degree turn inside the mountain, but it deposited us back into daylight several hundred feet higher and heading back to the east. The switchback and climb were so subtle that we were completely unaware that we had reversed direction.

The climbing continued until we finally pulled to a stop in Divisadero, the gateway to Copper Canyon. At the Divisadero Barranca—the canyon overlook—we got our first incredible views of the canyon, as we peered off the rim toward the Urique River many thousands of feet below. The view was very similar to that of the South Rim of the Grand Canyon, except that five Grand Canyons could fit inside Copper Canyon. Here, too, we saw the many Tarahumara—or as they call themselves, Rarámuri—who had set up their tables on the platform to sell their wares to the many tourists on board. But we were only interested in ice cream cones.

Zac had visited Copper Canyon a few months before, and had told us we might run into a crazy gringo called El Caballo Blanco—the White Horse—who is a virtual ghost often seen running along the narrow trails of the canyon wearing little more than sandals on his feet. But I forgot about him almost as soon as Zac finished his story, certain I would not run into this so-called ghost.

After crossing the Continental Divide, we pulled into Creel late in the afternoon. It was Saturday, the day before Easter, and I could see that the train was overloaded with travelers on the Semana Santa holiday. I told Van to get his pack and prepare to jump off, as I surmised that if the lone hostel in Creel wasn't already full, it soon would be. We raced across the street to learn that we had indeed secured the final two spots available at Casa Margarita's, located on the corner of the town square.

When the proprietor showed us where we would be bunking, however, we found that it was on the floor of the already overcrowded dorm room right in front of the bathroom and we could see water coming from underneath the door while someone was in the shower. Van and I looked at each other disapprovingly. We asked to look around for a few minutes before deciding—there was a long line of fellow backpackers at the door awaiting our decision. We spied a flat, cement rooftop over one of the other rooms and asked if we could simply pitch our tents there.

"No problema," we were told.

For Mex$50 a night—which included breakfast and dinner—we felt we had stumbled onto a bargain.

In spite of the constant barking of dogs throughout the night and being awakened early by the roosters, we enjoyed our rooftop digs. It was open to the clear night sky, and we were only a couple of nights removed from the full moon. It was considerably colder in Creel than it had been in La Fuerte, and it had even snowed in the previous few days, which was unusual for March, despite the elevation of 7,700 feet.

On Easter Sunday, we made the requisite hike up to a huge statue of Jesus that overlooks the entire town, and went for a 10-mile hike through places with names such as the Valley of the Mushrooms and the Valley of the Frogs, begrudgingly paying an entrance fee of Mex$15. Though sporting many natural rock formations that did indeed look like mushrooms and frogs, they were all little more than tourist traps set up by the local Tarahumara.

Mostly, though, it was just a chance to kill some time before Monday, when the banks would reopen and we could get the money we needed for our real goal: a trip to the bottom of the canyon for a multiday hike. When the bank finally opened, though, things were so complicated that we missed the only bus of the day to the town of Batopilas, and had to return to Casa Margarita's for another night on the roof. But this turned out to be fortuitous.

That day, we connected with a Canadian named Rich Patha, and we all went on a 15-mile hike into the Valley of the Monks, which was much better than anything we had seen the day before and cost Mex$5 less. Towering, monolithic rock pillars jutted into the sky in this valley. We were able to climb some of the smaller ones, and ate lunch atop one in the brilliant sunshine.

There, we agreed to team up for a four-day hike through Copper Canyon from Batopilas to Urique. We caught a bus at 7:30 the next morning for the 5-hour ride to Batopilas, located several thousand feet below at the bottom of the canyon. We quickly left pavement behind and began a dizzying descent down a narrow, rutted road into the depths of this immense canyon.

Several times we met cars coming up the road, and passing became a tight squeeze. Later, we rounded a corner that was so sharp that the driver—who appeared to be no older than 15—had to back the bus up until the rear tires were at the edge of the cliff to make the turn. Sitting in the back, I was looking down at nothing but air as the rear of the bus hung over the precipice. Below were the rusted hulks of other buses that had not successfully made the turn. But our driver appeared to be a seasoned veteran of these twisting, turning roads—did I mention he was barely out of puberty?—and we arrived safely in Batopilas shortly after noon.

The first person we saw when we got off the bus was a gringo with bronzed, weathered skin who appeared to be in his late 50s and was wearing frayed shorts, a holey shirt, a straw hat, and sandals called *huaraches*, many of which are made out of discarded tires by the local Tarahumara. He was leaning against a building in the town square waiting for the bus to arrive, hoping to find some wayward tourists to hire him as their guide. He stepped forward and we immediately recognized him.

"You're Caballo Blanco!" Rich and I said almost in unison. A crooked smile quickly broke out on his gaunt face.

"Yes, I am," he said, pleased that we had heard of him.

Caballo Blanco, in fact, had been living in a hut near Batopilas for months at a time over the past ten years. He'd paced one of the Tarahumara runners who had come to race Colorado's Leadville 100 in the early '90s and wanted to know more about their people. So he set out for Copper Canyon, hoping to learn what he could about these Rarámuri, the "Running People," who had been holed up in the canyon's depths ever since the Spanish conquistadors arrived.

Over time, he gained their trust and respect and forged an unspoken kinship. Wanting to give back to his hosts, he came up with the idea for an ultramarathon in Copper Canyon. It took until 2006 to convince Scott Jurek, the seven-time Western States Endurance Run champion and perhaps the best ultrarunner on the planet at the time, to come to Urique to run his race. Jurek finished a humbled second to a local Tarahumara runner in that first race.

Now, of course, almost everyone has heard of Caballo Blanco, or at least the entire ultrarunning community has. Caballo Blanco, or Micah True, which also wasn't his real name, became a cult hero virtually overnight after he was the focal character in the *New York Times* best-selling book *Born to Run* by Christopher McDougall, which was released in 2009.

Thanks to the popularity of the book, the race has grown into a huge event, with hundreds of Tarahumara and dozens of runners from all over the world descending upon Urique every March. We had missed the Copper Canyon Ultramarathon by just a few weeks when we arrived in Batopilas that spring day in 2008—and our trip preceded the book by a year.

Just a few weeks after the 2012 race, Caballo Blanco was in New Mexico and went for a run in the Gila Wilderness, one of his favorite haunts. When he didn't return, his girlfriend of two years, Maria Walton, whom I have since met and gotten to know, was notified. Ultrarunners from all over the country dropped everything and headed to New Mexico to help in the search. Many were not sure if Caballo Blanco even wanted to be found, as he was quoted at the end of *Born to Run* as saying he might just go wandering off when he felt his time was up—something his hero, the legendary Apache warrior Geronimo, had never gotten the chance to do, Micah often said. Geronimo instead died of pneumonia while imprisoned at Fort Sill, in Oklahoma.

"When I get too old to work, I'll do what Geronimo would've [done] if they'd left him alone," Caballo is quoted by McDougall. "I'll walk off into the deep canyons and find a quiet place to lie down."

That's not what happened in the end. While Micah was found lying down in a canyon, he had died of a heart ailment. He was only 58 years old.

On the day we met Caballo Blanco in Batopilas, he was hoping we would hire him as our guide. When we told him we were planning a self-guided trip from Batopilas to Urique—about 30 miles over three canyon rims—he tried to talk us out of it, since we had no map, no compass, and pretty much no clue about where we were going. Our plan was simply to navigate by the sun, as all we really knew was that Urique was northwest of us. We knew our venture was not the conventional way to do such a hike, but we felt confident in our abilities, and Caballo Blanco soon gave up trying to talk us out of it.

Realizing that we were intent on our decision, Caballo Blanco said we needed to follow the Manzano Trail, and told us roughly where to pick it up, just a short ways upstream from town. But, still hopeful that we would change our minds, he wasn't forthcoming with much additional information about the route. Seeing we each had a gallon water jug with us, and knowing we would require much more than that on the journey, he scratched his chin and said in a long, drawn-out sentence, "Well, you *might* find water out there *some*where."

This part was especially true; for the next four days, I am convinced that we located water only through divine intervention.

After eating lunch at the home of a woman named Claudita—whom Caballo Blanco recommended—we set off by following the river upstream for about 4 miles, where a tributary came in from our left and Caballo Blanco had said we would find the trailhead. Arriving late in the afternoon, we started up this sidestream a few hundred yards and camped for the night on a sandy riverbank. It was still hot enough that we went for a cool dip in the stream, but we expected it to get quite cold once the sun went down.

That night was pure heaven as Van, Rich, and I enjoyed one of the clearest night skies any of us had ever seen. There is no light pollution in Copper Canyon, and we could see many constellations, including Orion's Belt, which Rich pointed out. Then, suddenly, I noticed a satellite streaking across the sky, perhaps the International Space Station, we all agreed.

Packing up in the morning, we headed across a road where a trail led up the side of the mountain. The day before, we had asked a local farmer about the whereabouts of the trailhead, and, despite the language barrier, he had pointed in this direction. Perhaps we should have hired Caballo Blanco after all, because almost immediately, we were lost.

The "trail" we were on soon dead-ended, and we found ourselves on the bushwhack from hell. Blocked by a sheer cliff in front of us, we spent two miserable hours trying to climb up to a road that we could see several hundred feet above us. Getting to it required crawling through thick thorn bushes and overhanging branches that caught our oversize backpacks repeatedly. More than once I fell onto cactus bushes, turning my hands into pincushions. When we finally broke through to the road, we were so exhausted that we simply collapsed in the middle of it—the only flat ground we had been on all day—and took a nap.

It was after lunch before we started hiking up this road, covering about 8 miles before it led us into some high, open meadows, where it appeared that cows had been grazing. Out of water, we knocked on the door of a house we came upon, and, when no one answered, we unhooked the twisted piece of wire holding the door closed and went inside. To us it appeared that no one lived there, and since we found no water, we left, and continued on until we came to a place where a trail led off into the woods to our right. Following this trail, we promptly located a spring—the only water we had seen since leaving the river that morning. The only problem, however, was that this small pool was stagnant, with dead mosquitoes and green slime floating on the surface. Fortunately, Van had a water filter with him and began to fill our bottles, even though none of us wanted to drink this putrid water.

Suddenly, the apparent owner of the house—the first person we had seen the entire day—mysteriously appeared with his own bucket to fill, not from the spring, but from a secret hose that was hidden under some leaves. Picking the hose up from the ground, he uncoupled it and drank straight from the tap; no need to filter. He allowed us to fill all of our bottles and waved us good-bye. We would never have noticed this hose had he not happened along at that very moment.

Returning to the road, we hiked only another 5 minutes before we decided to set up camp next to it under some tall, stately oak trees. In the morning, we reached the end of the road and started climbing up a ridge, which led to a cliff to our west where the view was the most magnificent we had yet seen. In fact, we agreed that this view alone made the entire trip worth it. From our flat spot on the rim, we could not even count all the sheer cliffs we could see on all the canyon walls surrounding us, all different shades of reds and blues, depending on where the sun was shining.

Hiking over this ridge, by late afternoon we came to some more pastures and spotted some more houses. Like the one the day before, these rough-hewn structures appeared to be little more than abandoned shacks, perhaps used only in summer months when the ranchers brought their cattle higher up the mountainside to graze. Again, we were virtually out of water, and had seen no sign of any all day. But, once again, providence intervened. Walking along a trail in the woods, we were met by a man carrying his own empty water jug. And, just like the day before, the man reached into the leaves and pulled up a thin, black hose, uncoupled it, and fresh, sparkling water poured out. He was the only person we had seen all day. Another day, another coincidence that bordered on miraculous.

He spoke very little English, but we were able to discern that the trail leading past his house went directo to Urique, and we continued on. Moments later, the man's five children, all between the ages of 5 and 12, ran after us, and offered to guide us to Urique for US$50. We all laughed; we probably wouldn't have had to pay Caballo Blanco that much.

We hiked until we couldn't hear them following us anymore, but it was getting late, and there was no flat ground to be found. Finally, we came to a small, rounded pasture and decided to camp there, despite the fact that the place was littered with cow patties. I had to kick several out of the way just to create enough space to lay out my sleeping bag. The nights had been so warm that we no longer bothered with our tents. I might have wanted one on this night; sometime after midnight, we were awakened by cows grazing all around us.

Around midday the following day, we came to a sheer cliff face that was more than a thousand-foot drop. From this high perch, which appeared to be the top of a waterfall during the rainy season, we could see the Urique River far below, and what we thought must be the village of Urique on the far side, many miles away.

We wished that the waterfall had been running, as we were again low on water. Then, Van and I noticed another of those thin, black hoses snaking across the bare rock. There was no place we found where we could uncouple the hose as we had the previous two days, but knew there must be a spring nearby somewhere. Then suddenly I heard a gurgling sound coming from the ledge and discovered a flat rock covering a tiny well that had been chiseled out of the limestone rock by hand. It was just big enough to lower our Nalgene water bottles into, and, for the third day in a row, a miracle had delivered us life.

Several houses were perched hundreds of feet below this cliff on the only flat patches of ground we could see. We began picking our way down this cliff face on a rudimentary goat path that was difficult to traverse with our large backpacks. There was only one way to go, and it led straight into the backyard of one of the houses we could see from the waterfall. We had to walk through someone's garden and past their back door to get beyond their house, and apologized profusely to the woman who was sitting on the back steps. Her children or grandchildren—it was hard to tell her age—were running around playing in the yard, such as it was. The entire house sat on a little rocky outcropping on the cliff face, and the only access to the property was by another narrow path that hugged the cliff beyond.

Making our way slowly along this rocky path, we were startled when the three children we had seen in the yard—apparently between the ages of 3 and 6—came running and laughing past us on this narrow path as if they were on their way to the park on some city sidewalk. One of the boys was even barefoot, seemingly unaffected by the sharp, volcanic texture of the rock under his feet.

Finally, we reached a dirt road that led steeply downhill past a school toward what everyone we had met had told us was the town of Urique. When we finally got to the bottom of the canyon, we were much relieved to see a small town on the other side of the river, and assumed that this was Urique. Here the road simply crossed the river without a bridge, with trucks driving through the foot-deep water to the other side. (When I returned to Copper Canyon in 2015, a bridge spanned the river at this point.) We walked partway across and sat down in the cold, clear water and enjoyed our first baths in days. Locals walked by and stared at us as if we were loco.

Crossing the river, we walked into town and stopped at a small tienda and bought a couple of ice-cold Cokes. It was like drinking liquid gold, they tasted so good after four days on the trail.

Rich and I asked some locals if this was indeed Urique, as we surmised, and were told, "No, Guapalayna." Urique, we were informed by one man, was still another "5 kilometers" north. Another said it was "an hour-and-a-half walk." Unfortunately, the second guy was closer to the mark.

The look on Van's face was priceless when Rich and I informed him that we still had a few miles to go. I thought the soda in his mouth was going to shoot out his nose.

It was dark long before we three bedraggled hikers completed what was more like an 8-kilometer walk into the town of Urique. The sidewalks had pretty much been rolled up by the time we arrived, even though it was a Friday night. We easily found the hotel in the center of town that we had been told about, and the owner quickly let us in and rented us a pair of rooms. We noticed that the restaurant across the street was closed and inquired about any others that might still be open, and the man motioned for us to wait as he went across the street and knocked on the door. A man came to the door and they conversed quickly, and our proprietor came back and announced that his son-in-law owned the restaurant, and would reopen just for us.

He prepared for us an incredible steak dinner that probably tasted all the better because we had been eating freeze-dried foods for the past few days. I also downed three ice-cold Dos Equis. It was a very fitting conclusion to one of the most epic, unforgettable hikes ever.

The beers finally got Rich to open up a little, as he had been a bit secretive since we had met him. While he called Vancouver home, he said he was Czech by birth and about the same age as Van. On Facebook, he went by the name Ricardo Ofnolastname, and he had spent much of his adult life traveling the world. He had just spent a considerable time in Central America, and was headed off to Asia soon, he said.

In the morning our hotel owner held the bus for us, as we were a few minutes late finishing breakfast across the street. Then began the steep, 3-hour climb out of Urique back to the canyon rim on a winding road that was nearly as nerve-racking as the one we had taken down to Batopilas several days before. Arriving in the town of Bahuichivo, which we had been through on El Chepe the week before, we expected a 4-hour wait for the next train heading toward Creel. But a microbus was ready to roll when we got there, and we crammed in, even though I had to stand up, hunched over in the back with my head pressed against the ceiling, absorbing every bump during the dusty 2.5-hour ride to the town of San Rafael. There we were able to switch to a big coach for the remaining 55 kilometers back to Creel.

Rich said his goodbyes in Bahuichivo, as he was heading down to Los Mochis and the beach, and we never saw him again, though we've been in touch. The last I heard, he was teaching English in Taiwan.

Back in Creel, Van and I resumed our perch on the roof at Casa Margarita's, and were once again kept awake all night by the barking dogs. The next day was a Sunday, and Van and I had planned it as a rest day, but upon checking the bus schedules, we determined that if we were going to make it back to Tecate in time for my brother to pick us up on Tuesday, we needed to leave Creel on the afternoon bus to La Junta.

We were warned by a Mexican named Rodrigo, whom we had met at Casa Margarita's, that La Junta was not a friendly town, and it certainly seemed that way when we arrived and started looking for a hotel. The first one we came to was Mex$350—about US$35—which was more than we had paid on any night during our entire three-month trip. A shady-looking guy, who was considerably drunk, said there were some cheaper places down the street, and offered to show them to us, but they all turned out to be closed and finally we just gave the guy a few pesos to leave us alone. Then, just as it was getting dark, we relented and returned to the first hotel and paid the exorbitant price.

After a shower, we went out to get dinner, but we returned straight to the hotel afterward, as this was the first place during our entire trip in which we hadn't felt safe.

Rodrigo had told us that it would be an 8-hour bus ride from La Junta to Hermosillo, but I should have known better. He seemed to have a different concept of time. Twelve hours after leaving La Junta, we rolled into the terminal in Hermosillo, not knowing if there was an overnight bus going to Tecate or not. But when we pulled in, the bus next to ours said "Tijuana" on the front—I knew Tecate was on that route—and was just getting ready to depart. We had just enough time to use the *baños* and purchase our ticket before the bus rolled out for the overnight journey across the Sonoran Desert and into Baja.

At 8:30 the next morning, we were again sitting in the Parque Central in Tecate, where our journey had begun eighty-five days before. It was chillier than it had been then, probably because it was earlier in the day, and we sat in the growing warmth of the brilliant sunshine waiting for the Internet café to open so I could email my brother and let him know we had arrived.

Around one o'clock, Bryon's pickup truck pulled up on the American side, and just like we had done three months before, Van and I simply walked across the border.

Back at Bryon's house in Alpine, he and his girlfriend, Lynn, wanted to hear all about our adventures, but there were too many to recount. We spent the day washing dirty clothes and packing, and I discovered I had gained 10 pounds on the trip. Who else but me could gain weight eating Central American food for three months?

The next day, Van and I said our goodbyes at the airport, as we were on different flights. He was not the same shy, timid kid who had walked into Mexico with me three months before. I had watched him grow up before my very eyes. He was now a man.

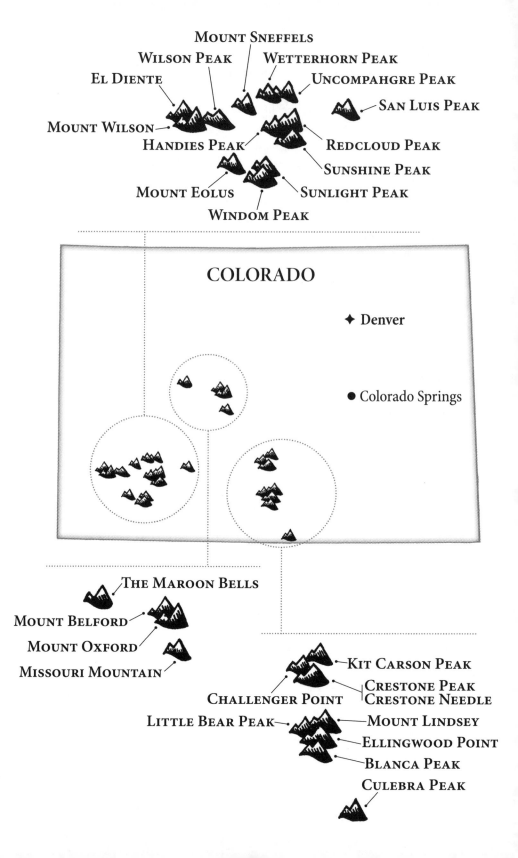

MOUNT SNEFFELS
WILSON PEAK   WETTERHORN PEAK
EL DIENTE   UNCOMPAHGRE PEAK
                                    SAN LUIS PEAK
MOUNT WILSON
HANDIES PEAK   REDCLOUD PEAK
                              SUNSHINE PEAK
MOUNT EOLUS   SUNLIGHT PEAK
WINDOM PEAK

COLORADO

✦ Denver

● Colorado Springs

THE MAROON BELLS
MOUNT BELFORD
MOUNT OXFORD
MISSOURI MOUNTAIN

KIT CARSON PEAK
CRESTONE PEAK
CRESTONE NEEDLE
CHALLENGER POINT
LITTLE BEAR PEAK   MOUNT LINDSEY
                                    ELLINGWOOD POINT
                                    BLANCA PEAK
                                    CULEBRA PEAK

Chapter 7
September 2008

RETURN
TO THE
ROCKIES

THE STORIES OF MY THREE-MONTH BACKPACKING TRIP QUICKLY TOOK ON EPIC proportions when I returned to New Hampshire and caught up with my friends. I spent most of my days that spring atop Monadnock and most afternoons sitting in the sunshine outside my favorite sidewalk café, Armadillos—a Mexican place where I was a regular—retelling those stories over cold beers. That summer, I drove for UPS waiting for my month-long layoff prior to the start of Christmas Rush in October. When September arrived, I was ready to finish my quest for the 14ers.

I returned to Colorado early in the month with immense anticipation to complete the Colorado 14ers over a span of the next twenty-one days. Unlike the previous two Septembers, I would be alone on this trip, and had mapped out an aggressive itinerary for knocking off the final twenty 14ers needed to finish the list. Among them were the dreaded Maroon Bells, as well as both of the Crestones. Daunting challenges awaited.

This time, my rental vehicle was a Nissan Pathfinder. I loaded up and headed for the Leadville Hostel, stopping only in the town of Frisco to purchase supplies. Unfortunately, I spent a miserable first night there, slammed by a head cold that threatened to derail my entire trip. I could not get out of bed the next morning, and burned one of the two rest days I had planned for the three-week stay.

Not feeling much better after that second night, I headed out early the next day, driving an hour south to the old ghost town of Vicksburg, near where Van and I had ended our trip two years before because of deep snow. After pulling into the Missouri Gulch trailhead, I noticed that my right rear tire was flat. Furthermore, I could not for the life of me figure out how to lower the spare tire from its location under the vehicle. With daylight burning, I decided not to worry about it until I got back, even if it meant spending the night in the parking lot.

The climb was beautiful—at least what I remember of it. I made my way into the grassy basin of Missouri Gulch, surrounded by the three 14ers I hoped to bag that day—Missouri Mountain, Mount Oxford, and Mount Belford. The aspens were just beginning to hint at changing into their golden brilliance. I headed for the summit of Missouri first, but I could tell right away that something was wrong. My breathing was heavy and difficult, and, for the first time ever, I was feeling the adverse effects of altitude. This, I guessed, was due entirely to my cold, but I soldiered on, intent on my mission.

Climbing the ridge of Missouri, I met a hiker coming down who said he was also doing all three peaks that day, but I was about an hour or so behind him. After summiting, I returned to the basin and headed for Elkhead Pass, the broad, open bowl separating the three peaks. But even that relatively gradual slope was taxing. I left the trail and climbed directly up a grassy ridge to the saddle between Mounts Oxford and Belford. When I reached the ridgeline, I couldn't believe how far away the summit of Oxford appeared, but I met that same hiker returning across the ridge, and he assured me it wasn't that far.

After crossing over and back, I headed for the summit of Belford and signed the register; my thirty-seventh 14er was now in the books. By the time I got back to the car, I was completely wiped out. I'd covered 15 miles, with 7,400 feet of climbing. With thunder rumbling overhead, I envisioned a long, cold rest of the day trying to figure out how to change that flat tire.

A welcome sight greeted me when I got back to the parking lot: that hiker I had met was sitting next to my car in a lawn chair waiting for me. He had seen my flat tire, had seen my debilitated condition, and had been kind enough to stay and help me out. A grad student from Seattle named Sean, he said he had previously owned a Pathfinder and knew how to change the tire.

Turned out, even with the owner's manual I would never have figured out how to perfectly connect the jack's handle to a hidden notch beneath the car and to turn the handle until the spare tire descended. Even Sean had trouble, and he'd known how to do it. But, after lowering the spare, he quickly changed the tire. He planned to climb nearby Huron the next day, so I told him about the idyllic campsite Van and I had found two years before—the same one where 8 inches of snow had collapsed our tent roofs. And I thanked him profusely.

My destination was Aspen and the Maroon Bells, sick or no. But when I arrived at the Maroon Lakes just before dark, a foreboding scene greeted me. The Bells were covered with fresh snow and shrouded in rain clouds and an ominous sense of dread. A local climber just coming off the trail advised me against any foolhardy plans to continue, as more snow was forecast for overnight. My cold was now accompanied by a high fever, and it was all a bit overwhelming. I resigned myself to reality: I would have to put off the Bells for another year and probably would need to hire a guide to get me through them.

So I got in my car and drove back to the only place where I felt safe, even though it was an hour and a half away over a rugged 12,000-foot pass: the Leadville Hostel. I arrived at 10 P.M., and woke the owner, Bill Clower, who promptly helped me to the only bed he had left and told me not to get up in the morning. I had no problem with that.

I did not return to the living until the next afternoon, by which time I was feeling much better. But I had also lost another day of climbing, and with all the fresh snow on the mountains, it was appearing that this trip was going to be over before it really got started. That afternoon, I headed south to the artsy little river town of Salida, home to my friend Kari—whom I had met in Belize. She took me on a 5-mile mountain-bike ride around town, and I had trouble keeping up with her, as much because I was under the weather as because she was in remarkably good shape.

I spent much of the next day recovering; my only real accomplishment was getting a new tire at Big O to replace the one that had gone flat.

By then, I had given up all hope of completing the remaining 14ers on this trip. I still had seventeen peaks to climb and only twelve days remaining before my return flight on October 2. I did the math; it seemed impossible. But all I could do was keep climbing and keep my fingers crossed.

Culebra Peak is the southernmost 14er, but climbing it requires advance permission and a hundred-dollar bill. The mountain is on private land, and the owner charges climbers to gain access to the trailhead. Others have told me they have climbed Culebra from the south, sneaking onto the Cielo Vista Ranch's property undetected, but I had an additional dilemma. My arrival in Colorado would coincide with elk-hunting season, and the ranch's guests flocked to the mountain's gentle slopes after Labor Day. I could sneak in, but I didn't want to get shot.

I had started trying to untangle this knot earlier in the summer. I called the Cielo Vista Ranch and asked to speak to the owner, to see if he might make an exception. I was told that the owner, Mr. Hill, lived in Texas. I refused to accept that it was a dead end. I asked for the owner's email address, and composed a carefully written note about my plans and my request. It dawned on me that he was likely a churchgoer, and having recently become a steady attendee of Sunday services for the first time since I was a child, I explained my request and said I was praying that he would relent.

When he didn't reply, I pretty much put it out of my head.

But then, the night before I left for Colorado, a phone call interrupted my packing. I didn't recognize the area code, but the voice on the other end of the line had a thick Texan drawl.

He said my prayers had been answered.

Mr. Hill told me to arrive at his gate at 9 A.M. on Saturday, September 20, and that he would pull his elk hunters off the high ridges to allow me to climb Culebra.

Later, when I told a friend how I had prayed on Mr. Hill to change his mind, she said, "No, you *preyed* on Mr. Hill to change his mind!"

The peak's name means "harmless snake" in Spanish, and that pretty much describes the open, barren mountain, whose ridgeline snakes around in a long, broad semicircle to a benign summit. After paying the $100 at the ranch house, I drove to the four-wheel-drive trailhead at 11,700 feet and started climbing. I threw Gerry Roach's guidebook into my small daypack only as an afterthought, since I certainly wouldn't need it on this glorious day. With so little foot traffic across the private property, there is no defined trail on Culebra anyway, just wide, grassy slopes leading up to the ridgeline. Dozens of marmots stretched out sunning themselves on the warm, flat rocks, enjoying the last vestiges of summer. Even if I couldn't finish all the 14ers that trip, days like that one made every step worth it.

Upon reaching the summit, I was unable to log into the register book. The last person there apparently had failed to tightly screw on the lid to the cylinder, and rain had turned all the pages to mush. I could see a couple of other high peaks nearby, so I reached for Roach's "bible" to identify them. To my horror, I had failed to zip the side pouch on my pack and the book was gone, having apparently fallen out at some point during the ascent. Since I had not followed a trail, I could only guess as to my path up the grassy slopes, and tried to return the same way, but did not see the book anywhere.

Then, just before reaching my vehicle, there it was on the side of the road. Crisis averted. My trip would have come to a standstill without it, and, being a Saturday, I might not have secured another copy until Monday, if then. But fate had cut me a break.

I spent much of the climb working out scenarios in my head, and convinced myself that if everything went as planned the remainder of the trip, I just might be able to complete the 14ers on this visit after all, though that would mean finishing on the dreaded Maroon Bells and having to attempt their deadly traverse. Not a comforting thought.

With renewed hope, I left Culebra and drove the 150 miles to the South Colony Lakes trailhead, where I had been snowed out the year before on my attempt to summit the Crestones. Of course, these two peaks would be no picnic either. The routes up Crestone Peak and Crestone Needle were listed as Class 4, and the traverse between the two is another of the four great 14er traverses in Roach's book. I had planned to climb each one individually, however, to avoid the dangerous traverse, since I again would be climbing solo. It wouldn't take any longer, I figured, to climb them separately, as the traverse would have been a time-consuming and unnecessarily dangerous proposition.

Cold rain and sleet greeted me at South Colony Lakes, and I set up my tent in the same spot as I had the year before, tucked in the shadow of Broken Hand Pass, which I would have to climb in the morning to reach the Crestones. But, unlike last year, I was here on a Saturday, and I expected there would be other hikers on the trail. Knowing I wouldn't be alone if anything serious happened was comforting.

I slept through my predawn alarm and got a late start over Broken Hand Pass in the morning. Crossing the pass, I descended into the valley on the other side and the turnoff for Crestone Peak, considered the harder of the two. Some call it the hardest of all the 14ers. At one point in its history, it had been deemed unclimbable. In fact, the Crestones were the last Colorado 14ers to be conquered. Crestone Peak withstood all efforts to be tamed until 1916 when a party from Colorado Springs that included a woman, Eleanor Davis—who would later be known as the most experienced female American climber of her generation—successfully summited both peaks in one day, after having been the first to conquer nearby Kit Carson a few days before.

As I started up Crestone Peak, low-hanging clouds descended all the way to the valley floor, mist was heavy in the air, and visibility was only a few feet. Before long I met two other hikers who said they were bailing because of icy conditions higher up, but that another couple had continued on above them. Following Roach's instructions, I stayed out of the gully in front of me and climbed to the right of it up a Class 3 ridge that should have taken me to the "red notch" just below the summit. But, with virtually zero visibility, I must have strayed off course. The next thing I knew, I was on an ice-encrusted ridge crest peering off into nothingness.

I was in a precarious position. Rime coated the rocks around me, and when I looked at my jacket, I was covered in ice as well. I could not see the summit, which I guessed was off to my left, but only some steep spires that jutted menacingly into the milky obliqueness that surrounded me. It took some careful downclimbing to safely extricate myself from my predicament. I was still considerably shaken when I returned to the safety of the valley floor, accepting that I would not be making another attempt at the summit in these conditions. Just as I reached the bottom, I rounded a corner and almost walked into two hikers standing under the protection of an overhanging rock and removing some wet layers of clothing. I immediately took them as being the couple the other two hikers had told me about.

Sure enough, the husband-and-wife team, Tom and Sandi Yukman from Colorado Springs, had just descended from the red gully after a successful summit. Pressing them for details, they said I should have stayed in the gully all the way to the notch; from there, the summit was just a short scramble up to the left. Feeling that another summit bid in these conditions was too dangerous, I dejectedly started to hike out with them back over Broken Hand Pass, explaining my quest along the way and how I would now surely have to come back again the next year to complete the list.

When we got to the top of the pass, they invited me to join them for the climb up Crestone Needle, but I declined. I had already resigned myself to having to come back another time to climb Crestone Peak; what difference would it make? But, thankfully, they talked me out of my funk.

The exhilarating climb with newfound friends turned the day around. For one thing, it was great not having to climb such an exposed route alone, though the clouds prevented us from seeing our airy perch. But the weather also cleared on the descent. When we reached Broken Hand Pass again, Tom pointed out that it was still only 1 P.M., giving me plenty of time to go back and retry Crestone Peak. This time, I stayed in the red gully all the way to the notch and was on the summit at 2:18 P.M. Tom and Sandi had saved my vacation.

I was back at my car by 4:30 P.M. to find Tom's business card on my windshield. I emailed them later and said that if I ever saw them again, I owed them dinner for saving me a return trip to Colorado—well, assuming I survived the Bells, that is.

Driving out, I met only one car. As we passed each other on the narrow road, I must have rolled over a sharp rock, because I punctured another tire. At least this time the spare was in the back, as I had not resecured it under the vehicle, and it took me only 20 minutes to change. It did, however, mean a return trip to Salida to get another new tire from the guys at Big O.

Then, it was off on US 50 over Monarch Pass to head for the San Juans, considered by just about everyone to be the most spectacular range in all of Colorado. My indoctrination began with an uneventful 12-mile slog on remote San Luis Peak, perhaps the least-visited 14er. This toothless peak did nothing to bolster the range's reputation as the finest in Colorado, but that all changed a few hours later, the moment I drove my rental car over the crest of Slumgullion Pass.

Unfolding before me was one of the most spectacular vistas I had ever seen. Rising majestically in front of me was the profile of Uncompahgre Peak, the top of which—at least from this angle—appeared oddly misshapen, with dramatic, blocky angles protruding skyward, making its summit look entirely inaccessible. Below Uncompahgre lay a beautiful alpine valley and the town of Lake City, which sounded like it was something out of a storybook.

All I had ever known about Lake City came from reading Peter Jenkins's book *The Walk West*, in which he raved about Lake City like no other town he walked through during his five-year cross-country trek in the '70s. When Jenkins crested Slumgullion Pass as the winter of 1977 approached, he too had been taken aback by its unparalleled beauty. "The mountains were as jagged and sharp as shark's teeth," was how Jenkins described Uncompaghre and the other 14ers rising majestically in the distance. "This was the first time in my life that I ever had my breath taken away by a turn in the road."

I found Lake City to be one of the more charming towns I had ever seen. Most of the houses dated to the late 1800s, when this was a bustling little mining town, but all seemed to be in excellent condition and freshly painted, telling me the 375 residents were quite proud of their little "city" by the lake.

Turning onto Second Avenue, I headed west toward the Matterhorn Creek trailhead to camp for the night. Another camper was already there, and his dog—a pretty little Australian shepherd with a cropped tail—came over to visit while I set up my tent down near the creek. I always tried to camp as close to running water as possible; not only did the white noise help lull me to sleep, but, I told myself, it would also block out the sounds made by any animals in the vicinity. If there was a mountain lion or a black bear stalking my tent site in the middle of the night, I didn't want to know about it.

After setting up camp, I walked the dog back over to the other tent, but that was just a ready excuse, since the camper had a roaring fire going that was overly inviting. He was sitting by the fire strumming his guitar, and I brought him a cold beer to break the ice. His name was Steve Till, he lived in Flagstaff, Arizona, and Pepper was his best friend. We both planned to climb Uncompahgre and Wetterhorn peaks in the morning, so we immediately decided to team up.

It turned out that Steve, who was 28, was a pretty interesting guy. For starters, he got *paid* for rafting through the Grand Canyon. A botanist, Steve tracked the plant life in the world's most famous ditch for the National Park Service.

"I know I've got the greatest job in the world," Steve told me. "It's pretty amazing."

He'd grown up near the Mexican border in Sierra Vista, Arizona, and when he graduated high school not knowing what he wanted to do with his life, had enrolled at Northern Arizona University in Flagstaff. But, he said, he soon found the classroom lectures boring. One day, staring out the window while daydreaming, he noticed another class doing fieldwork.

"I found out it was a class called the Native Plants of Arizona, which was an entirely outside class," Steve said. "Walking and hiking outdoors, that was for me." When he learned class members were going on a ten-day float trip down the Colorado River to remove nonnative tamarisk trees from the Grand Canyon, he told instructors he was available to join them, even though he knew he would have to blow off nearly two weeks of classes to do so.

But even though that eventually led to a degree in botany, he never expected it to amount to a career. All his volunteering for river and backpacking trips into the Grand Canyon led to his job and has allowed him to live a life many only dream of. For several years, he lived in his Chinook motor home, just traveling from job to job.

"I get paid by the National Park Service," he said, "but I don't even have a job title." One of his more recent jobs in the Grand Canyon was the removal of a nonnative species of trout from the Colorado River. The fish are "electro-shocked," he explained, using an apparatus that looks like something out of *Ghostbusters*. "We stun them and then scoop them up with a net," Steve said. "It's mandated that every fish we remove has to be consumed, so we give them to backpackers to eat, and the rest are packed in freezers and we fly them out.

"My friends all want to know what they have to do to get in on this," Steve said with a laugh. I did too.

"I'm getting paid to exercise and breathe fresh air," he went on. "It doesn't seem like work. It's always fun."

And sometimes dangerous. The month before, Steve had been with five friends exploring Surprise Canyon, located on the north side of the Grand Canyon's western end. One of them was somewhere downstream doing work in another side canyon.

"It was a vegetation-mapping trip," Steve said, "and we were in Twin Spring Canyon, which is a split from upper Surprise Canyon. It started raining steadily and we saw big clouds dumping on Mount Dellenbaugh to our north. At first, we were not alarmed."

But soon a second storm moved in from the southwest, merging with the storm already upon them. "It started raining really hard, and there was thunder and lightning all around us," Steve recalled. "We took shelter on a little overhang high above the creek. We weren't necessarily anticipating a flash flood; that was just an obvious spot out of the elements. The lightning was crashing all around us, so we spaced out about 20 feet apart so we wouldn't all get hit at once. It was terrifying."

Then they heard it.

"Finally, we heard a roar that sounded like the wind and got louder and steadier and then it came around the corner." A flash flood was upon them, and they were only 10 feet above creek level in a spot where the canyon was barely 50 feet wide.

"We just grabbed our stuff and started scrambling," Steve said. "A wall of water and mud came shooting at us, and if it had been any higher, we would've been caught. The water stayed that high for 7 hours."

As it was, they were lucky they were in a relatively safe place. They had been headed back to their campsite downstream, which would have taken them through a narrow slot canyon. "If we had been in the Narrows, we would have been absolutely dead."

Still, they knew they were in for a long, cold night in wet clothes, and they did not know the fate of the final member of their party, Glen. They feared the worst. "We thought he was dead," Steve said. "It wasn't until the next morning, when we were about to head out, that he walked into camp. We were all pretty lucky.

"It was one of the scariest, yet exciting, experiences I've ever had," he went on. "It was really thrilling."

It was a pristine autumn morning when we set out the next day on the trail, which led across a broad, grassy basin underneath Matterhorn Peak, a 12,000-footer separating Uncompahgre and Wetterhorn peaks.

Approaching Uncompahgre, we climbed straight up a scree slope to the ridgeline and then headed directly for the summit. The climbing was not as difficult as it had appeared it might be from my vantage point at Slumgullion Pass the day before. At the top, the main feature was the 700-foot cliff on the north face, one of the most dramatic reliefs on any 14er. Peering over the edge was enough to make my knees buckle, but not so for Pepper: she stood on the edge, and when Steve called her back, she leapt over a gap in the rocks as if it were nothing.

Heading for Wetterhorn, we contoured across the open slopes and a big boulder field underneath Matterhorn Peak and climbed up a grassy ridge to rejoin the path at ridgeline. Then, the real fun began. This trail was steep and true, leading around to the backside of the cliff to our right, ending at a huge, flat rock just below the summit.

In front of us was a 200-foot, nearly vertical wall that appeared to have perfectly placed hand- and footholds all the way to the top. But it was too steep for Pepper, who had shown incredible climbing prowess throughout the day. Instead of leaving her there, Steve emptied his backpack and carefully placed the 30-pound dog inside, cinching the drawstring so that just her head protruded. Incredibly, she remained perfectly still while Steve scrambled up the cliff face to the summit. I filmed the ascent with my camera and then followed, and we enjoyed lunch on the tiny, flat summit. It was the most gorgeous day of the trip.

It was tough saying goodbye to my new friend upon returning to Lake City, but Steve and I agreed to stay in touch. Steve and Pepper headed for Gunnison for some more climbing, while I continued on the road to Cinnamon Pass, where three more 14ers awaited me the following day.

The next morning, I made quick work of Redcloud and Sunshine peaks, two of the easiest 14ers. Then, I drove up the road to American Basin for an afternoon ascent of Handies Peak. I laced up my running shoes, summited, and completed this round-trip in less than 2 hours.

I was particularly excited about the next leg of my journey, which would include a train ride out of the historical mining town of Silverton. Who doesn't like a train ride? But after crossing over 12,640-foot Cinnamon Pass and descending into Silverton, itself situated at 9,300 feet, I was informed that the next train wasn't leaving until 2:45 the following afternoon. That gave me plenty of time, I reckoned, to drive to Ouray and climb Mount Sneffels the next morning.

The drive to Ouray is quintessential Colorado. There, US 550 goes over 11,000-foot Red Mountain Pass and is known as the "Million Dollar Highway" because it reportedly cost a million dollars per mile to complete in 1924. The 12-mile section from the top of Red Mountain Pass to the picture-postcard town of Ouray descends through the Uncompahgre Gorge and is perhaps the most stunning road in America, marked by sharp hairpin turns, sheer cliffs, and a conspicuous lack of guardrails. From the air, the road must resemble a piece of ribbon candy; it has more twists and turns than a Tom Clancy novel.

You won't find a more picturesque mountain town anywhere in the United States than Ouray, called the "Switzerland of America" by locals as it sits at the head of a narrow valley with steep mountains rising dramatically on three sides. Main Street in its entirety is a National Historic District. Once a wild and lawless mining town, Ouray has been a tourist mecca, especially in winter, since an ice-climbing park opened there twenty years ago, spawning an ice festival that attracts thousands each year.

My interest, however, was in Mount Sneffels, just one of the jagged mountains that rose precipitously above town. A steep, rutted dirt road—at times literally carved out of the cliff face—leads out of Ouray and climbs to Yankee Boy Basin at 10,700 feet, which I followed until it became impassable. I pitched my tent for the night underneath a sign that read, "No Camping Allowed," correctly presuming that no one else would be around.

Sneffels provided some of the finest climbing I had yet experienced. The trail led directly to the saddle between Sneffels and its smaller neighbor, Kismet. I then ascended a steep couloir reaching just below the top, where I had to lift myself through a crack in the rocks to gain access to the summit. The peak marked number forty-eight on my list; only six more to go.

Driving out of Yankee Boy Basin, I heard an all-too-familiar hissing sound coming from a rear tire, and knew it would soon be flat. I had to drive a considerable distance before I could find a spot that was flat enough for me to safely change the tire—on one of the hairpin turns. Even so, I worried about the vehicle sliding off the jack, which would have left me stranded and caused me to miss my train. But, it being my third flat tire of the trip, I was getting pretty good at the game. It took me only 10 minutes to change it this time, and I was soon on my way back over the pass to Silverton.

Arriving in town, I stopped to gas up and asked the attendant where I could get a tire fixed.

"Right out back," he said. "I own the company." What luck.

I left the tire with him and told him I would return in a few days to pick it up. I had a train to catch.

The Durango & Silverton Narrow Gauge Railroad is one of a kind. Built in 1882 to travel the Animas River gorge—which had proved too narrow for a standard-width track—the line hauled both tourists and more than $300 million of gold and silver over its history. The train has been in continuous operation ever since, and still uses the same steam locomotives that covered the 45.4-mile route in the 1920s. The only gold seen on the route today is the foliage of the brilliant aspen trees that line the banks of the Animas River.

My destination was desolate Needleton Station, where the train stops in the middle of nowhere to drop off hikers headed for some of the remote peaks of the San Juans. I was headed to Chicago Basin, where four more 14ers awaited my assault. I did not disembark until almost 4 P.M., and still had a 3,000-foot climb over 6 miles to reach the basin and my campsite. I double-timed it to beat the onset of darkness, arriving just in time to set up camp on the only flat spot I could find, as fellow hikers had already grabbed all the prime locations.

They had all just climbed one or more of the three ranked 14ers in the basin directly above us—Mount Eolus, Sunlight Peak, and Windom Peak. I intended to climb all of them, along with unranked 14er North Eolus, the next day so long as the weather cooperated. The best news: I heard that mountain goats were running all over the basin. The hikers reported that the shaggy, white critters were practically following them around like puppies. I felt certain I would finally get to see my first mountain goat in Colorado.

In the morning, I climbed into the basin to reach Twin Lakes, where a view of my day was laid out before me. Eolus rose abruptly to my left and was much more intimidating than I had anticipated. Sunlight, which sports one of the scariest summits of any 14er, was across the basin directly in front of me.

To my right was open, exposed Windom Peak, which I would save for last—despite it being the season for afternoon thunderstorms.

The crux of the climb to the summit of Eolus was a narrow path called The Catwalk, which Roach described as a 2-foot-wide ridge with sharp dropoffs on both sides. He was exaggerating a bit, I found, as the ridge was at least 6 feet wide. But, true to his word, the rest of the climb was classic Class 3 scrambling with plenty of exposure. It was a stomach-curdling type of climb. I gained the airy summit with much relief, but realized that I was going to have to retrace my steps and turn around in order to cross over and bag North Eolus. It may not have qualified as a true 14er by virtue of it not meeting the 300-foot standard, but it was over 14,000 feet nonetheless and since I was right there, I figured I might as well tag it too.

I returned to the basin, then headed for Sunlight, which Roach warned would also feature some hairy climbing. A 30-foot-high block of granite rests precariously on the summit, and Roach called the final move to gain this block the hardest move on any 14er in Colorado. It required a leap of faith as I stepped across an exposed gap and pulled myself up onto the rounded summit block. I did not find it particularly difficult, but, then again, I am 6-foot-1. While the step across the open chasm was intrepid, I would not have fallen too far had I slipped. Just far enough to break my leg, not kill me. Of course, considering how far I would have been from help, I probably would have preferred a quick death.

Returning quickly to the valley floor, I turned my attention to Windom Peak, the tamest of the three. But from the basin, I saw dark clouds moving in, so I knew I had to hurry. Forgoing the search for a trail, I simply scrambled up to the saddle between the summit and a nub called Peak 18. By the time I reached Windom Peak's summit, however, thunder rumbled and rain approached from the west.

Hustling off the summit back to the relative safety of the basin, I arrived back at an empty camp just as it started to rain. Only then did it dawn on me: I had not seen a single mountain goat all day. Denied again.

One consequence of the long day was that my cell phone died, and with it my only clock—I wasn't carrying a watch, as I have never owned one. So, when I awoke the next morning, I was unsure of what time it was, since all the other campers in this glade appeared to have left the day before. I knew the train arrived back at Needleton Station at 11:30 A.M. Not taking any chances, I packed up quickly and hit the trail. I arrived at the tracks to find two elk hunters also waiting for the train and they informed me that it was only 10:07. We sat and waited together as it began to rain again and, impressed by my quest, they announced that lunch was on them when we arrived back in Silverton.

The only 14ers remaining in the San Juans were the Wilson Group—

Mount Wilson, Wilson Peak, and unranked El Diente—west of Telluride, so that's where I headed next after picking up my tire at the gas station. When I reached the trailhead, I had just enough daylight left to hike the 5 rugged miles in to Navajo Lake. Two other hikers had set up camp near its outlet and I asked to join them. But they said they were just packing up for the hike out, having failed in an attempt to summit Mount Wilson earlier that day. Not because of all the snow they said they encountered, but rather because of a menacing lightning storm that forced them to abandon their quest just 50 feet shy of the summit.

They quickly left, and I was alone again. I cooked dinner in the dark, listening to rockfall off the slopes of El Diente behind me and looking at the thousands of stars. The clear night indicated that the weather the next day might not hamper my plans, as it had for the two other climbers.

The next morning, it was a grind to hit the trail. Having climbed fourteen peaks in the previous seven days, my legs were extremely tired. I was headed to the ridgeline leading past the old Rock of Ages Mine to the upper slopes of Wilson Peak. Just below the summit, I came to a spot referred to as "the crack" in Roach's book, and thought for a moment I would not be able to continue. Here, I had to downclimb around a large buttress and skirt around an exposed edge before climbing back to the summit ridge. This chute was full of fresh snow, and I feared sliding off the edge into the abyss. But the snow was firm, and negotiating the corner was easier than I expected. Soon I was on the summit, but I didn't linger. I could already see storm clouds approaching, and I still had two summits to go.

After returning to the ridgeline, I traversed underneath the shadow of Gladstone Peak—a Centennial 13er—and was headed for the slopes of Mount Wilson when graupel—what I call popcorn snow, little pellets of snow that aren't quite like ice, so they couldn't be called hail—began to fall more heavily. I thought it might just be a passing squall because patches of blue sky darted in and out of the dark gray clouds that had gathered around me.

But then it came out of nowhere, as lightning so often does. The brilliant flash illuminated everything around me, so close I could feel my heart flutter momentarily as the electricity seemed to pulsate through my body. Before I could even realize what had happened, the thunder exploded with such force it nearly knocked me off my feet, reverberating off the walls of the peaks surrounding me.

I froze in my tracks, momentarily unable to gather my jumbled thoughts. Quickly regaining my senses, I dived under the cover of an overhanging rock for what little protection it afforded.

Then I smelled it. The air reeked of a foul, burning sensation, similar to that of burning hair. It was noxious. I imagined it was the smell of death lingering in the air, and I cowered in my rock recess waiting for the end to come. But, eerily, all was quiet.

Around me, the snow got heavier, the clouds got darker, and the tension mounted, but there was no more lightning and no more deafening thunder. Perhaps it had been a one-time aberration.

I stayed motionless in my little tomb for what seemed like an eternity, but it was probably closer to half an hour. Finally, believing the danger had passed, I dared venture forth, and—cautiously—regained my feet in hopes of continuing my climb.

The moment I stood up, however, I was driven back into my refuge by a second flash of lightning and an instantaneous eruption of calamitous thunder, as if the storm had been lying in wait for me, like some demonic beast poised to spring its diabolical trap.

That was enough for me. I got up and ran off the slope back to the valley floor a few hundred feet below. Once I felt safer, I slowed to a defeated shuffle as I made my way back to my tent on the shores of nearby Navajo Lake. The snow changed to rain as I descended about a thousand feet. I was shivering from the cold as I crawled into my tent and dived into my warm sleeping bag. There was nothing to do now other than get some much-needed sleep. Later, I learned that the awful stench in the air that was reminiscent of burnt hair was actually the smell of the ozone burning.

I spent much of that afternoon huddled in my sleeping bag as wind and rain whipped the sides of my tent. But eventually the storm subsided, and I emerged from my cocoon. There was nothing to do now but wait for morning so I could take another stab at Mount Wilson. Thankfully, I had not had any similar delays since the Crestones. And thanks to my ambitious schedule, I even had an extra day in case I decided against the traverse of the Maroon Bells—the only peaks that would remain after I conquered Wilson.

The inside of my tent smelled horribly after all these days, and so did my gear, especially my socks and boots. I washed my feet in the lake, despite the ice-cold water. My feet were so foul, I was certain that if there were any fish in the lake, they would soon be floating on the surface.

It took about an hour the next morning to regain the thousand feet on Mount Wilson to the spot where lightning had ended my climb the day before. I was not on a trail, and the climbing was difficult through ever-deepening snow as I ascended the ridge. I had to stop about every 10 feet to catch my breath in the thin alpine air. Eventually, I topped out at a little walkway that led me out to a sheer cliff and the final 150 feet to the summit. I was about to find out what true mountaineering is all about: overcoming fear.

After climbing over an extremely exposed ridge crest and then downclimbing the other side, I reached a 50-foot vertical wall leading directly to the summit above, the same spot where the other two climbers had been turned back two days before. This wall had plenty of small, half-inch-wide hand- and footholds, but, being north-facing, the holds were all chocked full of ice and snow. Directly below was a drop of more than 2,000 feet. My insides curled in on themselves.

Taking my time, I slowly climbed up the cliff face to the summit. At the top, I was incredibly relieved. I'd just completed the most dangerous climbing I'd yet experienced. Then it dawned on me: I still had to get down! This proved even riskier, since I had to feel around clumsily with my boots for each foothold below me, not wanting to look down at the expanse of open air between my legs.

Safely back on level ground, I let out a huge sigh of relief as I peered out toward El Diente. The traverse there was as rugged-looking as the name implied—El Diente means "the tooth" in Spanish—and the many spires looming ahead of me did appear to be the fangs of some vicious beast lying in wait. Roach calls this crossing another of the four great 14er traverses, but I didn't figure it could be any worse than what I had just done.

In fact, I thought the climbing was easier than before. When I reached a 60-foot cliff that the book said to avoid by climbing around on one side or the other, I decided it looked safer to simply go straight over the top.

Gaining the well-guarded summit, I signed into the register book, which no one had signed in the past eight days. I could understand why: the day had required what were undoubtedly my greatest mountaineering feats yet and El Diente hadn't been a ranked 14er.

Only the Maroon Bells were left on my list of Colorado 14ers, and I was confident that I would be able to "ring" both Bells the next day. Even though I still had two days before my flight home, I was determined to complete the dreaded traverse and finish my quest the following day. And to do it without a guide, which now seemed unnecessary after my string of successes.

Coming down from El Diente proved no simple task, as it took conscious effort to safely retrace my steps until I was standing at the top of a dauntingly steep, snow-packed gully leading to the valley floor 2,000 feet below. Descending the 60-degree slope, however, felt more like going down a flight of stairs with crampons. Small avalanches helped carry me along. Fifteen minutes later I was at the bottom, and I was back in camp by 1 P.M. and at the car a couple of hours later.

I must have broken some speed records driving from the trailhead, located near the tiny town of Rico, to Aspen. It took me only 5.5 hours to cover nearly 300 miles, much of it on back roads. It was nearly 9 P.M. when I set up camp under a blanket of brilliant stars.

When I arrived at the Maroon Lakes shortly before sunrise the next morning, I thought a convention was going on. The parking lot was full. Not of hikers heading out to climb the Maroon Bells, but rather, of photographers there to shoot the iconic peaks. A continuous line of cameras on tripods stood sentinel on the shore of the lake waiting for the first rays of light to illuminate the red rocks that give the Bells their colorful name. Not one of them noticed as I headed for the trail, as all eyes were on the slopes that were about to reward them for their patience.

My plan was to climb the unranked North Maroon first, then to tackle the traverse from north to south, which I believed safer based on trip reports I had read. I found that the climbing from the base of North Maroon was relatively straightforward, not at all sketchy and exposed as it had looked from a distance. Near the summit, the trail moved around to the north side of the mountain, plunging me into shadows and thigh-deep snow. Before long, I topped out and returned to the brilliant autumn sunshine. I'd conquered the first Bell.

Nothing that lay ahead would be so routine. Looking out over the traverse toward the summit of South Maroon, I saw large spires jutting skyward that blocked the crossing and would require careful negotiation. As I progressed, I tried to pick a line where if I fell, I would tumble only 10 or 20 feet, not the entire 3,000 feet to the valley floor, as more than a few unlucky climbers have done. Twice, I came upon 4- or 5-foot gaps where I could see that most people had downclimbed on either side to get around, but that looked riskier than simply jumping them. Both times I tossed my backpack across the expanse, prayed that the rock on the other side was solid, and then leapt over a hundred-foot drop. Both times I got lucky.

As I neared the final saddle between the two peaks, my heart skipped a beat. I looked again to make sure I wasn't hallucinating.

Lying in the snow directly above me was a lone mountain goat, the first I had seen in three years of climbing 14ers. Ducking down, I carefully crossed underneath the ledge and climbed up a small snowfield on the west side of the ridge, hoping to poke up close enough to get a picture. The goat was too smart for me, though, and was long gone by the time I surfaced a few minutes later. I did not see it again. But I was gratified nonetheless.

Much of the rest of the climb to the summit stayed on the northwest side, meaning I had to deal with a lot of snow. But soon I was safely on the summit and had completed my fifty-fourth and final Colorado 14er.

Any celebrating had to wait until I got myself off the deadly peak. The two smaller summits ahead along the ridge posed plenty of sketchy climbing to navigate, but I finally found myself on familiar ground: the same tiny saddle from which the hailstorm had driven me the year before. It was a long, dreary descent of nearly 3,000 feet to the valley floor, and I was considerably tired when I finally got back to the car at 5 P.M. The photographers were long gone.

While there is an overwhelming feeling of euphoria when finally completing a list such as the Colorado 14ers, there is also a bit of sadness in realizing that the quest is over. I was in a bit of a conundrum about what to do the next day, the final day of my trip, without any more 14ers to climb.

Well, actually, there *was* one more: Conundrum, another unofficial 14er located opposite Castle Peak in the same Montezuma Basin where I had nearly killed Van with that dislodged rock the year before. Conundrum, at 14,060 feet, is high enough to be ranked, but its saddle with neighboring Castle Peak is too short to qualify. Still, climbing Conundrum would give me all fifty-nine Colorado 14ers, if you include the five unofficial ones.

I was more excited about the challenge of driving all the way to Montezuma Basin, something I had failed to accomplish in the Toyota Highlander the year before. But the Nissan Pathfinder performed brilliantly, as I bottomed out only once, and the climb itself proved to be a lark.

Just as I got back to the Leadville Hostel for my final night in Colorado, I got a call from Kari, checking in to see if I was okay and still in Colorado. Turned out, she was in Leadville herself, and we enjoyed dinner together with one of her friends that night.

The next day I found a car wash and spent a couple of hours erasing all evidence of the previous three weeks. When I returned the car to Enterprise the next morning, I was asked if I had had any problems.

I said, "Well, I did get a flat tire...."

"Oh, I'm sorry," said the agent, apologetically. "Let me take a day off your bill."

It was all I could do to suppress a laugh as I wondered whether I should mention the other two flats. I decided I should keep that to myself.

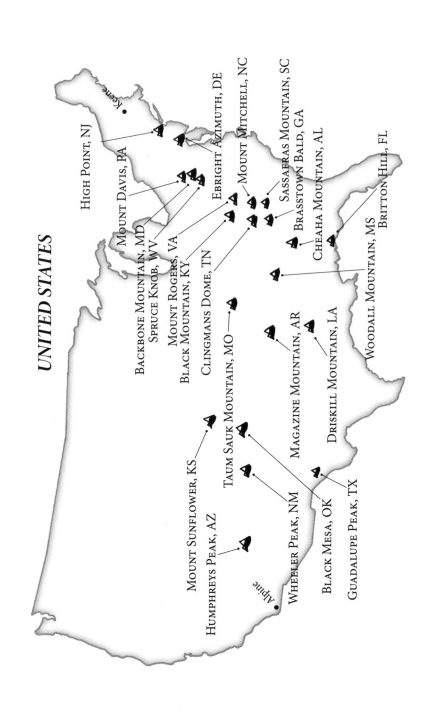

UNITED STATES

- High Point, NJ
- Keene
- Ebright Azimuth, DE
- Mount Mitchell, NC
- Sassafras Mountain, SC
- Brasstown Bald, GA
- Cheaha Mountain, AL
- Britton Hill, FL
- Mount Davis, PA
- Backbone Mountain, MD
- Spruce Knob, WV
- Mount Rogers, VA
- Black Mountain, KY
- Clingmans Dome, TN
- Woodall Mountain, MS
- Taum Sauk Mountain, MO
- Magazine Mountain, AR
- Driskill Mountain, LA
- Mount Sunflower, KS
- Wheeler Peak, NM
- Black Mesa, OK
- Guadalupe Peak, TX
- Humphreys Peak, AZ
- Alpine

Chapter 8
January 2009

THE THE
GREAT
HIGHPOINT
ADVENTURE
BEGINS

I HAD PLANNED TO SPEND THE FIRST THREE MONTHS OF 2009 IN CUENCA, Ecuador, immersed in a Spanish-language school, training for the Massanutten Mountain Trails 100-miler in May and climbing as many of the high volcanoes as I could. By the time I had left for Colorado in 2008, I had already contacted a mountaineering club and a Spanish-language school there. All my plans were set to go south for the winter.

But the economy went south instead. When the economy collapsed in the fall of 2008, UPS had proved susceptible to the downturn. As I was not a full-time driver, I was the first one laid off each day, and as Christmas came and went, I had worked just eight days over the final three months of the year. Without money in the bank, I had to call off the trip to Ecuador, and set about looking for other adventures closer to home.

That's when my brother, Bryon, invited me to come back to California to visit him for a while. He'd been researching that Campo gunfight that he and his Wild West team had been reenacting all those years and asked me to ghostwrite about it. He even offered to buy my plane ticket. But I quickly decided that I would drive instead. Along the way, I would visit as many state highpoints as I could, taking a southerly route on the way out and a northerly route on the way back later in the spring. I had always wanted to take a cross-country road trip, and since the price of gas had recently dipped to a low of $1.75 a gallon, I figured there might not ever be a better time.

Having previously climbed the highpoints of all six New England states, I had no need to climb them again on this trip. I had also climbed Mount Elbert on my 2006 trip to Colorado. Other peaks would be snowbound and would have to wait for future trips. The access road to Kings Peak in Utah's Uintas Wilderness would be closed until well after I'd passed through because of snow. Glacier-capped Gannett Peak, located deep in the Wind River Range of western Wyoming, is a serious mountain and not one lightly tackled in March. Oregon, Washington, Idaho, and Montana would have to wait for the same reason. That left thirty-four state highpoints to bag over the next three months.

It would be quite a hodgepodge of summits. Many were drive-ups, such as Delaware's, which is on a city street corner, one of several highpoints in the Southeast that can be "summited" without getting out of your car. Many of those would be a piece of cake. Others, such as Mount Whitney in California— the highest point in the contiguous United States—would require a veritable expedition. Checking a list of completers on the highpointers.org website, there were roughly 350 people who had finished the Lower 48 state highpoints.

Loading up my Volkswagen Passat, I left New Hampshire on January 12 and headed for the highest point in New Jersey, which, coincidentally, is called High Point, located in Sussex County, in the northwestern corner of the state. There is a huge obelisk monument on the top of High Point—it resembles the Washington Monument, but at only 220 feet tall is less than half its height. I arrived at the parking lot at the visitor center to find that a winter storm had coated the summit with a thick layer of ice, with long icicles hanging from all the signs. I cautiously hiked the mile and a half to the monument and back. One highpoint down.

The following day, I visited the Delaware state highpoint—Elbright Azimuth— which is on a street corner in suburban Wilmington and sits at 448 feet above sea level. Only Florida has a lower highpoint. I then headed for Cumberland Gap in Maryland, turning north into Pennsylvania as I drove through Amish country to reach Mount Davis, where a young George Washington had once led troops during the French and Indian War. A relatively flat, snow-covered road led to a 53-foot-tall wooden observation tower that marked the summit. Like at the other two highpoints so far, I had the place to myself.

It was cold, dark, and snowing again by the time I drove back across the Maryland border and headed for the town of Oakland, where I planned to camp at a state park, despite the failing weather. When I arrived, however, the park was closed. The gate was open and the road led to the ranger's house, where the lights were on and smoke wafted from the chimney. I turned my headlights off and idled in, making sure I wasn't spotted. I parked next to a cabin and went around to a porch in the back, where I found a broom and swept off all the snow that had been accumulating. I set up my tent out of sight and tried to sleep, which became more difficult as the night went on and the temperature dipped to just 5 degrees Fahrenheit.

I was absolutely freezing when my alarm went off at 6:30 the next morning. I decided to linger in my sleeping bag, not wanting to brave the new day. By the time I crawled out of my tent 15 minutes later, the headlights of the ranger's pickup truck were on; he must have been warming it up. He pulled out and I was certain I was going to get caught. I envisioned a long, cold day of shoveling snow to pay off my fine for illegal camping. He apparently didn't spot my car and drove out another way. I scrambled to disassemble my tent and get out of there before he returned.

The short drive to Maryland's highpoint crossed through West Virginia, and I enjoyed a 1.25-mile ascent up a logging road in fresh, powdery snow to the summit of Backbone Mountain. A mailbox on a tree near the summit marker protected the full register book, and there were certificates in the box to commemorate a successful visit. I thought that was a nice touch.

Driving on to the West Virginia highpoint later that day, I turned onto the road to Spruce Knob to discover that the road had not been plowed. I parked and hiked the final 2 miles in a couple of inches of fresh snow to the highpoint, which, like Pennsylvania's, was marked by a wooden observation tower next to the parking lot.

I spent Martin Luther King Jr. weekend training for the Massanutten 100-miler by joining in on two organized runs on parts of the racecourse itself. The first day, the temperature stayed below zero all day, and the second day wasn't much warmer. In two days, we logged 55 miles, which was exhausting, especially considering I had been recently sidelined with a hamstring injury. But I knew it would be crucial reconnaissance for the race in May.

On Monday morning, I headed south again on I-81 to reach the Virginia state highpoint; Mount Rogers, at 5,729 feet, would be the highest one on the trip so far. Driving up into the gap where the Appalachian Trail crosses VA 600, it was snowing heavily on top of the 8 inches already on the ground from the night before. Hiking in on the AT, I was making fresh tracks in the virgin powder when I came upon a group of four hikers on their way out who said they had camped at Thomas Knob Shelter the night before. I followed their tracks all the way to the half-mile spur trail that leads to the summit of Mount Rogers, which proved pretty unspectacular; the trail led me to a small clearing with a stump in the middle, which seemed to mark the highpoint.

I returned to the small town of Chilhowie with just $30 in my pocket and attempted to rent a motel room that had been advertised as $45 a night. Since it appeared I would be the only one staying there that night, I felt the manager should have jumped at my offer, but he hemmed and hawed for a considerable time. Thankfully, he relented and took the deal. But, he said, if he saw me bringing a second person into the room, he would evict me immediately. I just laughed, wondering where I would find another person in this desolate town. Perhaps he thought I was going to conjure up a prostitute. (Coincidentally, the term "hooker" is said to have originated in Virginia, the result of prostitutes being brought into the Army camps by Joseph Hooker, a major general in the Union Army during the Civil War, whose camp in Falmouth, Virginia, was said to resemble a "saloon and a brothel.") But since I had already spent my last thirty bucks, the prospects seemed unlikely, even if I had been so inclined.

My destination the next morning was Kentucky, one of only two states east of the Mississippi that I'd never been to (Wisconsin being the other). After topping out in a pass that marked the Kentucky border, I promptly came to a side road that would lead me to the state highpoint. Black Mountain sits atop the Tennessee Valley Divide and an old coal mine, and is also home to an FAA Long Range Radar facility, as well as several other abandoned towers, one of which appeared to mark the summit. If there was a benchmark on the true summit, it was either lost or stolen, as I couldn't find it.

Arriving at Gatlinburg, Tennessee, later that afternoon, I was surprised to see the place lit up like the Vegas Strip, and even more surprised to learn that the road leading to the summit of Clingmans Dome was closed—more than a foot of snow had fallen in the last 24 hours. And more was on the way.

Park rangers at the Sugarlands Visitor Center in Great Smoky Mountains National Park told me that it might be days before the road reopened. I was more than a bit dismayed; I had a schedule to keep. I pleaded with the rangers to let me pass, but they told me the only way I was going to get up that road today was to hike it, which elicited hearty laughter from everyone in the room. Except me, that is.

Heading back to the parking lot, I packed up every shred of winter gear I had with me. Fortunately, I was well prepared, but most of the items I was stuffing into my pack were things I didn't expect to need until Mount Whitney in California, not here in Tennessee.

When I returned to the visitor center 20 minutes later to secure my permit, the rangers there were no longer laughing. They were worried. An older ranger advised me against this suicide march, telling me it was more than 17 miles to the Mount Collins Shelter, where I was required to camp for the night, and it would soon be dark. Undaunted, I ignored the warning, having hiked in far worse conditions in the White Mountains on many occasions. In hindsight, I probably should have listened.

Like all crazy adventures, this one had seemed like a good idea at the time. But looking back, I'm not so sure.

It was 3:40 P.M. when I started up the road to Newfound Gap just as snow began falling with more serious urgency. It was not a hard climb, as the road had been plowed earlier in the day.

But snow was swirling around me in a veritable blizzard, and the temperature had dropped below zero. I wasn't particularly worried about my situation, however, as I was properly dressed—except for a pair of thin, cotton gloves with holes in two of the fingers—and I had on a headlamp to pierce the tempest that confronted me. Darkness overtook me as I was still climbing the main road—TN 441—to Newfound Gap, where I knew I had to bear right at a fork to continue on toward the summit. Along this road, I was supposed to find a signpost directing me onto the Appalachian Trail and to the Mount Collins Shelter, located a short distance off the trail.

But turning on my headlamp, I discovered that I could see nothing! Nothing but blowing, swirling snow inches in front of my face. The light was utterly useless against this raging blizzard and I realized with a bit of apprehension that I was essentially blind. Suddenly, my very survival depended on me finding a solitary signpost in the middle of a complete whiteout. I swallowed hard as I considered my predicament.

Rather than admit defeat and follow my tracks back to the visitor center, I turned off my lamp and soldiered on, using the complete blackness of the treeline on either side of the road as my only reference points.

Finally, the road leveled and I figured that I had reached Newfound Gap. I needed to find Clingmans Dome Road, which branched to my right somewhere in the darkness. Continuing to use the treeline as my guide, I found the unplowed road. The ranger had told me that I'd find a parking lot on my left about halfway up this road, and a sign opposite it leading to the Appalachian Trail and the Mount Collins Shelter. But I doubted I would be able to see any of this and knew I ran the disastrous risk of walking right past this trail in the darkness. I feared being found sitting frozen in a snowbank, like Jack Nicholson in *The Shining*, a maniacal grin etched permanently on my face. I realized sometime later that it was probably the same mentality that my friend Kenny Holmes had held before he hiked off to his death in the White Mountains that fateful day in 2004.

I checked the time. It was 7:45. I had more than 3 miles to hike to the trail-head at the parking lot. I calculated that I could reach it in an hour, so I began trudging up the road.

I kept an eye on my phone and looked for the parking lot, but the blizzard had apparently swallowed it up. I started hiking closer to the left side of the road in hopes of seeing something—anything. I knew if I missed this turnoff, I would have no choice but to keep hiking or. . . .

I didn't want to think about the "or."

It was still snowing hard when I saw something on my left that looked like a human-made object, rather than another tree. I walked over to it and leaned close. It was a trail sign! I turned on my headlamp and could just make out the name of the trail. This was it! I knew the spur to the Appalachian Trail and the shelter would be directly across the road from this sign.

Once in the woods, and under the canopy of the trees, the whiteout abated, and I found I could use my headlamp. I almost immediately noticed fresh footsteps in the snow and followed them straight to the shelter, where I arrived at 9:40—6 hours after I had started—cold and hungry. Two college-aged brothers from Massachusetts, who were thru-hiking the AT, were already in the shelter trying to sleep, but were mostly shivering. They would tell me in the morning it was the coldest night they had spent since they had left Katahdin back in August.

Only dumb luck—or, as I called it, superb intuition—had enabled me to find the shelter in the raging blizzard.

My hands were almost useless as I pulled everything I could out of my pack and prepared for a long, cold night. The wind was whipping into the open side of the shelter and I could barely light my stove, but I had no choice. I was famished and extremely cold. After melting snow for my prepackaged meal, I pulled on every bit of clothing I had with me, topped by a thick, down jacket.

I wolfed down my dinner and climbed into my sleeping bag, having already stuffed my snow-covered boots into the bottom in hopes of drying them out. As I zipped myself in, though, I noticed something disconcerting. Two of the fingertips on my right hand—which had been exposed to the cold through the holes worn in my thin, cotton gloves—were frozen completely solid. My fingers felt like rocks.

Struggling back out of my bag, I somehow relit my stove and painfully thawed out the fingertips before they were entirely lost to frostbite. Thankfully, this worked, and I was soon inside my bag again. All the layers I had on were just enough to keep me toasty. In fact, my hands got so hot in the heavy mittens I had put on that they started to sweat and get cold, so I spent the night comfortably without any gloves on.

The next morning dawned clear and cold. Later, I was told it had dipped to 8 degrees below zero Fahrenheit on the summit that night, but with the brisk wind whipping into the enclosure, it had felt much colder. I pulled my boots out of the bottom of my sleeping bag to find that none of the snow that had bonded to them had melted. Not a smidgen.

The brothers had broken camp ahead of me, heading south toward Clingmans Dome, still nearly 4 miles away. I thought I would catch them, but they got to the summit—the highest point they would hit during their entire journey—and were back on the trail before I arrived, with just the final 199 miles to go before reaching the Appalachian Trail's terminus at Springer Mountain, Georgia.

Clingmans Dome, at 6,643 feet, may be one of the highest points east of the Mississippi, but there is still a road to the top. From a distance, the spiraling, cement observation tower that marks the summit looks like a flying saucer. Upon reaching it, I took out my camera, only to discover that the battery was dead. All this work and no pictures; who would believe I was ever there?

From the deck of the observation tower, the views were amazing on this perfectly still morning. The Great Smoky Mountains were indeed smoking, with mist seemingly rising from every valley from here to the horizon. The blue of the cloudless sky stood out in absolute brilliance against the pure-white mountaintops all covered in another 6 inches of immaculate, glistening fresh powder. It was one of the most pristine views I had ever seen, and worth every step of the dangerous trek the night before.

It was a long, unpleasant hike down the road through all the new-fallen snow. About halfway down Clingmans Dome Road, I came upon the trail sign that had saved me the night before, and saw no parking lot next to it. I had been in search of an illusion; I knew then that finding that sign by pure chance had probably saved my life.

When I got back to Newfound Gap, I felt much better, but I still had 13 miles to go to get back to the visitor center. The constant downhill turned into an excruciating ordeal. My feet were wet, and it became almost torturous to continue. I stopped twice to take my boots off, airing out my wrinkled feet and changing into a pair of socks that were only slightly drier.

With about 5 miles to go, I heard the sound of an engine somewhere down in the valley. A snowplow, perhaps? Could I speed up enough to get to it before it left for the day, as it was now getting to be late afternoon again?

Reaching a side road just as a snowplow was driving out, I was never so thankful to see someone in my life. I faked a limp to make sure the driver would stop; he let me throw my pack in the back and gave me a ride the final 4 miles to my car.

Then, I hobbled inside the visitor center and told the rangers my story. All they could do was shake their heads in wonder and be thankful they hadn't been called out to rescue me.

Tennessee now checked off my list, I got into my car and headed for North Carolina and Mount Mitchell, stopping at the first hotel I could find in Gatlinburg. After having spent a surprisingly comfortable night in below-zero temperatures on top of the mountain the night before, I went out to eat at a local Applebee's and, as I was sitting at the bar, I started shivering uncontrollably. Maybe it was just the events of the previous 24 hours catching up to me.

Especially sore the next day, I looked forward to drive-up summits in North Carolina, South Carolina, and Georgia, all of which I had hoped to get that day. Coming over the top of a pass on I-40 just inside the North Carolina border, I got caught daydreaming and did not see the speed limit sign where it dropped to 55 MPH. Clocked at 70, I was handed a $151 ticket by a state trooper who had a permanent scowl etched on his face. The officer did not see any humor in my comment about being only a half-mile from my exit.

Although Mount Mitchell, at 6,684 feet, is the highest point in the United States east of the Mississippi, it also has a road to the summit, just like Mount Washington in New Hampshire. There is a large observation tower on the summit, with great views of the nearby Black Mountains, which contain nine peaks over 6,000 feet, and the Smoky Mountains beyond.

While Mount Mitchell and Brasstown Bald—Georgia's highpoint, which I would visit later in the day—had well-kept summits, showing the pride these states have in their highpoints, the summit of South Carolina's highpoint was a dump in comparison. Sassafras Mountain, located just across the border from North Carolina, had a large, wooden sign to mark the location, but it was all busted up, with large holes through it—perhaps the result of shotgun practice. There was a fire pit on the actual summit, where it looked as if local high school kids had held a recent party. I didn't stay long, as there was nothing to see, and quickly crossed back into North Carolina and then into Georgia, where I was surprised to find such rugged, mountainous terrain that I might have mistaken it for my native New England.

Brasstown Bald, at 4,784 feet, also had a road to the top, and has had a tower on its summit since the 1920s. It was a steep, 3-mile drive up to the visitor center, which was closed, and another half-mile hike on a paved path to the observation tower. There was about an inch of fresh snow near the summit. My feet were very happy that this was the only hiking I asked them to do today.

The next day, I left the snow behind and headed for the highpoint of Alabama. Getting off the interstate near Talladega, I drove south to pick up AL 218, which I expected would deliver me to Mount Cheaha. I must have made a wrong turn, because without warning the road dead-ended in the middle of nowhere.

There was, however, a trailhead here, and I decided to go for a run, as my legs were feeling better after a day's rest. This trail was part of the Pinhoti National Recreation Trail, a 335-mile trail that stretches into Georgia and connects with the Appalachian Trail. It was fun to run on, with lots of rolling hills and then a steep ascent to Silent Gap and back—about 12 miles total. It was nice to be able to run in shorts and a T-shirt after all the cold days I had experienced farther north.

Cheaha Mountain, another drive-up, was another disappointment. The stone lookout tower on the summit seemed outdated and unkempt.

Getting back on the road, it was dark by the time I got off I-65 south of Montgomery, but since it was warm, I kept driving. I reached the Florida border, just a half-mile from the state highpoint, which was located in a town park in a flat area ironically called Britton Hill, just outside the village of Paxton.

My guidebook said Lakewood Park was always open, so I drove in, only to be greeted by a sign that said it had closed at sunset. I walked over to the plaque—located right next to the bathrooms—marking the state highpoint at just 345 feet above sea level, and just as quickly walked back to my car. In 2015, it would be determined that the actual state highpoint is located about 200 yards farther into the woods, but at the time I was there, the plaque was the recognized location.

I was hungry, though, so I dug my stove out of my trunk and cooked myself some dinner in the parking lot. I had hoped to finish before any cops discovered me, but I was about three bites away from that when a county sheriff rolled into the parking lot and pulled up beside me.

Thankfully, he was not as dour as the North Carolina state trooper, and seemed quite interested when I told him about my highpointing quest. We chatted and I was on my way.

Crossing back into Alabama and badly in need of a shower, I broke down and paid $54 for a motel room in Andalusia. I was hoping it would be the last one I would need for a while—a motel room, that is, not a shower.

The first rain I had seen on my trip fell as I left southeastern Alabama to retrace much of my route from the day before. But it had turned into a beautiful, sunny day by the time I had gotten to the northwestern corner of the state. Crossing into Mississippi, both my car and I were soon on the state highpoint. This one was literally a drive-up, as I was able to position my Passat directly over the stone marker signifying the highest point. Like South Carolina, this highpoint was pretty lame, as I imagine not many people besides fellow peakbaggers bother with the 860-foot summit of Woodall Mountain.

From there, I needed a route to Jackson, and there was no interstate route available. I had seen the Natchez Trace on my map the night before, spotting it only with the help of a magnifying glass.

I knew nothing of its history or of its status as one of the oldest roads in the nation. Which road is the oldest in the United States has been debated. Some sources state that it is the Old Mine Road, built by Dutch settlers in the early 1600s in the Delaware Water Gap, which forms the border between New Jersey and Pennsylvania. But the Natchez Trace Parkway, deep in the South, has been in use, in some form, for perhaps as long as 10,000 years.

The road, which stretches nearly 450 miles from Nashville, Tennessee, to Natchez, Mississippi, follows a historical pathway through the wilderness first used by American Indians to follow the large game, including bison, which roamed the corridor in search of salt licks. French maps dating to 1733 show the Trace as a distinct path bisecting what would become the state of Mississippi. Around the turn of the nineteenth century—a time when Americans were expanding into the lands beyond the Appalachian Mountains—the Natchez Trace became an important trading route, the most heavily traveled road in what was then known as the Southwest. By 1809, the route was fully navigable by wagon, but within three years, the arrival of the steamboat on the Mississippi made river travel quicker and cheaper. Long before the Civil War broke out, the Natchez Trace had become little more than a memory.

In the 1880s, however, interest in all things nostalgic began to seep into American culture, and local members of the Daughters of the American Revolution began to push for the commemoration of the "Old Natchez Trace." Not long after, the invention of the automobile fueled the need for a more-efficient road system, and many "national" roads were being built. Those in Mississippi pushed Congress for just such a road to roughly parallel the route of the Natchez Trace, but political debate stalled this project until the mid-1930s. Resurrected by Mississippi Congressman Thomas Jefferson Busby as a "parkway," the proposal finally passed in 1937 and construction began a year later. The road would not be completed until 2005, though it has been designated a National Scenic Byway since 1995.

When I started out, I simply saw it as the most expedient route on my map. Few roads I have ever driven, however, have left such an indelible imprint on my soul.

The Natchez Trace Parkway is a limited-access, two-lane road that cuts straight through the wilderness. No commercial vehicles are allowed. Driving this road was like traveling through a time warp. No one seemed in a hurry on the Trace. I felt completely detached from the outside world, as thick, dense forest lined both sides of the roadway—everything from tall, majestic oaks to lazy cypress trees covered in Spanish moss, swaying in the breeze—blocking out all semblance of civilization. I almost expected to see DeSotos and Ramblers slowly passing alongside me. Occasionally, I would go over a bridge and, looking left or right, could see modern society's infringement, such as the golden arches of a

McDonald's. But on the Trace, I felt immune to these intrusions, the way I used to feel standing atop Monadnock, peering down on the workaday world below.

About halfway to Jackson, on the east side of the Trace at Milepost 193.1, I pulled into the Jeff Busby Site, named for the senator responsible for the parkway. Here, there were eighteen campsites—all of them vacant except for one inhabited by a church group of Boy Scouts—and a short trail system leading to the summit of Little Mountain, Mississippi's sixth highest. I ran the short 1.75-mile loop three times before dinner.

Driving the 100 miles to Jackson the next morning, I came upon only two other cars going in my direction, though it was a Sunday, and I imagined everyone else was at church. I also saw my first-ever armadillo scurrying across the road in front of me; well, I had seen several others on the road the day before, but none had successfully made the crossing. Heading west on I-20, it wasn't long before I crossed the Mississippi River—two full weeks after I had left New Hampshire. So far, thanks to my foolish exploits in Tennessee, my trip was right on schedule.

Driskill Mountain—the highpoint of Louisiana—is only 585 feet above sea level, but it did require a hike of about 0.8 mile up an old dirt road from the Mount Zion Presbyterian Church to get there. The summit, such as it is—just a pile of rocks in the woods—did have a register book, the first one I had seen since Maryland. But other than that, the place was unremarkable. I looked forward to getting back to some true mountain highpoints as I continued west.

From here, I headed due north across the Arkansas state line and made such good time that I arrived at Hot Springs National Park with enough daylight left to go for a run. I was going to camp again without paying, since it appeared I was the only person there, but there was a sign that read, "Camping Strictly Enforced," so I figured a ranger would be patrolling during the night, and paid the $10 fee. I found myriad trails in the park, all impeccably well groomed. For the first time on the trip, my legs did not feel sore. Getting back to my campsite, I was greeted by a park ranger, who was indeed checking my registration card.

For the first time since I had left home, I woke up the next day with a sense of urgency. A huge ice storm was forecast, and I hoped to stay ahead of it. I got an early start and arrived at Magazine Mountain—the Arkansas highpoint— for a half-mile hike to a stone cairn in the middle of the woods that marks the summit. From there, I continued north, and then did something I didn't necessarily want to do: I turned east. Mapping out my route weeks before, I had determined that the only expedient way for me to get Missouri's highpoint was to backtrack after having checked off Arkansas. Taum Sauk, located in the Ozarks of southeastern Missouri, would be easier to reach with an early detour than it would be in a couple of months on my return trip, when I would be as far north as the Dakotas.

It had already started drizzling by the time I got onto I-44 for the 3-hour drive to St. James, but I was able to stay just ahead of the storm as I drove the remaining 70 miles on back roads and arrived at Taum Sauk Mountain State Park just as it was getting dark, about 5:30 P.M. It was a quarter-mile walk to the highpoint, but by the time I got back to the car, it had started sleeting heavily. I had originally contemplated camping here, but the road into the state park had been very steep, and I did not want to attempt driving off the mountain in the morning. By then it would be a veritable bobsled run.

Slowly making my way off the mountain, I had to drive with one tire on the right shoulder to maintain traction. At the bottom, I discovered that the junction with the main highway was already a disaster area: multiple cars had piled up, and police cars and an ambulance were on the scene. One car was over an embankment and another was head-on into a tree. As I tried to turn left onto the main road, I slid straight across the highway until my tire caught dirt on the far shoulder. These roads were not the kind I was used to driving in New England; they were very smooth, with very little texture, and they did not respond well to ice. Narrow grooves had been cut into the road surface to channel away water, but ice had built up in them as the road had frozen over.

I had only a short drive back to the town of Ironton, but en route I saw several more cars off the road—including one on its roof—and I think I was the only driver to avoid going into the ditch. I slid into the parking lot of a motel and holed up for what I hoped would be just one night. But the storm proved to be one of the worst in history. A state of emergency had been called, as the entire region was coated with 2 inches of ice, knocking out power to 1.3 million customers and causing more than fifty deaths from Arkansas to Kentucky. In fact, the governor of Kentucky soon declared it the worst natural disaster in state history.

In the morning, I warmed up my car to melt the thick coating of ice and contemplated an escape. The TV was telling people to stay off the roads, but a lull in the storm had been predicted for 9 A.M., and when it indeed did stop raining just after breakfast, I went for it. The roads actually weren't that bad by New England standards, but I found there was no one out with a Missouri license plate. In fact, I saw only about a half dozen cars on the road during my entire 3-hour drive to Jefferson City; it was eerily apocalyptic. It soon started raining again, even though the temperature was in the midteens, and my defroster soon was unable to keep pace with the ice buildup.

The rain didn't abate until I reached Kansas City, and from there, I drove another 3 hours to Salina, Kansas, where I was to stay for the night at the home of my friend Linda Lawrence, an ophthalmologist whom I had met in Guatemala in 2004. In fact, Linda had just gotten back from Guatemala the day before and was heading to Nigeria the following week. She is always traveling somewhere, performing eye exams and cataract surgeries as part of her charitable organization, the Amaranth Foundation. I was extremely fortunate to have found her at home.

I had not seen Linda since the day I had met her purely by accident on the lancha on Lake Atitlán, but we had been in touch from time to time. It was great to see her again, even if it would be for only one night. In the morning, I awoke at 7:15 just as she was returning from a workout at the gym, and then she proceeded to cook me *huevos rancheros* for breakfast. I thought I was back in Guatemala. I'm not sure where she gets her energy. Last time I checked in with her, she was in Spain doing a pilgrimage on the El Camino de Santiago.

Leaving Salina, I continued west on I-70 across some of the most boring land I had ever seen. I could see why Dorothy was so anxious to get out of Kansas; I couldn't wait, either. Turning south in Oakley, I headed for the state highpoint, which is about a half-mile from the Colorado border. Don't let Mount Sunflower's name fool you: there are no mountains in Kansas. Though the elevation of Mount Sunflower is more than 4,000 feet, so is all the surrounding prairieland. The highpoint is merely a rise in the middle of a farmer's field. It proved a bit interesting, as there was a large metal sculpture welded into the shape of a sunflower—the state flower—with the words "Mount Sunflower" and "4039" spelled out in wrought iron. Next to the sculpture was a mailbox with a register book inside, which I signed. It is one of the few state highpoints on private property; the owners keep it open to the public even though vandals trashed the place a few years after my visit.

I drove due south for well over 100 miles toward the Oklahoma border on a road that was so straight I didn't need my hands on the wheel, except to dodge all the sagebrush blown across the road by the gusty winds. Just as with Kentucky and Arkansas, this was my first visit to Oklahoma, and I could immediately tell that after bagging the highpoint—Black Mesa—I likely would never have any reason to return. I did go back again a few years later when I accompanied a peakbagging friend as she checked Black Mesa off her list, but I can't imagine what would necessitate another return visit.

Pulling into Black Mesa State Park, I could see right away that I wouldn't be stealth camping that night. A park ranger was on duty and seemed overly eager to pocket my $10. I was probably the first camper they had had all winter. After a 5-mile run and a shower, during which I had to awkwardly hold the knob with one hand in order to make the water run, I cooked dinner and went to bed expecting a nice, warm night. Instead, it was one of the coldest I endured during the entire trip. I hadn't felt that cold when I had slept in the lean-to atop Clingmans Dome. It got down to about 2 degrees Fahrenheit that night. Sometime after midnight, I ran to my car and pulled some more clothes out of the trunk. In the morning, I had on my snow pants, a down jacket, and the felt liners to my Dunham boots.

The guidebook said the hike to the Black Mesa highpoint was an easy 8.6-mile round-trip with less than 800 feet of elevation gain, but every step was a struggle as I tried to run to the top the next morning. After gaining all the elevation to reach a broad plateau, which stretched 40 miles into New Mexico and Colorado, making it one of the largest mesas in the world, it didn't take long to find the highpoint, which was marked by a 10-foot-high granite obelisk that seemed bizarrely out of place among this desert landscape. The guidebook warned of rattlesnakes here, but it being January, they were all still hibernating.

Returning to the car, I drove back to the town of Kenton, which I might have mistaken for a ghost town had not my guidebook suggested stopping at the Kenton Mercantile and asking owner Allan Griggs for a certificate to commemorate my highpointing achievement. As it turned out, Allan didn't own the grocery store/post office/restaurant/gas station anymore, but the nice ladies inside said that while they didn't have any certificates for me, they could offer me a slab of blueberry pie. It was delicious.

There might not be a more desolate road in America than the one that leaves Kenton and heads west across the New Mexico state line. Straight as an arrow, I cruised at 90 mph until the pavement suddenly ended at the border, leaving me with a 17-mile stretch of dirt road to contend with—probably the same "road" the early settlers used to get to Santa Fe. Soon, though, I could see high mountains in front of me, all covered in snow and glistening in the midday sun. My heart raced at the sight.

I inquired at the ranger station in the town of Questa as to the hiking conditions near Wheeler Peak, at 13,161 feet the first big mountain I would be tackling on this trip. The rangers put me in touch with Nate at The Boot Doctor's in Taos Ski Valley, near the trailhead. He told me the trail had been hiked out to the lake underneath the peak, and that the weather forecast was favorable for the next few days. Avalanche danger was minimal. When I told him I was camping, however, he warned against it: the temperature that night was supposed to drop to 14 degrees below zero Fahrenheit. Instead, he suggested staying in nearby Arroyo Seco at a hostel called the Abominable SnowMansion, and it was a great call.

Driving into Taos Ski Valley the next morning, I had no problems negotiating a road with a sign that read, "4WD Only" to get to the trailhead parking lot. From there, it was an easy 2.5-mile hike on a broken-out trail to Williams Lake, which sits in a huge bowl surrounded by several tall peaks, all of which seemed to be roughly the same height to me. I was unsure of which one was Wheeler Peak, so I pulled out my guidebook. It said to hike northeast from the lake and then east up a steep gully, but I couldn't see anything that looked like a gully, so I started up the mountain to my left, not certain if I was climbing the right one. I eventually found a steep gully, which was full of snow, making for difficult climbing. About two-thirds of the way up this unrelenting slope, I turned back to see another climber behind me, so I was either on the right peak after all, or this guy was going to be pretty pissed when he discovered he had followed some idiot up the wrong mountain.

Upon reaching the ridge crest and looking around, I could now see I was indeed on the highest peak, so I turned to my right and hiked a short ways to the summit, which was marked by an engraved plaque and what looked like a large shell casing sticking out of a rock wall. This was actually a piece of steel piping with a cap on the end; unscrewing this, I found the trail register inside.

It had turned into a brilliant bluebird day, a perfect day in the mountains, and I sat and ate my lunch in the sunshine waiting for the other climber to arrive. It was the first time on any of the twenty highpoints so far that I had had company on the summit, even on the drive-ups. His name was Dave Dyess, from Taos, and he said he had climbed Wheeler Peak about fifty times. Incredibly fit

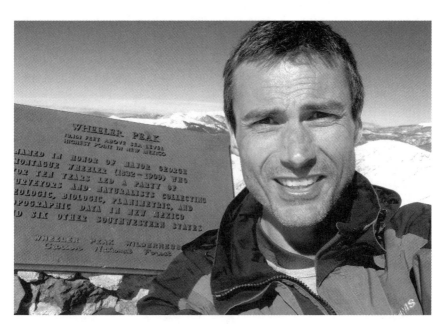

A bluebird winter day welcomes me upon reaching the summit of Wheeler Peak, the highpoint of New Mexico.

for a man who was probably in his 60s, he said I had pretty much been on the trail the entire way up, even though I admitted I wasn't even sure I had been on the right peak.

We hiked out together, and he offered to buy me a beer at the Bavarian Haus, located at the base of the ski area's Kachina Chairlift. We sat down in the brilliant afternoon sunshine on the front deck, but before we had even taken a sip, the sun dipped below the ridge, and I was instantly shivering. The hot shower later at the Abominable SnowMansion was a godsend.

The next morning, I headed south for what would be a nearly all-day drive to my next stop—Guadelupe Peak, the Texas highpoint. The drive into Guadelupe National Park was breathtaking, as the escarpment that followed me down from New Mexico abruptly ended with a sheer drop off El Capitan, the last mountain in the range and the one next to Guadelupe Peak, one of several 8,000-foot peaks in the vicinity. All of these peaks soared dramatically more than 3,000 feet above the floor of the Chihuahuan Desert of West Texas.

As soon as the sun dipped below the ridge at about 4:30, the temperature instantly plunged and the wind picked up. I anticipated another long, cold night. I had to put large rocks in all four corners of my tent to keep it from blowing away; the ground was far too hard to use my tent stakes.

The wind blew so hard that night that I barely slept at all; the constant flapping of my tent kept me awake. When my alarm went off the next morning at 6:30, I at first ignored it, but then the first rays of the sun filtered over the horizon and I unzipped my tent to have a look at the new day. I was shocked: the ground appeared to be covered with fresh snow. It had not been *that* cold. Once I put in my contact lenses and looked again, however, I realized it was just the light color of the Texan sand.

It was a cold, hour-plus run to cover the more than 4 miles up the Guadelupe Peak Trail to the 8,749-foot summit, and I had to put on a jacket upon arriving at the three-sided pyramid-shaped marker at the top. This 6-foot-high, stainless-steel object appeared more out of place than the obelisk atop Black Mesa, but the views here were incredible in all directions, and I would not have guessed I was in Texas had I not known better. The pyramid was erected in 1958 by American Airlines to commemorate the hundredth anniversary of the Butterfield Overland stagecoach, which ran past the base of these mountains from 1857 to 1861.

Back at the campground, I found my tent upside down and stuck on some tree branches, as the wind had proven too powerful even for the rocks I had put in the corners. I quickly broke camp and headed for El Paso on what was the straightest and most desolate road I had yet driven. But the views back toward El Capitan were stunning.

Driving as far as Deming, New Mexico, I pulled off and found a motel; it was

Super Bowl Sunday, and while the Patriots had missed the playoffs despite an 11-5 record, the game between the Pittsburgh Steelers and Arizona Cardinals proved one of the greatest ever, though I was disappointed when the Steelers pulled out a last-second 27–23 victory. I watched the game at the Butterfield Stage Inn, also named for the famous stagecoach route. The only other people watching with me were other travelers who had pulled off I-10 just to see the game. Fortunately, none of them were Steelers fans.

Back on I-10 in the morning, I headed for the outskirts of Phoenix, where I would stay with my cousin Rick for the next few days. I had not seen Rick in many, many years, and we spent our first evening reminiscing while drinking Coors Light straight from a tapped keg he kept in his kitchen.

The next day, I headed for Lost Dutchman State Park east of the city and had a great run up into the Superstition Mountains, climbing a steep, narrow gully to reach a bluff, where I was able to run for several miles along the mesa ridge. Later, I sat on the edge of the rim looking out over the vast Valley of the Sun for an hour or more, talking with a young man named Keith, who was from Phoenix but was being deployed to Afghanistan in a few days. He told me the terrain there would be much the same as where we were right now.

Saying goodbye to Rick the next morning, I headed for Sedona, but I kept stopping to take pictures every chance I got, and it seemingly took me forever to get there. Sedona is nearly impossible to describe; it's a place you really need to *feel* to understand. Nestled among some of the most beautiful red sandstone formations on Earth, Sedona is a haven for spiritual-minded people, as it's said to have one of the highest-energy vortexes on the planet, akin to Lake Atitlán in Guatemala.

One of the first things I noticed when I drove into town was a sign that read, "Marathon This Weekend," so I drove to the race office and immediately signed up. I knew the race would be difficult, and I'd run only two marathons in my life, so I treated it like a training run. I started slowly, hoping to enjoy the experience. The course was tough, but I felt good when I hit the turnaround at the halfway point, and slowly increased my pace, picking off ten runners on the way back, to finish twenty-fourth overall in 3:41:07. Later, I discovered that I had finished first in the men's 45-49 age group. I was starting to feel that I could actually run the upcoming 100 miles.

I was sporting a wide smile when I drove up Oak Creek Canyon to Flagstaff that afternoon and pulled into the driveway of my friend Steve Till, whom I had met, along with his dog, Pepper, climbing 14ers in Colorado the September before. Though I had just run the marathon and despite the fact that 6 inches of fresh snow would fall overnight with more in the forecast, we planned to climb Humphreys Peak, the Arizona highpoint at 12,635 feet, the next day.

In the morning, Steve checked the forecast and learned that there was supposed to be a window of good weather before a second storm moved in late that afternoon. So we ate a quick breakfast and headed for the Arizona Snowbowl, one of the oldest continuously operated ski areas in the country, located in the San Francisco Peaks north of Flagstaff. We were hiking up through lofty pine trees in fresh virgin snow when a man came swooshing down through the trees on a pair of skis, stopping right in front of us. He had long dreadlocks and used the word "dude" a lot. He said he had been camping in a snow cave high on the mountain for the past eight days, and had run out of supplies. He said the cave he had dug was tall enough to stand up in, and we decided to follow his tracks to check it out.

But, soon thereafter, we came upon two others hiking out after having camped at 11,000 feet the night before, and Steve said we should follow their tracks instead, since they went more directly to the ridgeline. He said he thought he knew the whereabouts of this snow cave, and we could drop off the ridge on the way back and find it. The snow deepened as we started breaking trail above their campsite, and it was difficult to gain the ridge, especially for poor Pepper. By the time we got there, the wind had become ferocious; the second storm had come in earlier than predicted. Battered by the wind, we staggered the half-mile along the ridge to the barren summit, snapped a couple of photos, and quickly retreated.

Pepper was now completely white, covered in a thick coating of snow. Steve lost his bearings in the whiteout, and we abandoned the ridge a little too soon, missing the snow cave and also our destination, as we came out below the parking lot and had to hike back up to reach our car.

I was fortunate that Steve had agreed to climb with me—he had done Humphreys many times—as nearly 2 feet of additional snow would fall in the next 24 hours, and the avalanche danger would have been too severe for me to have attempted the climb by myself over the following days. The roads weren't much better, and leaving Flagstaff on I-40 the next morning, I quickly came upon an accident in which an eighteen-wheeler had somehow hopped the guardrail and ended up on its side at least a hundred feet from the road.

It took just over 8 hours to drive to my brother's house in California, much of it on some more desolate highways, such as US 95 from Needles to Blythe, with beautiful scenery on both sides of the road vying for my attention. So much so, that I didn't see the sign dropping the speed limit from 65 MPH to 55 MPH when I crossed the Imperial County line, and soon I was talking to a California Highway patrolman about my oversight. I really didn't have a valid excuse, since he said he clocked me at 78 MPH, but he agreed to reduce the ticket to 65, meaning I would be eligible to take an online driver's safety course and keep the ticket from showing up on my insurance. I already feared what UPS was going to say about the ticket I had gotten in North Carolina.

I picked up I-8 in El Centro, which is a few feet below sea level, and started the long drive back to 4,000 feet, where I found it was snowing again, even though I often was within site of the Mexican border. Cars were off the road as I took the Descanso exit, and I pulled into my brother's yard at five o'clock sharp, just as I had predicted when I had spoken with him that morning.

I spent the next five weeks helping Bryon write his book about the Campo gunfight, and training for the 100-miler I would run in May.

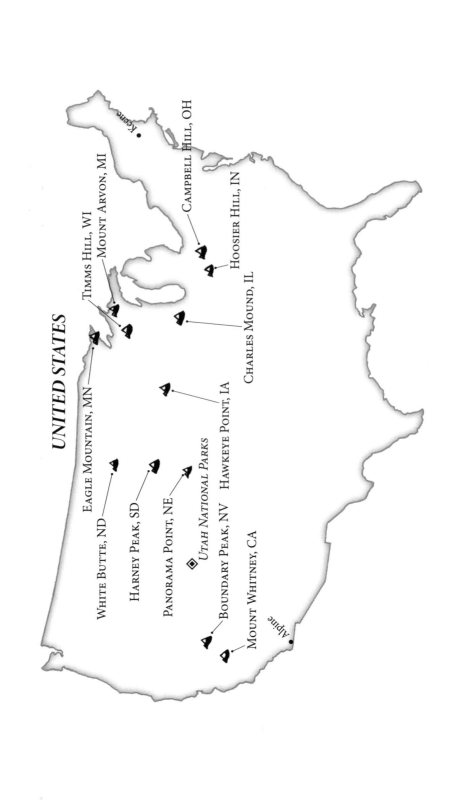

UNITED STATES

Keene

Campbell Hill, OH

Hoosier Hill, IN

Timms Hill, WI

Mount Arvon, MI

Charles Mound, IL

Eagle Mountain, MN

Hawkeye Point, IA

White Butte, ND

Harney Peak, SD

Panorama Point, NE

⊕ Utah National Parks

Boundary Peak, NV

Mount Whitney, CA

Alpine

MOUNT WHITNEY AND THE LONG DRIVE HOME

PEAKBAGGING IS NOT ONLY THE DOMAIN OF ADULTS. IN 2004, THIRD-GRADER Jordan Romero of Big Bear Lake, California, began dreaming of the world's high peaks. It was five years later when I met him by chance on Mount Whitney. There, he and his parents told me about the mural that had started it all. Gracing a hallway of his elementary school, it depicted the Seven Summits: the highest points on each continent, capped by Mount Everest, the highest of them all. While other kids never gave the mural a second glance on their way out to the playground to play kickball at recess, Jordan would stop and stare at it for so long he was probably often late for class.

On the first day of fourth grade, Jordan went home after school and announced to his father, Paul, that he wanted to climb the Seven Summits. Not someday, when he was older, but now. He was 9 years old.

Any other parent might have laughed and dismissed this as mere folly. But Paul Romero wasn't any ordinary dad. He was a well-known adventure racer, competing in crazy races all over the world along with his then-girlfriend, Karen Lundgren, and whose motto hung on a sign over the front door of their house: "Go Fast. Take Chances." He saw that his son was serious.

Paul knew that Jordan would not be easily dissuaded from this quest, but the preparations to climb some of the highest and most dangerous mountains in the world would test Jordan's dedication. At first, Jordan had trouble climbing some of the high peaks around Big Bear, which lies at 7,000 feet in the San Bernardino Mountains of Southern California. But he got stronger and his climbing improved, so they decided to see what he could do. The next summer,

Paul and Karen took him to Africa to climb Mount Kilimanjaro, the highest freestanding mountain in the world at 19,341 feet. Jordan even sold lemonade to help fund the trip.

Jordan so impressed the Maasai porters, who accompanied them to the summit, that they nicknamed him the "Little Lion" for his flowing blond locks. He climbed in three days what it takes regular clients up to six days to hike. At 10, he was the youngest person to ever stand on the summit. When he got home, he soon found himself a guest on *The Martha Stewart Show.*

Next came a trip to Australia, to climb Mount Kosciuszko, the smallest of the Seven Summits at 7,310 feet. A few months later, they went to Russia and climbed Mount Elbrus, the highest point in Europe at 18,510 feet, which he summited the day before his eleventh birthday, setting another record as the youngest ever. But both those peaks were relatively easy compared with the ones that remained.

Aconcagua, on the border between Argentina and Chile, is the highest mountain in the world outside the Himalaya, at 22,837 feet. It was also a mountain that no one under the age of 14 was allowed to climb. But Jordan didn't want to wait three more years. So, they petitioned the Argentinean courts in hopes a judge would grant him a special waiver to obtain a climbing permit, as another young climber had recently done. Jordan impressed the judge with his maturity and she granted his request. Their elation, however, quickly turned to dejection when they arrived at the permit office and the ranger there refused to abide by the judge's order, saying the court had no jurisdiction over his office. A lengthy, heated exchange ensued, which ultimately resulted in the park ranger relenting and granting the permit. But when they arrived at the trailhead, they were again denied passage despite the permit. Not until after a doctor examined Jordan were they finally allowed on the mountain. The doctor had probably never seen such a hale and hardy 11-year-old.

But in the deep snow and bitter cold near the summit of Aconcagua, Jordan nearly broke down and quit, questioning, for the first time, why he was climbing. Encouraging words from Karen, and a sudden parting of the clouds that they took as a sign from above, enabled Jordan to summit, becoming the youngest person to climb Aconcagua. Returning to the bottom, Jordan suddenly found he had become a celebrity, as even the park rangers who had attempted to deny him passage now wanted their pictures taken with him. He was front-page news in the Buenos Aires daily paper the next day, and the story was all over national TV.

The next June, Jordan, Paul and Karen summited Denali together in Alaska, tackling North America's highest peak at 20,310 feet. While he was not the youngest ever—he was four months older than the record—the quickness and assuredness of the ascent and descent gave Jordan a resounding confidence that he could climb the peaks that remained, including Everest. He was incredibly fit, having spent months dragging an SUV tire up and down the street in front of his house to get in shape. Jordan had now climbed five of the Seven Summits before he had turned 12.

As with other mountaineers seeking the Seven Summits, Jordan's plan had to tackle some geographic controversy. Some consider the entirety of Oceania, and not just the Australian mainland, a continent. Under this definition, 16,024-foot Carstensz Pyramid in New Guinea would be on the Seven Summits list rather than Mount Kosciuszko at 7,310 feet in Australia. So, Jordan decided to remove all doubt by climbing Carstenz Pyramid, too, setting another record as the youngest ever.

Up until that point, Jordan's quest had become well known within the climbing community, but not beyond. That quickly changed when Paul announced that they were not only going to take Jordan to the top of Mount Everest, they were going to do it on their own, not by hiring one of the many Western commercial climbing outfitters to guide them there. Not only did they plan to climb using just three hired Sherpas, but they were going to climb from the more difficult Tibetan side, not wanting to subject Jordan to the dangerous Khumbu Icefall on the standard route from the Nepalese side. Karen had almost died there when she fell into a crevasse during a scouting mission the year before.

The critics lined up hard against Paul, labeling him an irresponsible parent. They looked at Jordan's age and opened fire, never considering Jordan's abilities. David Hillebrandt, the medical adviser to the British Mountaineering Council, summed up what many were thinking when he questioned whether any 13-year-old had the mental maturity for such an undertaking, saying such a stunt was "verging on child abuse."

Many others made similar remarks, and popular opinion was running well against them when they boarded a flight to Kathmandu in April 2010. Anything short of success would see Paul get excoriated in the press. But Jordan was undaunted, and undoubtedly was more fit than almost all of the climbers being guided by the commercial outfitters on the other side of the mountain. At 5-foot-10 and 160 pounds, Jordan had grown into a man's body; he was certainly bigger than the Sherpas who would be assisting them up and down the mountain.

Their critics were nearly validated in the first days of the climb. During an acclimatization hike, Jordan was caught in an avalanche, which tragically killed another climber. A Hungarian man, who had just said "Hi" to Jordan seconds before while descending, was swept thousands of feet to his death, having not been clipped into the fixed rope at the time of the mishap. Jordan was saved only because he had been securely tied in to an anchor and the rope held. While trying to extricate himself from the snow, however, Jordan accidentally kicked Paul in the head with his crampons, opening up a scalp wound that would require stitches back at base camp. The expedition was almost over before it started.

Undeterred, they stayed on the mountain and continued the climb, reaching the summit on May 22, 2010, along with one of the Sherpas.

They had done what no one said they could.

When they returned to Nepal, they were met at the border by a horde of reporters from all over the world. Jordan returned to Kathmandu to a reception befitting a rock star. At home, he made an appearance on *The Tonight Show with Jay Leno*, and was featured on several other shows, including *20/20*.

But his quest was not over. He still had Vinson Massif in Antarctica to climb. At first, there was a logistical problem they couldn't find a way around; the only outfitter with permission to fly climbers to the continent had a steadfast rule that no one under the age of 18 was even allowed on the plane, let alone the mountain. Jordan did not want to wait another five years to complete his quest. Fortunately, Jordan's mother, Leigh Anne, had some connections, which Karen pursued. The company relented. On Christmas Eve 2011, Jordan stood with Paul and Karen atop the 16,050-foot summit of Vinson Massif. He was just 15.

Jordan's record may never be broken. Subsequent to his climb on Everest, Nepal adopted a rule that requires a climber to be at least 16 to acquire a permit, and China was expected to follow suit. However, in 2014, a 13-year-old Indian girl, Malavath Poorna—just a couple of months older than Jordan—summited Everest, setting a record as the youngest female ever.

Since then, Jordan has been on a mission to bring his message of "Find your own Everest" to schools around the country, encouraging and motivating kids, as well as adults, to follow their dreams, no matter how impossible they may seem. "Don't ever let the size of your dreams overwhelm you," Jordan tells them.

I couldn't have been prouder of Jordan had he been my own son. While my own kids were now all in their 20s, they weren't quite sure what to make of their father's wanderlust. While none of them is particularly interested in running or mountain climbing, they have many friends who are, and I have heard that they have spoken of their "old man" with pride when recounting some of my adventures.

I have been asked many times if I would ever want to run the Badwater 135, the grueling, brain-broiling ultramarathon from Death Valley to Mount Whitney. The 135-mile race—which starts at Badwater Basin at 282 feet below sea level and usually finishes at the Whitney Portal at an elevation of 8,300 feet—dubs itself as the world's toughest race. In fact, it was originally even tougher: runners continued on from the Whitney Portal to the summit of the highest mountain in the Lower 48. The race is held in July, when the area's average high temperature is 116 degrees Fahrenheit, and Death Valley is home to the highest temperature ever recorded on the planet—134 degrees Fahrenheit in 1913. The asphalt gets so hot—upward of 200 degrees Fahrenheit—that runners have had the soles of their shoes literally melt out from under them. Many run directly on the road's painted white lines, which are considerably cooler than the blacktop itself.

I've had the pleasure to spend time with Bart Yasso, chief running officer for *Runner's World* magazine, who once ran Badwater on assignment. Amazingly, he finished second, but it was an ordeal he said he would not wish to do again. Bart wrote in his book, *My Life on the Run,* that at one point in the race, he kept seeing banana bread baked on the roadway and thought he might be hallucinating, a common occurrence in any long ultra race. But, he later discovered, the race leader ahead of him was eating bananas and kept throwing up, unable to keep them down. The bananas were baking on the pavement, appearing to Bart as little pancakes of banana bread. He said he knew he was gaining ground when the banana bread droppings were no longer fully cooked.

One of Badwater's most famous competitors is Marshall Ulrich, from Idaho Springs, Colorado, who has famously had all of his toenails removed, as "they kept falling off all the time anyway," he said. These are some hard-core runners. Marshall, whom I have also gotten to know, has run Badwater nineteen times. He said running in Death Valley is harder than climbing Mount Everest, which he has also done.

Would I ever want to run the Badwater 135? My answer: not a chance.

I arrived at Badwater Basin in mid-March 2009; it was 82 degrees Fahrenheit, and that was hot enough for me. I cannot imagine being able to endure the heat confronting those who run in this annual race. The parking lot marks the lowest spot in the Western Hemisphere, and high above, on the cliff face opposite the road, a sign reads, "Sea Level." Some boardwalks in the basin jut into an expanse of endless salt flats; stepping off them was like walking on snow-covered ice as it crunched beneath my feet.

I'd left my brother's that morning to begin my journey home. I planned to climb Mount Whitney and tackle the eleven other continental state highpoints remaining on my return trip.

Driving through the national park, I stopped at places with such names as Furnace Creek and Stovepipe Wells, conjuring up images of what hell must be like. There are giant sand dunes just off US 190 in Stovepipe Wells, and I walked out onto them, feeling the intense heat reflecting off the light-colored sand.

Crossing Emigrant Pass the next morning, my first views of Mount Whitney and the glorious Sierra Nevada greeted me across the Owens River Valley like a splash of ice-cold water to the face. They got my attention in a hurry. I can only imagine the reaction the first settlers had when they topped this pass and were confronted by the impenetrable wall of the Sierras. I figure they must have been the ones who founded the nearby town of Lone Pine at the foot of the Alabama Hills, deciding this was as far west as they were going to go.

After picking up my climbing permit in Lone Pine, I had the rest of the day to relax while waiting for my friend Zac Bookman—whom I had met the year before in Mexico while climbing Izta—to arrive from Los Angeles, where he now lived. He had agreed to join me to climb Mount Whitney, but would not be able to get away from his job at a law firm until after 5 P.M., and had a nearly 4-hour drive ahead of him.

I spent the afternoon hiking up the main trail to Mirror Lake, locating the turnoff to the Mountaineers Route, the trail we would ascend the next morning. The Mountaineers Route is more than 4 miles shorter than the standard route, which we had planned to descend, and a lot more interesting, as it includes an exhilarating scramble up a steep gully from Iceberg Lake, located directly under the striking east wall of Whitney's lofty summit. This route was first climbed by none other than John Muir, the famed naturalist and Sierra Club founder, called by his biographer "the patron saint of American environmental activity." Muir completed the climb solo on October 21, 1873, when the peak was the tallest mountain on American soil. Had he ventured south from his home in the Yosemite Valley a few months earlier, he would undoubtedly have been the first to summit Whitney.

That honor was thought to have belonged to Clarence King of the California Geological Survey, who claimed to have summited Mount Whitney in June 1871. He'd left a silver half-dollar with his name etched on it at the top. No one disputed this fact until two years later, when W.A. Goodyear and M.W. Belshaw climbed what would later become known as Mount Langley, 6 miles to the south of Whitney, and discovered a silver half-dollar with King's name on it. King had clearly climbed the wrong mountain.

When Goodyear reported this finding to the California Academy of Sciences on August 4, 1873, King was back east. Upon learning of his folly, King hastened back to the Sierras to rectify the mistake, but he was too late. By the time he got there and summited the correct mountain on September 19, three other parties had beaten him to the top.

The first was a group of three fishermen, who had retreated into the Sierras to beat the summer heat of the valley below, intent on two weeks of "fishing, drinking, and enjoying the cool air of the high country," according to an article that later appeared in the *Inyo Independent*. But, after climbing Langley (then still known as Whitney) and seeing a higher mountain to the north, they resolved to climb that one, as well, and were on the summit the following afternoon, August 18. Some wanted to call the new highpoint Fishermen's Peak, but King quickly bestowed it as the new Mount Whitney, named in honor of his boss at the California Geological Survey, Josiah Dwight Whitney, and the "old" Whitney eventually became Mount Langley, named for Samuel Pierpont Langley, the director of the Allegheny Observatory in Pittsburgh, who would conduct scientific research in the Sierras in the 1880s.

Despite his gaffe, King went on to become the first director of the U.S. Geological Survey.

Muir, of course, was America's first conservationist and would eventually become known as the "Father of the National Park System," having lobbied through his many letters and newspaper articles on environmental issues. As for his first Whitney climb on what would later become known as the Mountaineers Route, Muir wrote, "For climbers, there is a canyon which comes down from the north shoulder of the Whitney peak. Well-seasoned limbs will enjoy the climb of 9,000 feet required for the direct route, but soft, succulent people should go the mule way."

Zac and I didn't consider ourselves the soft and succulent type, and we looked forward to the challenge of using our well-seasoned limbs on the Mountaineers Route. We hit the snowy trail at 6:20 on a beautiful morning—the first day of spring—and made good time as we climbed over large granite slabs into a high basin. Approaching Upper Boy Scout Lake, we came upon another party camped in the basin. Walking over, we introduced ourselves to Paul Romero, Karen Lundgren, and Paul's 12-year-old son, Jordan, who was lounging in the tent, resting up for the summit push ahead of them.

Paul and Karen were acclimatizing before leaving for Everest on a scouting mission ahead of Jordan's record-setting ascent the following year. Zac and I were blown away by the stamina and maturity of this 12-year-old, and we posed for several pictures. When I explained my highpointing quest, Jordan turned to his dad and said, "I want to do that next!" A couple of years later, when I watched Jordan on *The Tonight Show* following his successful Everest summit, Jay Leno asked what he planned to do next. Jordan quickly exclaimed, "I want to climb all the state highpoints!" I smiled, knowing I was the one who had introduced him to highpointing.

We hiked with them as far as Iceberg Lake, where the Romeros rested again; Zac and I continued up the steep 1,500-foot couloir, reaching a notch that leads to the west side of the mountain for the final scramble to the summit. Here, we ran into a traffic jam. Several climbing parties were going both up and down this final 300-foot section, and their fixed ropes were getting in our way. Zac and I simply strapped on our crampons and walked right up the steep snow slope to the broad summit plateau. A storm forecast for later that day was apparently coming in early; we saw it rolling in as we looked out over the vast expanse of the John Muir Wilderness to our west. We abandoned plans to descend via the standard route, which would have kept us up high and on the west side of the mountain, and would have needlessly exposed us to the oncoming storm. Returning the way we had come, we crossed paths with the Romeros, all roped up and still climbing. It would be their first-ever summit of Whitney, and being experienced climbers, they obviously were undaunted by the approaching storm.

It was a long, agonizing, 6-mile hike out, as Zac and I spent a lot of time postholing in the deep snow, which was now quite soft, as the day had become very warm. My feet were killing me from being scrunched inside my new La Sportiva mountaineering boots, which I was wearing for just the second time. The narrow toe box pinched my feet, making every step excruciating, and I could hardly walk when we got back to the Whitney Portal, by which time it was snowing. Fortunately, Eastern Mountain Sports allowed me to return these boots for a full refund upon my return home.

Still, Zac and I had made the round-trip in just 10.5 hours, a remarkable time given the snow. But then again, we weren't soft or succulent. We headed back to Lone Pine, where the falling snow had changed to rain, and booked a room at the Dow Villa Motel—the same place where John Wayne and many other Hollywood stars used to stay while shooting any of the dozens of Westerns that were filmed in the nearby Alabama Hills.

That night, Zac and I ventured out to celebrate our successful climb and somehow wandered into a dive called the Double L Bar. In reality, we had unwittingly walked into an episode of *The Twilight Zone*.

All the requisite characters were in place: There was Tony and his wife, Caroline, a couple of local drunks who spent half the night arguing and the other half making up. Caroline must've smoked four packs of cigarettes while we were there. Young Eric, a stumpy-looking construction worker, sported a frayed Red Man baseball cap, worn backward, and sat at the bar bopping his head to the music, or maybe nodding off. There was Tony's friend Ed Montana, who wore a big cowboy hat and carried two tins of chewing tobacco at all times, and kept telling Zac and me to beat Tony at pool "like a redheaded stepchild." And there was Ray, the only "normal" person in the place—despite an overgrown goatee that made him look like he might be in the Witness Protection Program—who told us he had just arrived from South Carolina the day before, but later changed the story to Florida. And I almost forgot about the little old man, whose name escaped us, with a cowboy hat and a bladder-control problem; he went to the bathroom every 10 minutes like clockwork the entire

5 hours we were there.

But no one seemed more out of place than Cedric, a black man from Jamaica with an affable personality that was belied only by his Popeye-esque forearms. Amid this sea of whisky-drinking hillbillies, Cedric preferred to drink rum with a smooth sophistication that transcended this backwoods honky-tonk. He reminded me of Michael Clarke Duncan, the guy who played "Frankie Figs" in *The Whole Nine Yards*. Cedric was the epitome of cool, right down to his tinted sunglasses, which he never took off despite the bar being so dark it was hard to see through the thick haze of cigarette smoke. He interrupted the constant twang of country and Western music by playing reggae on the juke box every chance he got, dancing by himself in a corner while constantly holding his crotch. He wore a button-down shirt with only one button done, exposing a belt buckle that was the size of a dinner plate, with Bob Marley's picture on it.

This place, to be sure, was beyond surreal.

Zac and I must have beaten Tony and Ray at pool more than thirty games in a row. And that's being conservative. But they kept pumping quarters into the table, asking for more punishment. We had been joking and clowning, when suddenly everything got serious: Tony decided he didn't like Zac anymore and wanted to fight him. A tiny little fellow with buck teeth, Tony was shaking with rage as he charged Zac with a pool cue and then invited him outside where he said he was going to "wipe the sidewalk" with him. Zac, who is 6 feet and a burly 180 pounds, would have destroyed him, but that became moot once Tony saw that Cedric, who seemed to be the bar's enforcer, wasn't going to back him.

Cedric swelled his chest, and in his best Bob Marley imitation, told Tony: "We practice one love here. Don't make me break your face."

Tony calmed down, ending the tension as quickly as it had begun. He profusely apologized, blaming it on the whisky. The rest of the night played out as if the incident had never happened.

We must've been the first outsiders to venture into the Double L in years. At some point during the night, every one of these characters bought Zac and me a beer. Some of them bought us more than one round, especially Tony and Ray, who, thanks to their losing streak, also paid for us to play pool all night.

When we finally left, there was such an emotional scene that Caroline had to give us each a big hug and might even have started crying, and everyone else shook our hands a couple of times and acted as if we'd all known each other for years. Zac and I could only laugh uncontrollably at this insanity as we staggered up Main Street on the way back to our motel.

In the morning, Zac left to return to L.A., and I headed back to the Whitney Portal, where I discovered 4 inches of new snow. I returned down the hill to the Lone

Pine Campground, intent on climbing the standard route the following day in an attempt to bag Mount Muir, another ranked 14er on the Mount Whitney Massif. The campground was nearly deserted; there were three guys I had met the previous Friday who had said they were on their way to go bouldering in Joshua Tree, but didn't seem to be making any progress on that assertion, and also a family from Oregon staying in their RV camper. After the husband and wife had lost their jobs in the economic collapse, they had embarked on an extended vacation so they could rent out their home rather than lose it to the bank.

The next morning, I awoke before the sun came up and looked out of my tent, thought there was fresh snow on the ground, and went back to sleep. Muir would have to wait for another trip. Only later did I realize that once again I had been fooled by the reflection of the starlight off the light-colored sand because I did not have my contact lenses in.

Without a mountain to climb, I was in no real hurry the rest of the day, and slowly drove north on US 395, headed for Boundary Peak, the highpoint of Nevada. In the town of Bishop, the sign in front of the Mountain Light Gallery caught my eye, so I stopped. I am glad I did; no trip to the Sierras should be considered complete without a visit to Mountain Light Gallery. Inside are thousands of photos of the Sierras and from all over the world, all taken by noted outdoor photographer Galen Rowell.

In the 1970s, Galen may have been the greatest photographer in the world; but at the same time, he was also one of the greatest climbers in the world, logging more than one hundred first ascents of new climbing routes in the Sierras. His stunning wilderness photographs would adorn covers of magazines such as *National Geographic*, and there are several best-selling coffee table books published of his work. I have given several as wedding gifts to my friends in the years since I first stumbled into this studio. Tragically, Galen and his wife, Barbara, were killed in a plane crash flying into the Bishop airport in 2002 on their return from a photography workshop in Alaska.

Leaving Bishop, I crossed into Nevada, another new state for me, and headed south on NV 264. I found a nice campsite with a fire pit off of a muddy dirt road and thought I might try to light a fire that night, since at 3 P.M. it was so cold that I could already see my breath. But the stack of wood at the campsite proved too wet to ignite, and I had to endure another cold night in my tent.

The next day, Boundary Peak proved a lot harder to climb than I had anticipated. First, there was a lot more snow than I had bargained for, and I had to use my snowshoes more than I would have liked. Second, once reaching the ridgeline, there was a lot of scree to deal with, which, as I have said, is not my favorite surface. Finally, let's face it, I was still pretty wiped from climbing Whitney in those uncomfortable boots three days before. Thankfully, I had a more comfortable pair of boots on for this climb.

Gaining the summit, I thought I had pulled a Clarence King and climbed the wrong peak; the mountain next to me was definitely higher than the one I was on. But then I remembered that the state border runs directly through the saddle between 13,146-foot Boundary Peak and neighboring Montgomery Peak—300 feet higher—which is on the California side. In fact, a survey conducted in 1873 placed Boundary Peak on the California side, as well, but a subsequent survey in 1899 established the current boundary, though even that borderline was not finalized until 1980. Had the 1873 border stood, Wheeler Peak in Great Basin National Park near the Utah border would be the highest point in Nevada.

Upon opening the metal Army footlocker that doubled as a register canister, I discovered that I was the first person to sign into the logbook since the previous October, six months before. Winter summiters, however, might not have been able to find this box, as it would have been buried under deep snow.

Crossing back over the saddle between Boundary's summit and a subsidiary peak along the ridge crest, I emerged at the top of a steep, snow-filled gully, which I could plainly see led down to the trail I had ascended earlier in the day. I decided it would make a great shortcut, enabling me to avoid reclimbing this ancillary peak, which was littered with scree.

As soon as I stepped off the ridge and past an overhanging cornice, I found myself on rock-hard crust. I slipped and sped down the icy slope on my butt. Several small boulders protruded from the snow and I frantically grabbed at them as I sped past, but I just bounced off, bruising my backside. About 2,000 feet below, huge boulders the size of cars stretched across this gully like the bumpers of a giant pinball machine. I panicked. There was apparently nothing to keep me from rocketing down this steep slope directly into them.

Then, almost as suddenly as it began, my slide stopped. The icy crust gave way to deep powder, putting the brakes on my rapid descent. The hard crust had been exposed only at the top of the gully, where wind had peeled away a blanket of snow.

Disaster averted, I safely glissaded to the bottom in just a matter of minutes. My clothes, however, were now soaked. I stripped naked on a large, flat rock and put on shorts and a T-shirt for the hike back to the car, as it was now much warmer at this lower elevation.

Getting back on US 6, I continued east for another 50 miles to the junction of NV 375, better known as the Extraterrestrial Highway. I drove until almost dark, when I pulled off the road into a little wash below an earthen dam and set up camp out of the wind and out of sight of any passing cars, had there been any. I later read that only about 200 cars a day travel the road, making it one of the most desolate routes in America.

It's called the Extraterrestrial Highway because of its proximity to Area 51. In 1989, an engineer named Bob Lazar, who claimed to have worked on alien spacecraft at Area 51, became a local media sensation, and, in 1996, the Nevada Commission on Tourism decided to capitalize on the publicity by renaming NV 375 as the "Extraterrestrial Highway." They erected a sign to that effect in the tiny oasis of Rachel, the only town on the 98-mile stretch of blacktop. While tourism didn't increase much, the area reportedly still generates two or three reports of UFO encounters every week.

The following morning, I thought I might have had one myself. Getting back onto the highway, I drove no more than a quarter-mile before the Passat's engine suddenly quit, leaving me stranded more than 100 miles from the nearest service station and a long way from any cell phone reception. I sat there for quite a while, with the hood up, before a cable company van finally happened by and the driver stopped to assist me. Upon leaving, he promised to call the state police as soon as he had phone service, but that might not be for hours, I reckoned.

Fortunately, about 15 minutes later, I tried the key again and the car started right up as if there had never been a problem. That's when I started to wonder if I had just had a close encounter of my own. I had no further problems the rest of the day, driving all the way to Zion National Park to begin my whirlwind tour of Utah's five national parks, skipping the state's snowbound highpoint, Kings Peak, as planned.

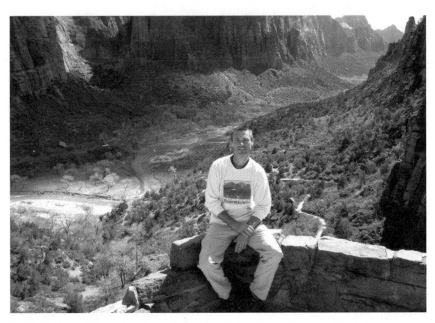

Not for the faint of heart, Angels Landing in Zion National Park offers breathtaking views.

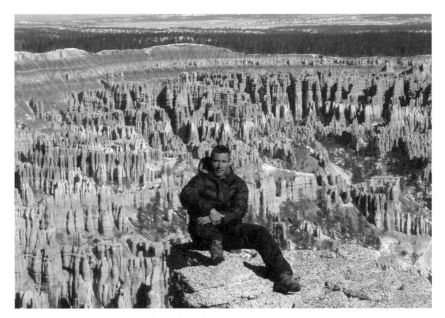
A stunning vista, Bryce Canyon National Park features distinctive rock formations called hoodoos, formed by frost weathering and stream erosion of the river and lake bed sedimentary rocks.

In the morning, my car would not start again. I called AAA, had it towed to the city of St. George, and paid $190 to have a new coil installed. Turned out it wasn't aliens after all, but I had to consider myself extremely lucky that my car hadn't quit for good in the middle of nowhere, as it nearly had the day before.

I was back in Zion by early afternoon and figured I had enough time to visit just one of the many attractions in the park. The woman at the tollbooth said I should make that Angels Landing, and she was right.

The climb to Angels Landing was spectacular. The 2.5-mile trail, cut out of solid rock in 1926, heads straight up the side of a cliff to a narrow canyon and a promontory, then zigzags on some more narrow switchbacks to an airy summit. But this was just the beginning. From there, the path continues along a knife's-edge ridge that drops nearly 1,400 feet on either side. It then works its way along a shelf system of slippery ledges that tilt out over the canyon. Steps chiseled into the slickrock and chains bolted to the wall offer firm hand- and footholds, but it is still a very dangerous place. The park's website says that five people have died from falls off Angels Landing; another site listed at least eight names.

Once at the top, I was greeted by stunning 360-degree views up and down the canyon. It started to snow, so I quickly retraced my steps back to safer ground. I had wanted to hike through the Zion Narrows, a popular slot canyon where one hikes right in the ice-cold river, but that excursion would have to wait until 2012, when I returned to Zion. Instead, I headed for Bryce Canyon National

Park, exiting Zion through a mile-long tunnel built in 1920 that had windows cut out of the rock every quarter-mile so I could look out from the cliff face as I drove along.

Near the entrance to Bryce, I pulled up a side road and found a nice campsite out of view of any passing cars, and prepared for another cold night. Bryce is at 9,000 feet, and several inches of snow fell on my tent overnight. I couldn't even cook anything for breakfast in the morning, as my water jug had frozen solid.

After stopping at all the obligatory viewpoints along Bryce's 15-mile, dead-end road the next morning, I headed for the Grand Staircase-Escalante, a road that slowly climbed up a narrow ridge—and by narrow, I mean it was no wider than the road at times, with harrowing drops of more than a thousand feet on either side—before topping out and abruptly dropping through a series of switchbacks into the tiny town of Boulder, Utah.

There, I turned off on the Burr Trail, an incredible drive through a narrow canyon with steep red cliffs shooting up hundreds of feet on both sides. This road followed this canyon for more than 30 miles before dropping through another series of switchbacks to the Waterpocket Fold, the back door to Capitol Reef National Park. This uplifted warp in the Earth's crust runs for more than 100 miles to the north. Driving this dusty dirt road through the middle of the fold, I went more than 40 miles without seeing another car, and so much dust made its way into my trunk that even my pots and pans were filled with dirt— and they had lids on them. I wanted to stop and take pictures, but pretty soon everything started to look the same—it was all gorgeous.

Later, at Canyonlands National Park, I found that all the campsites in the park were taken—it being a Friday night—but, at the last site, I saw two guys cooking dinner and asked if I could share their site with them, reimbursing them the full $10 fee.

I had just enough time before dark to get to the Grand View Overlook to partake in the daily sunset extravaganza along with several other sightseers. It was much like watching the daily sunset celebration at Mallory Square in Key West, which I have done a few times, only Grand View had fewer street performers. As the sun set, shadows crept across the deep Colorado River basin below me, with only the tops of the hundreds of spires lit up by the remaining sunlight, like so many birthday candles. The guys whose site I was staying at were there too, and they snapped some pictures of me standing on the edge of one of the cliffs, with the Colorado winding gracefully far below.

Getting back in my car, I noticed that everything—especially me—smelled horribly. I had not taken a shower in five days since leaving Lone Pine. It was a good thing I was traveling alone.

The next day, I headed straight for Arches National Park, just down the road toward Moab. Just the drive in to Arches was mind-numbing, as the roadway switchbacked up onto a broad plateau, where a chorus line of fluted rock fins jutting into the brilliant blue sky saluted me as I passed. It was all sensory overload.

At the tollbooth, I was informed that I needed a permit to hike alone in what is known as the Fiery Furnace, a trail-less labyrinth of sandstone walls hiding a maze of narrow passages, which I had hoped to visit. Only seventy-five permits a day are issued, and I was lucky to snag the final one at the visitor center. After eating lunch at the arch-filled Devils Garden and checking out several other arches, I headed into the Fiery Furnace, where people reportedly have gotten lost for days. I could see why: there were no trails or signs anywhere—just row upon row of parallel passageways that all seemed to lead to dead-ends at cliff faces or sheer dropoffs.

I promised myself not to downclimb anything that I couldn't climb back up, since I didn't know if I would have to return the same way. I came to one such place with about a 12-foot drop and was about to turn back when I heard voices coming from farther down the canyon, which I guessed to be from a guided tour group. So I jumped down—assuming I could find a way to continue in the direction they were traveling—and went around the next corner, only to see the group standing 30 feet below me in a wash. There was no way for me to climb down to them without a rope.

Hiking back to the 12-foot cliff I had jumped down, I didn't see any way for me to get back to the top, and began wondering how long I could last on the small bottle of water I was carrying and a couple of Clif Bars. The walls were smooth, but then I noticed there was a hole in the roof of the overhang above me, just big enough for me to slip through. I shimmied up the corner of the wall like I was climbing a chimney and pushed my backpack up through the hole first. Then, somehow, I pulled myself up through this hole, wondering where my sudden upper-body strength had come from. I guess I had gone into survival mode.

I explored several narrow slot canyons, having to crawl on my hands and knees through the soft, cool dirt to get through some of the tighter squeezes.

Once safely back at the car, I headed for the park's signature landmark: Delicate Arch, the 65-foot freestanding sandstone monument that is depicted on the Utah license plate. The hike to Delicate Arch is a mile and a half along more slickrock, and the final part crosses a narrow shelf that winds around the side of a bluff, hiding views of the famous arch until the last possible moment. After hiking up to it, through it, and around it—getting pictures from all angles—I climbed up on a flat rock bench opposite the arch, which was basking in the late-afternoon sunshine.

After shadows began creeping in, I headed out, driving into Moab, an adventure paradise. It was exactly as I had pictured it to be: a mountain bike or a kayak (or both) on top of every car, most of which were either Jeeps or Subarus. Someone suggested I spend the night at Kings Bottom, a campground 4 miles south of town right on the Colorado River, and that sounded just about perfect.

Arriving there, however, I found the place completely full. But a young woman motioned me over and told me they were leaving to get a motel room, since they had forgotten their tent poles. I offered to loan them my big tent if they let me share the site in my one-man tent, but they bequeathed the entire site to me instead. After a dinner of beans and franks, I considered hitting some of the hip-looking bars I had seen in town, but I remembered how bad I smelled. Instead, I went to a store and bought a six-pack of Coronas and hung out with my neighbors—Ken and John, a couple of mountain bikers from Denver— making sure I sat downwind. They had a nice fire going, and we sat up drinking beer and listening to loud music until 2 A.M. I can't believe that none of the other campers complained about the ruckus we made.

Crossing the Colorado border the next morning, I turned south on US 550 at Grand Junction and headed for my favorite hostel in Leadville. Fortunately, I would not have to reclimb Mount Elbert, the Colorado highpoint, as I had already done that on my first visit to the Rockies, in 2006. I had hoped to hear from my friend Kari, but it turned out she was still wintering in San Felipe, Mexico. Missing her, I got to Leadville with plenty of daylight remaining. Five inches of snow was forecast for the night, and I didn't want to get trapped if the storm shut I-70 down, so I decided to drive on.

When I got to the interstate, I found traffic at a standstill, the lanes clogged with urbanites returning to Denver after spending the weekend skiing. It was nearly dark when I descended the Front Range and turned north onto I-25. At some point during the day, I passed my trip's 10,000-mile mark. I made it as far as Boyd Lake State Park in Loveland, where I camped on a muddy cement slab within direct view of the caretaker's RV, though he never came out to collect a fee, and once again I snuck out in the morning without paying. This campground was quite disappointing, but it was off-season, so perhaps they planned to clean it up and do something about the smell of raw sewage before opening for the season.

The next morning, I crossed into Wyoming, but that state highpoint was not on my agenda for this trip, either; I'd need to come back to get Gannett Peak sometime in the future. Heading east again, I crossed into Nebraska and drove to Panorama Point, the highpoint tucked into the corner of the panhandle only a mile from the Colorado and Wyoming borders. I was able to drive to within a hundred yards of the "summit," which like Kansas was just a slight bump on an endless prairie, and then walked to a stone monument that looked more like someone's gravestone.

It started to snow as I got on NE 71 and headed north toward South Dakota. The roads were especially slippery, though mostly devoid of traffic, as whiteout conditions persisted until late afternoon. I drove into Custer State Park around 3:30 P.M. and found the trailhead to Harney Peak. I figured I had just enough time to bag another peak today, as the guidebook said the round-trip to Harney Peak, South Dakota's highpoint, was only 6.8 miles on an easy trail.

It snowed hard throughout the climb, however, and the wind was blowing at near gale force when I reached a set of metal steps leading up the side of a rock escarpment. I ascended, and out of the gloaming emerged a medieval-looking stone fortress. I had not expected it, as I had failed to read beyond the trail info in my guidebook. This large stone tower, built on Harney Peak by the Civilian Conservation Corps during the Great Depression, was used as a fire tower until 1967. I felt like I was in an abandoned castle as I walked around the place, which had snowdrifts piled up in every corner. The book also said there were magnificent views of the surrounding Black Hills, but I could barely see my hand in front of my face. At 7,242 feet, there isn't a point higher than Harney Peak east of there until you reach the Pyrenees in Europe.

It was dark long before I got back to my car, and I was cold, wet, and hungry by the time I found a motel room in the town of Custer a short distance away. Once in my room, the TV weatherman revealed that the snow, still coming down, was just the front end of a blizzard that was supposed to shut down the western part of the state overnight. The roads I needed to take in the morning to get to the North Dakota highpoint were the same ones that were expected to be closed because of the weather. And, worse, there could be more snow just about every day that week. As much as a foot was expected by morning.

I'd spent my summers umpiring softball for the past ten years or so. I can imagine the uproar it would cause on the field if my calls were only as accurate as that weatherman's forecasts. By morning, the roads were clear and the storm left only a couple of more inches on the ground. I stopped at the Crazy Horse Memorial on my way to Mount Rushmore, and even though the visitor centers at both places were closed because of the storm, the parking lots were being plowed and the presidents' heads were still up on the mountainside, though they all looked like they had dandruff problems.

The only other people I saw at Mount Rushmore were a couple in a pickup with Alaska plates. When they saw my New Hampshire plates, they gave me a knowing smile; only hardy folks from cold-weather states would consider this a good day for sightseeing.

From there, I drove back into Wyoming and headed for Devils Tower, a place that intrigued me even before *Close Encounters of the Third Kind*. The tower is sacred to more than twenty American Indian tribes, including the Arapaho, Crow, Lakota, Cheyenne, Kiowa, and Shoshone. Many stories are told about the tower, but a common thread among them is an origin story about a giant bear scratching the deep grooves into the steep sides of the 1,200-foot butte. Noted Kiowa author N. Scott Momaday once wrote, "There are things in nature that engender an awful quiet in the heart of man; Devils Tower is one of them."

Deemed "inaccessible to anything without wings" by geologist Henry Newton in 1875, Devils Tower was climbed for the first time in 1893 by two local ranchers who built a 350-foot wooden ladder by driving stakes into the cracks running between two columns. More than a thousand people were on hand that Fourth of July to witness this achievement.

Thousands of people have climbed it since, most notably climbing legend Jack Durrance, who, in 1938, pioneered the most popular route to the top. In 1941, a man named George Hopkins parachuted onto the summit, but lost the rope he jumped with and was stranded on the top for six days. Goodyear offered to send a blimp to rescue him, and the Navy offered an untested helicopter, but in the end Durrance climbed up and brought Hopkins down. The incident gained worldwide publicity and caused a spike in tourism, just as *Close Encounters* later would.

I drove into the closed visitor center and snapped a few pictures. Any climbing I might have wished to do would have to wait for better weather. Back in South Dakota, I turned north on dead-straight SD 85 for a 150-mile drive through barren countryside; there was not a tree to be seen anywhere. Crossing into North Dakota, another new state for me, it wasn't long before I was driving down a dirt road toward the trailhead for a short 2-mile hike to the summit of White Butte.

The trailhead was down a half-mile-long driveway that led to a farmhouse. I noticed a snowdrift blocking the road ahead of me, but it did not appear that deep. I gunned the engine, thinking I could simply plow through it. I was wrong. I got about halfway across this hundred-foot-wide drift and got stuck tighter than a fly in a spiderweb. I couldn't move. Getting out, I cursed the owners of the farmhouse, which I could see in the distance, for failing to plow their driveway after the most recent storm. Later, though, I would realize that apparently no one lived there anymore, so it was no wonder it hadn't been plowed.

As luck would have it, my brother had given me a mountaineer's snow shovel— the kind with the short handle—for a birthday present while I was visiting him in California. I fished it out of my overloaded trunk and started shoveling. It took me more than an hour to dig the car out, and I must have stripped 5,000 miles of tread off my tires spinning back and forth trying to free it. And, once done, I still had the damn mountain to climb.

That part wasn't so hard, as it was a short stroll down an old farm road and then a short climb of just 400 feet to the summit of White Butte, whose elevation is 3,506. I could have benefitted from bringing my snowshoes, as the drifts were deep on this farm road too. It being March, at least I didn't have to worry about rattlesnakes; my guidebook cautioned that the place can be crawling with them in summer months. I can't say when the last visitor had been on White Butte's summit; the logbook had not been properly stowed in the metal case and was ruined by water and dirt.

Because of my mishap, I didn't cross back into South Dakota until it was too dark to look for a campsite, so I resigned myself to getting another room. I stopped in the town of Belle Fourche, which, I was soon corrected by the motel proprietor, is pronounced, "Bel-Foosh." In 1959, after Alaska and Hawaii were admitted to the union, it was determined that the new geographic center of the United States was located just north of Belle Fourche. I stopped at the monument commemorating this the next morning, then attempted to leave South Dakota. But, try as I might, I couldn't seem to accomplish this. I hadn't realized that South Dakota was such a big state. It seemed to take me all day to cover the 400 miles on I-90, though I did detour through Badlands National Park, which I thought paled in comparison with its counterparts in Utah that were still fresh on my mind.

I took another short detour into Iowa to bag Hawkeye Point, which was just a couple of miles over the Iowa–Minnesota border and next to a silo near some farmer's cornfield. At least this highpoint had a protected register book.

I pulled into Myre–Big Island State Park near Albert Lea, Minnesota, about an hour later, surprised to see the gate open, since no one else was there. Once again, I got away without paying, though it had long since become more of a game than about the money. Even though I had lost an hour by crossing back into the Central Time Zone for the first time since Oklahoma two months before, I had enough daylight left at 8 P.M. to set up camp and eat dinner without using my headlamp. The days were getting longer, as it was now April 1, and I would be home in a week.

But, I still had six more state highpoints to bag before then.

The next day, I turned north again, driving 300 miles to the Minnesota panhandle above Lake Superior. The interstate ended in Duluth, leaving me with a 90-mile drive up the north shore of the lake, which appeared as broad as an ocean from here. The same storm that had caught me on Harney Peak had dumped 2 feet of snow on this part of Minnesota, and I was worried that the back roads I needed to take to get to the trailhead for Eagle Mountain might still be snowbound. I stopped at the Lutsen General Store to inquire about this and was given detailed directions to the trailhead, which I might not have found otherwise. In rural areas, I always found it best to ask the locals for directions, but this never seemed to work in the cities; urbanites seem to have no sense of direction whatsoever.

It was a 21-mile drive on dirt roads to the trailhead parking lot, which had yet to be plowed, so I had to leave my car precariously in the roadway, hoping it wouldn't hinder the plow drivers. It was a glorious 3.5-mile hike through fresh, deep powder to the summit, and my snowshoes handled it well. The trail ended in a clearing that appeared to be the highest ground around. I could not find any marker designating the exact spot, and ended up trekking all around this clearing trying to find the highest point. The guidebook said there was a plaque attached to a rock, but it was likely under several feet of snow, and I never located it. I am sure the next person who visited this spot wondered why I had tracked up the entire clearing, probably thinking I was drunk.

After hiking back to my car and driving back to the main road, I did not hold out much hope of finding a campground open in northern Minnesota on April 2, what with spring still weeks away. Sure enough, the Split Rock Lighthouse and Gooseberry Falls campgrounds were both closed, and I figured I would just have to bite the bullet and get a motel room in Duluth. Approaching the town of Two Harbors, however, I saw a state police car parked next to the road and stopped to ask him if he knew of any place I might be able to camp that night, explaining to him my highpointing quest. He made a quick call and told me that the road leading to the county fairgrounds had been plowed out, and, if I wanted to, I could throw up a tent on the pavement at the end of the road. I had no problem with that, and spent a cozy night camped in the middle of a city street.

If the early settlers of Michigan had been better shots, the state highpoint would likely be on the Mitten—Briar Hill near the city of Cadillac—rather than Mount Arvon on the Upper Peninsula.

There is, if you are unaware, a blatant animosity between the states of Ohio and Michigan. Most people know about the intense college football rivalry between their teams and their legendary former coaches, Woody Hayes and Bo Schembechler, respectively. The Ohio State Buckeyes and the University of Michigan Wolverines met annually in what was known as the "Ten-Year War" from 1969 to 1978. In 1973, both teams were undefeated when they squared off in the final game of the season, with the winner earning a trip to the Rose Bowl. When the game ended tied 10–10, the remaining members of the Big Ten were left to select the Rose Bowl participant by secret ballot. Michigan's Schembechler and the Wolverine fans were infuriated when they didn't get the nod. Lawsuits were threatened, claiming an Ohio conspiracy.

Most people don't know that the discord between the two states actually dates all the way to 1835, when they took up arms against each other in the little-known Toledo War. A dispute had arisen over the exact geographic boundary between the state of Ohio and the territory of Michigan. Both parties laid claim to the Toledo Strip, a 5- to 8-mile-wide swath of land that might have seemed insignificant, except that it included the port of Toledo, located on Maumee Bay on Lake Erie. It was an important port at the time, since shipping was still the most expedient means of getting goods to market, as the steam train had yet to replace water travel. The Harris Line, a more recently surveyed border between the states, became the front of the tensions.

Both states raised militias. On April 26, 1835, a group of Ohio surveyors refused the Michigan militia's orders to withdraw from the Harris Line. The soldiers fired shots and started what became known as the Battle of Phillips Corner. No one was injured, as apparently all the shots missed their targets. The Michiganders later claimed they had not aimed at the Buckeyes, but instead had fired "forty or fifty" warning shots over their heads.

Either way, the escalating situation forced President Andrew Jackson to step in. In June 1836, he put the arm-twist on Michigan by signing a bill that would grant Michigan statehood, making it eligible to receive much-needed federal funds—the militia had virtually bankrupted the territorial government—but only if it ceded its claim to the Toledo Strip. In return, Michigan would receive compensation in the form of the Upper Peninsula, though at the time the land was considered worthless wilderness. Michiganders felt they had been dealt a bad hand. At first, they refused this consolation prize, but later acquiesced under additional pressure from Washington.

Within ten years, however, vast deposits of copper, and later iron, were discovered on the Upper Peninsula, and for nearly 100 years this region was the only place on Earth where copper was found in such extensive quantities. The area produced more than 90 percent of the copper in the world at the turn of the century. Vast fortunes were made before more economical findings in Arizona and Chile put many of Michigan's mines out of business.

In retrospect, considering the current reputation of Toledo, it certainly appears that Michigan was the real winner of the Toledo War, even if it couldn't shoot straight.

Which was why I was heading to the Upper Peninsula after crossing the top of Wisconsin along the shores of Lake Superior on this chilly April morning. Mount Arvon, at 1,979 feet, is located about 12 miles east of the town of L'Anse, which itself is tucked at the base of the Keewenah Peninsula, which juts into Lake Superior like the horn of a rhino. Spring comes late there, and I was worried that the long approach to Mount Arvon over several dirt roads might not yet be passable.

And that's exactly what the guy at the next pump told me when I was gassing up after arriving in L'Anse. The roads were still snow-covered and being used only by snowmobiles, he said, and I was looking at a hike of several miles to reach the summit. I said I didn't have time for a long hike; I needed to get to the Wisconsin highpoint later that day. He joked about giving me his cell phone number so I could call him to come pull me out after I got stuck, but then laughed and said there was no cell service in there anyway. "Good luck," he said, as he pulled away.

Leaving L'Anse, I had a 14-mile drive on the main road before I turned onto a dirt road that was easily navigable for the 5 miles needed to reach Ravine River Road, the turnoff to Mount Arvon. Here, things looked sketchy: the road was plowed only to the width of one car, and after 2 miles it dead-ended at a snowbank. But I could see that the road continued beyond and was covered by hard-packed snow from extensive snowmobile use. Not relishing a round-trip hike of 12 miles from this spot, I gunned the engine and held on tight.

The Passat plunged through the snowbank onto the snowmobile trail like I was competing in the Winter X Games. Fortunately, it was firm underneath, sort of like slushy ice, as the snow had apparently melted and refrozen many times. The trail was relatively flat, and I drove 4 miles on this path until I reached a T junction, and dared to drive no farther. The snow was now soft underneath and I feared getting stuck, what with nearly bald tires, the treads now virtually bare after getting stuck in that snowdrift in North Dakota. In fact, I did get stuck momentarily while turning my car around at this intersection, but after a few tense moments, I was able to get it pointed in the right direction for the drive out.

Leaving the car, I followed the snowmobile trail, which was marked by blue diamond-shaped markers on the trees, and it led me directly to the summit of Mount Arvon. Until I saw the sign for the highpoint, however, I was unsure I was in the right place, since all the surroundings looked the same. This had previously caused confusion: until a 1982 survey, nearby Mount Curwood, and not Mount Arvon, was considered the state's highest spot. The 4-mile round-trip took me little more than an hour, and, thankfully, I had no problem driving out on the snowmobile trail back to the main road.

It had been a foolhardy gamble, but it was one that paid off. I reached Timm's Hill, the highpoint of Wisconsin, later that afternoon, and then pulled into Cooper Dam Campground with just enough daylight to set up camp and cook dinner. I would not have to sneak out of this campground in the morning, as the local Westboro Conservation Corps provided it for free. Once again, I had the place to myself, and it was deathly quiet, except for the sound of the rushing Jump River, swollen from snowmelt, just a few yards away.

I had only a short drive the next day to the town of Galena, Illinois, in the extreme northwest corner of the state, where I would be going to church the following morning and climbing the state highpoint in the afternoon.

Charles Mound, the highpoint of Illinois, is on private property owned by Wayne and Jean Wuebbels, about 11 miles east of Galena and within a stone's throw of the Wisconsin border. The Wuebbelses open their property for two or three weekends a year for peakbaggers to come and check Charles Mound off their list. Unfortunately, April 4-5, 2009, had not been one of those weekends.

Prior to my trip, I had contacted the Wuebbelses and explained my quest and my schedule, in hopes they would relent and let me come in April, sort of like when Mr. Hill allowed me to climb Culebra Peak in Colorado. But Jean Wuebbels's return email was determined. Basically, it read like this: "We have gone out of our way over the years to accommodate you peakbaggers who want to climb Charles Mound, but we cannot make exceptions for those like you who want to come here whenever it suits your schedule, and not ours. Unfortunately, I will have to decline your request. You can come back during the two weekends in the summer when we will open Charles Mound to the public."

Then, she added a P.S.: "Unless you want to go to church with us."

I laughed out loud. I didn't care if they were a bunch of Bible-thumping rattlesnake handlers; come Sunday morning, I was going to be in the front pew with them.

Once, Galena had been one of the biggest cities in Illinois, as lead mining swelled the population to more than 14,000 in the mid-1800s, but now fewer than 4,000 people lived here, and tourism has long since become the main industry. Located tight on the banks of the Galena River, just a mile or so from the Mississippi, the town has endured several destructive floods in its history, including one in 1828 in which the water rose so high that steamships were seen traveling on Main Street. Because of the continued danger, huge floodgates were erected at both ends of the downtown district in 1951, and they have successfully prevented millions of dollars in damage since.

I drove to the Galena Bible Church at 10:20 on April 5, and met Wayne and Jean Wuebbels, a couple whom I guessed to be in their late 50s. Everyone welcomed them when they arrived. As it was Palm Sunday, a week before Easter, the sermon was about the persecution of Jesus leading up to the Crucifixion, and I thought the pastor did a good job. Afterward, we went to lunch with another couple from church at a place called Happy Joe's, and I appreciatively bought the Wuebbelses their meal. It was the least I could do, since they were making such an exception for me.

Before leaving to drive to their house—the Wuebbelses were headed to Walmart to do their weekly shopping—Jean told me that they often get requests from peakbaggers such as me who want to climb Charles Mound out of season, but they routinely offer the same terms I'd been extended. So far, she said, I had been the only person to take them up on their offer.

It was quite windy, with some snow flurries in the air, when I walked up their driveway and into their backyard, where a benchmark and a register book marked the highpoint.

Leaving Galena, I began the final leg of my journey to my trip's final two state highpoints—Indiana and Ohio, both drive-ups. Crossing Indiana, I got off the interstate just before the Ohio state line and headed north for an 11-mile detour to Hoosier Point—the Indiana state highpoint, marked by a stone cairn at the edge of some woods.

It has been reported that a landfill in Randolph County may, in fact, be higher than Hoosier Point, but for peakbagging purposes, only natural highpoints are considered; otherwise the roof of the Four Seasons Hotel in Miami would be the highest point in Florida. Likewise, some believe that the Rumpke Sanitary Landfill, also known as Mount Rumpke, is the highest point in Ohio. Located just north of Cincinnati, this landfill stands at 1,075 feet above sea level, but that is still nearly 500 feet lower than Campbell Hill, where I was headed that afternoon.

Campbell Hill is not the most natural of highpoints either, as it sits on the campus of the Ohio Hi-Point Career Center near the town of Bellefontaine, and was once a Nike missile site owned by the Air Force. It was raining slightly when I arrived, and I was gone again within minutes, heading northeast for the drive home.

Late that afternoon, I slipped silently into a deserted Geneva State Park, located about 45 miles east of Cleveland and only a short distance from the shores of Lake Erie. I drove to the most sheltered site I could find at the end of a cul-de-sac and hoped I wouldn't be spotted, as I once again was in "stealth mode." Cooking dinner, I saw what appeared to be a police car stop at the end of this cul-de-sac, but it continued on, and I spent my final night in my tent very comfortably despite snow flurries that left a dusting on the ground by morning.

It was hard to keep my speed under control during the 500-mile drive back to New England the next day, as the horse could smell the barn. I was fortunate not to have gotten another speeding ticket. Had New York's Mount Marcy been my only remaining lower 48 state highpoint, I might have made the detour north to finish the list. But since I still had several more remaining in the Pacific Northwest, I decided that a trip to the Adirondacks could wait for another day. I saw my first New Hampshire license plate just as I was getting off I-787 in Troy, New York, and then drove familiar roads across southern Vermont to arrive home in Keene, New Hampshire, by late afternoon.

The first thing I did after collecting three months of mail at the post office was to drive straight to City Tire. My state inspection had expired while I was away, and there was no way my completely bald tires would pass.

Getting to my apartment, I checked the odometer on my car and did the math: 14,321 miles and thirty-four state highpoints. It had been an incredible trip, an experience never to forget.

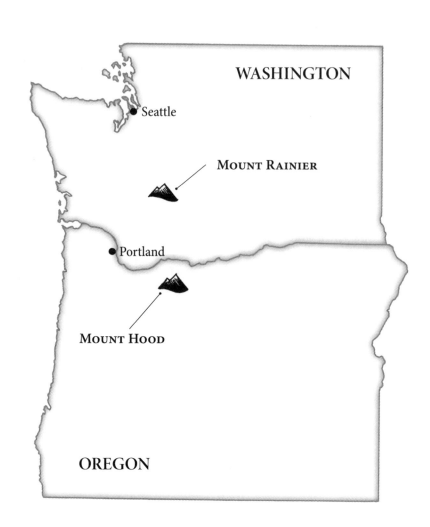

WASHINGTON

Seattle

MOUNT RAINIER

Portland

MOUNT HOOD

OREGON

THE PACIFIC NORTHWEST

Chapter 10
Summer 2009

AFTER THE THREE-MONTH BACKPACKING TRIP TO CENTRAL AMERICA IN 2008, I HAD come back to New Hampshire without a place to live for the first time. It was then that a former coworker told me about an assisted-living arrangement that had provided him free housing, and I looked into it. I was approved as a housemate for a man with Down syndrome, and in May 2008, I had moved into his apartment, where my "job" was to look after him through the night while we both slept.

The arrangement worked so well that when I had announced plans to go on the three-month cross-country trip in 2009, the agency allowed me the freedom to go on the trip and return to the assisted-living situation upon my return, just as I had done that previous September during my final trip to climb the Colorado 14ers. I was quite fortunate that my roommate enjoyed my company and that the agency continued to grant me great liberties for other excursions.

For example, in May 2009, I drove to Virginia and completed the Massanutten Mountian 100-miler. The running I'd done earlier in the year—on the course, during my travels, and when I got home—proved invaluable: when I came back a few months later, I finished in just over 25 hours, taking eleventh place overall.

That same month, I got an email from Tom Yukman, whom I had met, along with his wife, Sandi, on that climb of the Crestones during my most recent trip to Colorado the previous September. They had booked a trip to climb Mount Rainier in Washington and invited me to join them. I jumped at the chance, even though the trip would be guided and would cost almost $1,000 just for the outfitter. Having summited so many technical peaks solo, the idea of joining a group that would be guided at the pace of the slowest hiker did not appeal to me. But Rainier was one of the seven remaining state highpoints to check off my Lower 48 list, and was a 14er to boot. Plus, it is one of the most coveted climbs in North America. And we would be on the summit on the Fourth of July. It was an exciting opportunity and worth forsaking my usual preference to climb alone.

While there, I figured that I might as well climb Mount Hood, the highpoint of Oregon, too. My friend Dave Targan, the park ranger from Mount Monadnock, had climbed both peaks, the latter with Van just the year before. He was glad I would be using a guide service on Rainier, and warned me against attempting to climb Hood by myself. While the danger of falling into a crevasse was minimal, falling debris dislodged by other climbers above had contributed to many of the roughly 150 recorded deaths on Hood and to countless more injuries. When Dave and Van climbed Hood, they had been roped together on the steep crater wall when someone above dropped a water bottle. It rocketed down the slope and passed directly between Van's legs before striking another climber far below, breaking the man's shoulder. It was lucky no one was killed, Dave said.

Though the Massanutten 100-miler had been perfect endurance training for the mountains ahead, I came out of the race with a nagging Achilles problem. But all of the other pieces fell into place. UPS granted me time off in late June, and I headed to the Pacific Northwest.

My trip began in Seattle at the home of Charles Bookman—whom I had met in Mexico soon after meeting his son Zac. I planned to stay with him and his wife, Andrea, for a couple of days before heading to the mountains. Charles, too, said he was quite concerned about my intention to attempt Mount Hood by myself. So I called Doug Seitz, a local climber and a friend of a woman I had briefly dated in New Hampshire. She'd given me the impression that he would likely be busy, so I asked if he could recommend a climbing partner. But Doug immediately said he was free and would love to join me.

I picked Doug up at his apartment near the University of Washington campus a couple of days later. The massive shadow of Mount Rainier loomed over us as we headed south on I-5 for the 4-hour drive to Oregon. Soon, Mount Hood was clearly in our view, a massive behemoth, though seemingly not the feared dragon that I had been expecting. I mean, several of the peaks in Colorado looked more sinister from the same distance—the Maroon Bells immediately came to mind.

We camped under the open sky in a glade beneath some ponderosa pines a couple of miles from the ski area where we would begin our ascent. I think I was still awake when our alarm went off at 1 A.M. We broke camp and were at the parking lot to begin our climb just 40 minutes later.

More than 10,000 people climb Mount Hood every year, making it the most-climbed glaciated peak in North America. Perhaps the only glaciated peak in the world that sees more climbers each year is Mount Fuji in Japan.

We climbed steadily past the ski area on ever-steepening slopes. Now, normally I am setting the pace. Not on this day. Doug led the hike the entire time, not because he knew the way, but because I couldn't keep up with him. I could have blamed this on the nagging Achilles problem or on the tight-fitting and uncomfortable mountaineering boots I had borrowed for the trip, or on the fact that I hadn't slept a wink, or on the twenty years I had on him. All of these were true, but even on a good day, I would not have been able to match Doug's pace. It was one of the few times I have felt humbled with a backpack on.

As for being my usual organized self, my pack was ass-backward; when we stopped an hour or so into the climb to put on crampons, I had to dig everything out of it in order to reach mine on the bottom. I had about six items in my hands when I finally dug them out, then accidentally dropped my helmet. The thing went skittering down the steep slope like a turtle on its back until we couldn't hear it anymore in the darkness.

"Crevasse," Doug announced. I suspected he was right; my helmet had evidently disappeared over the lip of one of the gaping fissures we had skirted on the way up, lost for eternity.

All I could do was shrug my shoulders and try to get it together. I managed to strap the crampons on, but I was still struggling. When we reached a flat spot at about 10,000 feet, Doug said we should also put our harnesses on in case we needed to rope up later. I got out my harness, also borrowed, to find that I couldn't step through the stirrups without taking my crampons off first. More lost time. At home, I consider myself an accomplished hiker, but here I was coming across to Doug as an embarrassing beginner.

Despite my plodding, we reached the summit in just 4 hours 45 minutes, the first two climbers to stand on the summit on that glorious July 1. Two other climbers promptly arrived from the other direction—having come up the east side of the mountain—and three of the four climbers we had passed on the final slope also soon joined us on the summit. After eating our "lunch" at 7 A.M., we headed back down, meeting others who were ascending and overtaking still others who had taken one look at the final slope and chosen retreat.

When we reached an elevation of about 8,900 feet, Doug said we were at the place where I had dropped my helmet, so we detoured to our left to take a look into some of the crevasses clearly visible below us. I had long since given up hope of retrieving it and was prepared to buy a new one later that day at Second Ascent, an outdoor outfitting store not far from Charles's house, since I had to return to his house anyway, having forgotten my camera there.

We peered into the first crevasse and saw nothing, then made our way to the second one and looked over the edge. Far below, under the lip of a 50-foot wall, was my helmet. But how to get it? Doug noticed that the top end of the crevasse rose up, creating a possible path down into its depths. I put on my harness again and Doug roped me in and belayed me into the maw of the crevasse. The helmet was lying on a little snow bridge, with open gaps on either side that led farther into the depths of the abyss. Walking gingerly, I crept out onto the snow bridge, which, thankfully, held as I retrieved my helmet. I then explored around inside this crevasse for a little while before climbing back out. I think it was the highlight of the day for me; after all, I have climbed hundreds of mountains, but it was the first time I had ever been belayed into a crevasse.

We got back to the car after what had seemed like a full day of climbing to find that it was only 9:30 in the morning. We had completed the round-trip in less than 8 hours, despite my dragging pace for most of the trip; not a record, but a very respectable time nonetheless.

We took the scenic route back to Seattle, going through Hood River, where we had a beer at one of the many brewpubs there. Then we ate a real lunch at a hilltop restaurant overlooking the Columbia River, which is usually teeming with kiteboarders and windsurfers. But not on this day, as the weather was so perfect that not even a wisp of a breeze could be mustered

Back in Seattle, we picked up my camera at Charles's house and then went to Second Ascent anyway, where I bought a new pair of Koflach plastic double-boots, which I hoped would be kinder to my aching feet on Rainier. I was lucky to find them on half-price clearance at a mere $150. Doug and I struck up a good friendship during our two days together, despite our twenty-year age difference, and I told him I looked forward to climbing with him again sometime.

On a clear day, standing at Kerry Park Overlook, a city park in the hilly Queen Anne section of Seattle, the view is perhaps the most incredible I have ever seen in an urban environment. Framed perfectly behind the Seattle Space Needle is the towering presence of Mount Rainier, so massive and so high that I almost swore that the glistening white volcano was a mirage.

Rainier so dominates the horizon that it almost defies description; locals simply refer to it as "the mountain." There is no other like it. Rainier rises more than 13,200 feet above the surrounding plain, giving it a prominence greater even than that of K2, the world's second-highest peak. Cut it off at the base, and it would be the most massive mountain in the United States, greater even than Alaska's Denali, which has connecting ridges.

Dormant, but not extinct, Rainier supports twenty-six major glaciers, and is by far the most glaciated peak in the lower 48. Rainier was thought to have once been much taller—perhaps as high as 16,000 feet—until about 5,000 years ago, when the top of the mountain is believed to have sloughed off in a huge avalanche. The last reported eruptions occurred prior to 1900, but if Rainier were to explode and lose a face in similar fashion to what happened in 1980 at nearby Mount Saint Helens, there would be considerable loss of life and property. Even Seattle might be in its path if the eruption was big enough.

Rainier can be an extremely dangerous mountain to climb, as well. The deaths of six climbers on the Liberty Ridge section of the mountain in May 2014 brought the number of fatalities during summit bids to eighty-nine since 1897, with eleven of those having perished in an avalanche on the Ingraham Glacier in June 1981—the worst climbing accident in U.S. history.

While we would not be attempting the dangerous and technical Liberty Ridge route, we would be crossing the Ingraham Glacier, which is part of the standard route that all the outfitters use to ferry their clients to the summit.

I arrived at Rainier Mountaineering's headquarters in Ashland, Washington, on Thursday afternoon in time for our three o'clock meeting with the entire team and our main guide, Mark Falender. The Yukmans—Tom and Sandi—arrived soon after and it was great to see them again, having climbed with them just that one time on the Crestones the year before. After watching a slide presentation about the climb, Mark took us all outside and had us dump the entire contents of our packs on the ground. He then went over every item on his checklist to make sure we were all properly equipped.

Satisfied, he dismissed the three of us, and we headed up the road to the Copper Creek Inn. I had promised Tom and Sandi dinner would be on me the next time we met; after all, if not for them, I would not have summited the Crestones that day, and would have had to return to Colorado, at great expense, to finish the 14ers. Since then, they had completed the Colorado 14ers themselves while training for our Rainier climb. I couldn't convince Sandi to order anything more than a hamburger, but Tom enjoyed a delicious salmon dinner, and I had the pork tenderloin, which was exquisite. Then came dessert: Copper Creek's famous blackberry pie topped with a big scoop of vanilla ice cream. Normally, I never eat dessert at a restaurant, but this pie was not to pass up.

After spending Friday in "school," learning how to hike a big mountain while roped together, on Saturday we began our ascent, climbing the 4,600 feet or so from the Paradise Jackson Visitor Center to Camp Muir, located at 10,000 feet. The climb is considerably steep, and it's mostly on open snowfields. That day, because of nearly 70-degree temperatures, the snow was soft and slushy. I even got sunburned up the sleeves of my T-shirt from sunlight reflected off the bright, white fields.

We took nearly 6 hours to climb to Camp Muir, named for John Muir, who climbed Rainier by this route in 1888. Once there, we threw our sleeping bags onto one of the eighteen foam pads in the stone hut and then prepared our packs

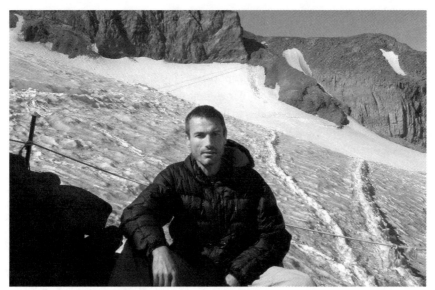

I relax after arriving at Camp Muir on Mount Rainier before an early morning summit bid the following day.

for the summit climb, making sure that they were packed in the reverse order of when we expected to need certain pieces of gear and clothing. Had I properly done this on Hood, I would not have lost my helmet into the crevasse.

Our guides brought out boiling water so we could eat our freeze-dried meals before going to bed—even though it was only 6:30 P.M. and it wouldn't get dark until at least 10. Our wakeup call came at 11:10 P.M., but I had yet to sleep a wink, just like on Hood earlier in the week. We all ate breakfast and waited for the guides to call us out for departure. We left the camp with crampons on and roped up in two groups of nine, each split into three teams of three with a guide at the head of the rope. We crossed the top of the Cowlitz Glacier to Cathedral Gap on then on to Ingraham Flats, where we took our first break after about 90 minutes of constant climbing. Other groups had camped on the snow here to shorten the distance of the summit push. As we passed their vacated tents in the dark, we could see their headlamps on the steep slope above us.

From Ingraham Flats, we crossed a few narrow crevasses by stepping across some and walking on metal ladders stretched across others. We then reached the crux of the climb: Disappointment Cleaver, a rocky ridge that juts out from the mountain, where a lot of tired climbers disappointedly turn around. After traversing under the steep face of the outcropping—this would not be a place to linger later in the day after it warmed up, as rocks often fall here—we zigzagged our way up the rock and dirt slope, glad to get back onto firm snow at the top.

Several more gaping crevasses had to be negotiated before we were beyond the danger and the steepness of the slope lessened.

By now, dawn was breaking, and our pace seemed to be slowing. Mark had put the two least-experienced climbers—Brian and Ryan—on his rope, with me as the fourth person pulling up the rear. I understood why he did this; he put his strongest climber as anchor on the rope behind the two weakest ones, which made for a frustrating experience for me. But I had known when I signed up for this expedition that we would be moving at the pace of the slowest climber, so I should not have been surprised.

That person happened to be Brian. As we approached 13,000 feet, he was about spent. He could barely move and was often incoherent when asked a question by the guides. But they assessed his condition continually and prodded him up the mountain, even though I once urged our third guide, Tyler, to take him back down. While I admit that I was a bit concerned that Brian might keep us all from summiting—especially me, I must selfishly add—I truly felt that Brian was completely exhausted and would have trouble descending.

But the guides apparently knew what they were doing. We arrived at the summit crater at 7:30 A.M., a little later than planned, but all nine of us in our group made it to the top. Later, we learned that two members of the other group of nine had turned back shy of the summit. Finally, we were let off our leashes and everyone scurried to various places on the open crater to pee. But in order to turn my back to everyone, I had to stand facing a 30 MPH wind, so it was a bit of a tricky maneuver that was not entirely successful, as the wet stains on my climbing pants would attest.

Then, some of us crossed the expansive crater and climbed the far rim to the actual highpoint. On our way, we stopped to log into the register book, and then hit the summit of Columbia Crest, the highest of three summits on the peak. It marked my forty-third state highpoint, and it was great to see the elation of the others in the group, some of whom had never climbed a mountain before. Like Ty and Jason, who had hatched the plan to climb Rainier over a bottle of whisky with Ryan a few weeks before. Tom and Sandi each took a can of Rainier beer from Ty, who had carried up a six-pack, and broke one open, toasting the summit in style.

We then all headed back to where we'd left our packs and roped up for the descent. This time, Mark put me in the front and told me to set a strong and steady pace on the way down. This, I liked. It was my reward, I guessed, for being on the end of the slowest rope team coming up. Tyler had already started back down with Brian, and we caught them partway down the mountain. The hardest part was descending the steep and rocky Disappointment Cleaver, which was even harder to climb down than it had been to come up. I have never liked the feel of crampons on dirt and rock; it is so easy to turn an ankle.

We had to scoot quickly under the lip of the cleaver, hoping the warming temperatures wouldn't dislodge any ice or rocks and rain them down on us. Safely across, we approached the many crevasses that now appeared even more massive and threatening in the daylight than they had in the darkness of night. Some appeared bottomless.

After what seemed like an eternity, we were back at Camp Muir and could finally take our crampons off. I can tell you that my feet are never happier than to have crampons removed from them. At least my feet were feeling much better than they had on Hood, thanks to the pair of Koflach boots I had purchased in Seattle a few days earlier. I was very pleased.

While we were all relieved to be back at camp, we still had to pack everything up and hike the couple of hours back to Paradise. But this was the most fun we had on the trip, as there were several steep slopes where the softening snow made for some excellent boot skiing. We arrived at Paradise with sore, wet feet and wide smiles. It had all been worth it.

After a 45-minute bus ride back to Ashland and RMI headquarters, we had a short awards ceremony where we all received certificates of achievement for summiting Rainier. And Brian was now feeling much better—so much so that he announced that the beer was on him, since he felt bad for having slowed us down so much on the ascent. The beer was greatly appreciated, though I could only have a couple: I still had to pack up my gear and drive back to Seattle to catch a flight home the next day. I went to say goodbye to Tom and Sandi, who were sticking around to hike the 93-mile Wonderland Trail that circumnavigates the entire mountain, but they apparently had already gone to dinner, and I missed them.

I spent the night on Doug's couch again and then caught my flight in the morning. Taking off, the specter of Rainier seemed to rise above us as the plane banked to the left and turned east. It was an amazing sight, and one hell of a mountain that I was glad to have checked off my bucket list.

In the early days of Facebook, every time one logged on, there would be a picture of "Someone You Should Know" in the top right-hand corner of the screen, based on mutual friends and common interests. In late July, after I had gotten back from Rainier, the photo of the same woman appeared on my screen four days in a row; her name was Nancy Hobbs, and she lived in Colorado Springs. Thinking Facebook must know something that I didn't, I decided to send her a friend request. It seemed pretty innocuous.

A couple of days later, I received confirmation that she had accepted my friend request. No big deal. I was adding new friends daily, most of them fellow runners and mountaineers. Nancy and I started chatting on Facebook and found that we did have a connection through running and that we were the same age. Soon, we exchanged numbers and started talking on the phone as well.

After a few weeks of this, one night she announced that she didn't want to talk to me on the phone anymore. I immediately thought, "Oh, well, that was fun while it lasted," but then she added, "I want you to come out and visit me. I'm sending you a plane ticket." I was dumbfounded. No woman had ever wanted to meet me that badly before.

Toward the end of August, I flew to Colorado Springs the Thursday before her birthday, and she picked me up at the airport for a weekend enjoying the running world and celebrating with friends. On Friday, we packed up her Toyota Tundra and headed for the mountains. We drove to the town of Winfield, near the turnaround for the Leadville 100 ultramarathon, which was being held that weekend. We drove in to the broad valley underneath Huron Peak, the 14er that I had climbed with Van back in 2006, when we awoke to fresh snow collapsing our tents. We camped at that same campsite and sat up late into the night watching shooting stars streak across the jet-black sky.

The next day, we climbed the trail to Hope Pass, the high point of the Leadville 100 course, then sat down on the cool grass and waited for the runners to arrive.

Later that day, we drove to nearby Buena Vista, where several of Nancy's friends were getting ready to start the next day's Trans-Rockies Run, an annual, multiday stage race. Standing outside their cabin, I noticed a familiar-looking guy at the next cabin, who also appeared to be looking my way. Just about the time I realized it was Dean Karnazes, author of *Ultramarathon Man* and perhaps the most famous ultrarunner in the world, he looked past me and exclaimed, "Nancy?" Then he ran over and gave her a big hug. Not only did Nancy know just about everyone in the running world, they knew her, too. I was understandably impressed.

It wasn't until later that I learned of Nancy's full résumé and her passion for the sport of running, particularly trail running. Before I met her in person, I had not been aware that she was such a tiny woman—barely 5 feet tall—but I certainly hadn't known that she was a giant in the running world. She has worn so many hats I can't remember them all: executive director of the American Trail Running Association, an organization she created out of her home; membership director for Running USA, a trade organization; chairperson of the Mountain/Ultra/Trail division of USA Track & Field; U.S. liaison to the World Mountain Running Association, accompanying the American teams to the World Championships each year, usually held in Europe. And she literally wrote the book on trail running, as she is co-author of *The Ultimate Guide to Trail Running*, a how-to guide on the sport. Her credentials put me to shame.

We spent the remainder of 2009 flying back and forth to see each other, thanks to all the frequent flyer miles she had racked up traveling the world, principally to attend races. Our relationship moved quickly, and before long I was telling my kids that I was planning to move to Colorado after the holidays. Though they would miss me, they said they were happy for me.

Nancy came to visit me in early November, and before she left, we finalized plans for me to move to Colorado Springs as soon as my Christmas season at UPS ended at the end of the year.

On Christmas Day, I achieved another milestone on the trails of Monadnock: I climbed to the summit for the 1,000th time. With me was my old friend Larry Davis, as he had been on that first day in 2000. By his count, I was only the twelfth person to record a thousand Monadnock summits, though no one knows for sure. We brought champagne to celebrate, though Larry did not take a sip. He took only pictures.

On December 29, I loaded everything I owned into my Passat and headed west again. I arrived late the next day, only to discover that Nancy had entered me in the annual Rescue Run 10K on New Year's Day. My lungs nearly burst trying to acclimate to the altitude change, but somehow I managed to finish without collapsing.

I spent my first few months in Colorado training to run the Massanutten 100 again in May 2010, where I once again placed eleventh and broke the event record for the 50–59 age division. I worked up to that race by taking a quick trip to California that March in Nancy's truck, where I ran in a pair of 50K races. During the week in between the races, I tried unsuccessfully to climb two more 14ers in the Sierras, only to be turned back by a storm on one peak and by deep snow on another. I had borrowed her Tundra in hopes of getting to these remote trailheads, but the climbing itself proved to be the problem. No worries, I thought. The Sierras weren't going anywhere and I knew I would be back. I chalked it up as a scouting mission.

I had moved to Colorado without a job, though I was not overly concerned. I knew I could umpire softball there that summer—just as I once had in New Hampshire—and, hopefully, would be able to hire on with UPS in Colorado Springs that fall for another Christmas rush. I did spend the summer umpiring, but I wouldn't get the chance to contact UPS until the following year.

Early that summer, I got a call from a Facebook friend, Andy Garza from Bozeman, Montana, asking if I might be interested in a job. His roommate had just made a film and was looking for someone to promote it. I laughed and replied, "What is it, porn?"

After he stopped laughing, he said, no, that it was a cycling film and a pretty good one at that. I asked him to send me a copy.

When I watched *Ride the Divide* for the first time, I could see that it was an exceptional film. In the documentary, Andy's roommate Hunter Weeks teamed up with fellow filmmaker Mike Dion of Lakewood, Colorado, to film a little-known bicycle race called the Tour Divide, considered the toughest mountain-bike race in the world. The 2,700-mile unsupported race runs from Banff, Alberta, along the Continental Divide, to the Mexican border in New Mexico. Only sixteen riders began the 2008 race when the movie was filmed.

The film had instant appeal. While I didn't know the first thing about promoting films, I agreed to give it a try. Nancy and I were heading to Europe for the World Mountain Running Championships in September, so, after a few successful shows in early August in Colorado, I planned an extended tour with the film starting in October. I set up a tour that would stretch from Idaho to the Mexican border near where the race ends, and hoped for the best. I had no clue what I was getting into.

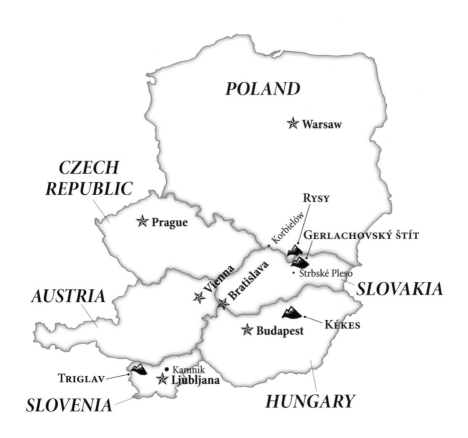

POLAND

☆ **Warsaw**

CZECH
REPUBLIC

☆ **Prague**

RYSY

Korbielów

GERLACHOVSKÝ ŠTÍT

• Štrbské Pleso

AUSTRIA

☆ **Vienna** **Bratislava**

SLOVAKIA

KÉKES

☆ **Budapest**

TRIGLAV • Kamnik
☆ **Ljubljana**

SLOVENIA

HUNGARY

Chapter 11
Summer 2010

EUROPEAN VACATION

PRIOR TO THE SUMMER OF 2010, I HAD BEEN TO EUROPE ONLY ONCE—DURING THAT trip to the Canary Islands with Larry Davis in 2001—if changing planes in both Paris and Madrid can be considered as having been to Europe.

In 2010, Nancy invited me to travel with her to two major races, the World Masters Mountain Running Championships in southern Poland, then the World Mountain Running Championships, which Slovenia was hosting in the picture-postcard village of Kamnik. We flew into Vienna, rented a car, and then drove through Slovakia—and briefly into the Czech Republic when we missed a turn—before arriving in the tiny village of Korbielów, Poland, located in the High Tatras region along the Polish–Slovak border.

We had no more than arrived in Poland when Nancy prepared me for some startling news: I was going to become a grandfather. My son, Evan, and his girlfriend were expecting. They had informed Nancy, wisely entrusting her to break the news. I was not entirely excited about the announcement, but I was excited for my son; I mean, for me becoming a grandfather meant I was getting old, though at 50 I considered myself too young for the role.

Nancy placed fourth in her World Masters age group despite a bone-chilling rain, then we had most of the next week to get from Poland to Slovenia for the WMRA championships. Nancy indulged my obsession with highpointing by agreeing to go to the village of Štrbské Pleso, Slovakia, from where I could climb the high-points of both Poland and Slovakia. A popular health resort in summer months and a ski area in the winter, Štrbské Pleso has been a tourist destination since it was first settled in the 1870s.

The weather had improved considerably by the time we arrived and we found a great, modern-looking hotel not far from the Rysy trailhead, which led to the Polish highpoint. We rented a very pleasant room from the Hotel Crocus for less than €100. The hotel was so modern we needed someone from the front desk to come up to show us how to turn on our futuristic stove. Then we had to have him come back a while later to show us how to turn it off. It looked like something out of *The Jetsons*. The hotelier must have just thought we were haughty Americans, unused to cooking our own food.

The next morning, I headed for Rysy, which my guidebook said was a 4.5-hour ascent. I made the entire round-trip in that time, but then again, I've never found guidebooks to be even remotely accurate in regard to hiking times. The ascent took me first to Popradské Pleso, the famous glacier lake that draws many tourists to the region, then north toward the border. A series of switchbacks on a well-trod trail led to the Chata pod Rysmi hut at nearly 7,400 feet. It being a Sunday, there were hundreds of hikers on the trail and dozens more at the hut when I arrived. It started to snow, and I soon was in a full-scale blizzard; heavy, wet snow swirled all around me. I had to remind myself that it was summer.

The final ascent to the summit was a bit tricky on the now wet and slippery rocks—and compounded by so many others scampering about—but I made it to the saddle between Rysy's two main summits, one of which is in Slovakia and the other the highpoint of Poland. The Polish summit, at 8,199 feet, was several feet lower than the Slovakian one, but seemed to attract just as many of the ascending climbers, many of them probably fellow peakbaggers in search of the official white cement post with the red top. I asked someone to snap a couple pictures of me, and then I immediately headed down, as I wasn't particularly prepared for snow in August.

The next morning, I planned to climb Gerlachovský štít, the highpoint of Slovakia at 8,707 feet. Nancy wasn't particularly pleased with this decision after she heard from someone at the information booth next to our hotel that no one is allowed to climb the Slovakian highpoint without a paid guide because it is too dangerous. I tried to explain to her that my guidebook said that anyone who was a member of a mountaineering club in their home country could climb without a guide. Our hotel's desk staff later confirmed this, and since I was a member of the Appalachian Mountain Club, I qualified.

Now, I can imagine how silly me flashing my AMC membership card would have been had a guide stopped me on the trail and demanded to know why I was climbing alone. Well, silly if he knew that anyone who purchases a membership can carry the card. The nonprofit does offer mountaineering education and trips, but its mission more broadly serves Northeastern outdoorspeople, regional conservation, and outdoor education. The card says nothing about a member's skill set.

But no one was likely to see me anyway. The most accessible trailhead for Gerlach štít was from the tiny village of Vyšné Hágy, which was not the same town from which the guided trips left, the book said. I did, however, run the chance that I might meet a guide after the three main trails converged at Batizovské Pleso, the tiny alpine lake not far below the summit that marked the start of the serious climbing.

After waiting for the hotel to prepare me a breakfast bag, I had to run to catch the 6:43 A.M. train to Vyšné Hágy. The trains in Slovakia are modern—as are their roads, spectacular in comparison with those in the United States, as I didn't see a pothole anywhere—and they run on a tidy schedule. I got off in Vyšné Hágy 17 minutes later and quickly found the trailhead, which ran directly past the station, up a side road, and then disappeared into the woods. The trail climbed steadily, and after a couple of hours I emerged onto rocky, more open terrain set among stunted high-alpine fir trees, called krummholz, that reminded me of almost every above-treeline hike in the White Mountains of New Hampshire. I could have easily been doing a Presidential traverse.

Once at the lake, I sat down and checked my breakfast bag to see what the hotel had prepared for me, since I had grabbed it without looking as I dashed for the train. An apple, some bread, and a box of orange juice hit the spot and then I hit the trail, which curled around the lake and headed up the edge of a waterfall toward a towering headwall that was still in shadows even at 8:30 A.M. The trail led me directly to the solid rock wall of Batizovské Zlab—at first glance, an apparent dead end that left me wondering if I had misread the directions.

There was a narrow chute running up from the bottom at a near-vertical angle, but it seemed too sheer to climb. As I got closer, I could see a series of heavy chains hanging down from above that were to be used to climb up the smooth cliff face. It appeared that they had been dangling there for more than a century.

Once above this section, I scrambled for a few hundred feet to a second set of chains, which were required to get past an even steeper section. Farther up, I came to a spot where iron rungs had been hammered into the rock face—these, too, looked to be more than 100 years old. I climbed them like a ladder to get past a protruding overhang. Once beyond the ledge, I was in the safer confines of a narrow gully, but the severity of the ascent did not slacken. I carefully climbed up the gully, switching from side to side to follow the path of least resistance, until after a seeming eternity I arrived at the top of the chute and found myself staring over the lip of the ridge into a gray, shapeless abyss. A thick cover of clouds shrouded any possible views. It had started to snow.

An unexpected storm was rolling in from the north over the top of the mountain while I still was looking back into relative sunshine to the south. The snow was immediately melting on the warm rocks, making them exceptionally slick. I didn't have a lot of time to waste, so I looked around for the summit, which I guessed was somewhere to my left. And then about a hundred yards away, in the swirling fog, I saw the apex of the mountain—a 4-foot-high metal crucifix embedded into a stone slab pointing skyward.

Getting there required some scrambling over the razor-thin ridgeline, with the very edge of the abyss to my right, which could easily have been a drop of several thousand feet, for all I knew. I made my way up the final push to the summit and found a metal box bolted to the side of a rock that housed the most impressive register book I had ever seen—it was even hardbound with embossed lettering on the front. There was no digging around under a rock or cairn to locate a poorly closed PVC tube wired with a nut to a rock. There was no disappointment to find a wet and soggy register "book"—a rolled-up notebook—and a pen that wouldn't write crammed into the spiral webbing. In contrast with the American summit registers I'd encountered, this book looked like it belonged in a church, it was so pristine.

Quickly scanning for any entries in English, I found none, so I logged in and,

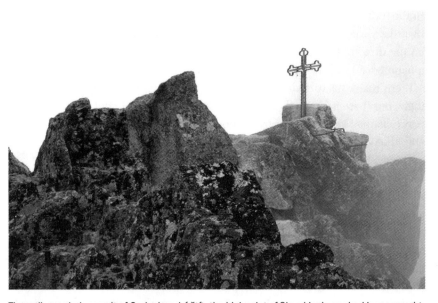

The well-guarded summit of Gerlachovský štít, the highpoint of Slovakia, is marked by a wrought-iron crucifix sticking out of the rocks.

just as quickly, put the book away. The summit itself was still ahead of me.

The crucifix was at the end of a 10-foot-long catwalk that was barely 2 feet wide, with exposed dropoffs on both sides, and the steel cross cemented to a 1-foot-square block. The block constituted the entire summit. I peered out at the ornate crucifix as if I were Harrison Ford in the closing scene of *Indiana Jones and the Last Crusade* when he looked across the "leap of faith" chasm. A large lump rose in my throat.

I swallowed hard and eased out toward the crucifix and grabbed hold of it like it was a life preserver. Nothing was going to pry this thing from my hands. I swung around and actually stood up on the block—just for a second—before I quickly sat down and snapped off a few selfies. That done, I figured it was time to get off this mountain.

Starting down, I noticed a series of chains that was supposed to have guided me to the summit; I had apparently missed them by going up the right-hand chute instead of the left one when the gully had split about a hundred yards below the ridge. I rappelled down these chains and back into the chute I had climbed up—a steep gully whose rocks now glistened from the wet snow that was falling. I picked my way down the gully with extreme care, knowing that one slip would result in a fall that would leave me far from rescue.

I descended the ladder and carefully rappelled down the next sketchy series of chains; I thought I was home free. But I had forgotten that the first climbing I had done after leaving the waterfall had been on that series of heavy chains. A cliff of more than 100 feet separated me from safety. I was dismayed to discover that the chains were now entirely wet and difficult to hold on to. With trembling knees, I rappelled off this final section and let out a huge sigh of relief when I touched down at the bottom of the cliff face.

From there, it was an easy hike down the edge of the waterfall to the lake, and from there just another 1.5 hour back to the train station in Vyšné Hágy. I arrived just in time to see the next train for Štrbské Pleso pulling out. Damn efficient Slovakian trains.

Turned out the next train didn't come for another hour, so I hunkered down in the now steady mist and staved off shivers until the next train arrived exactly 60 minutes later, right on schedule. Soon, I was back in Štrbské Pleso, safe and sound, despite perhaps the most adrenaline-pumping climb I'd ever done.

Nancy and I left the next morning for Slovenia, via a circuitous route well to our east over Hungary's highpoint. Like so many state highpoints I'd bagged before, "climbing" Kékes, at just 3,326 feet, was a misnomer. We drove up the winding, dreary mountain road to the parking lot of a ski area, and I strolled 3 minutes up a slope to the summit, which had a large hotel perched beside it. The only trouble we encountered was the unexpected fee at the entrance; a hunchbacked old man appeared from a little tollbooth that jumped out of the thick, eerie fog that had suddenly turned day into night.

He spoke no English, but wrote the number "200" on a slip of paper and shoved it toward me through the open window. I thought he was looking for €2, about $2.60, so Nancy handed me a €20 bill—the smallest she had—and I handed it to the man. He gave me back two coins, which I passed to Nancy, and was about to drive off when she exclaimed, "What are these?" Seems he had handed us back 300 of whatever the currency of Hungary was, and since we had no clue as to the exchange rate, we were left at the mercy of the old man.

Not until we stopped for dinner later that day did we find out that €20 was the equivalent of 2,500 Hungarian Forint, and he had given us an exchange of only 500 Ft. The old geezer had taken us by a factor of five to one. I felt like Jim Carrey in *Dumb and Dumber* when he entrusted his groceries to an elderly woman riding a power scooter, and she ripped him off. *"And I never saw it coming!"*

We passed through a corner of Croatia, spent the night in the charming town of Maribor, the second-largest city in Slovenia, and arrived in Kamnik, where the World Mountain Running Championships were to be held that weekend. My "job" that weekend was to shuttle some of the American athletes to and from the airport in Ljubljana about 15 miles away, but I would also get to climb, as majestic peaks burst from the valley floor right behind town, appearing more like paintings than real life.

Before the race, I met up with Tomo Šarf, one of Nancy's colleagues and friends and the Slovenian delegate to the World Mountain Running Association's council. We had plans to summit Triglav the Monday after the race, but Tomo was understandably reluctant to take a stranger along.

He has a long history with Triglav and has been climbing it for more than thirty years. About twenty-five years ago, when he said he was about 25 years old, he was drinking with some cycling friends at a bar when it was proposed that no one could climb Triglav in less than two days. Tomo scoffed at the idea and insisted he could climb it in a single day. In addition, he said he would bicycle the nearly 50 miles from Ljubljana to Triglav, climb the mountain, and ride home. A few friends joined him, and soon their challenge became a national sensation. A local TV station got wind of it and filmed the entire adventure and they all made national news. Tomo completed the entire expedition in just 11 hours.

But though he had conquered the mountain himself, he had also watched people fall to their death on his country's highpoint. So he had to test me first.

The day after I arrived, Tomo and I met at the trailhead for Šmarna Gora, a smaller, well-hiked mountain outside the capital city of Ljubljana that has a large restaurant on the summit. Hundreds of Slovenians make daily treks up the road to the summit, but, to test my resolve, Tomo took me up the technical route, which was littered with iron rungs, pegs, and bone-crushing drops. I scampered up the route right behind him and he was satisfied that I had the ability and nerve to handle such a serious endeavor as Triglav.

On Saturday, the day before the race, I climbed nearby Grintovec, which at 8,329 feet is the eighth-highest mountain in Slovenia and the tallest outside Triglav National Park. Tomo had been largely responsible for bringing the world championships to his homeland, which did a remarkable job hosting the event. And it was a great weekend for the Americans, as the U.S. men surprised even themselves by claiming the silver medal, their best team finish ever.

Monday morning dawned cold, at least on Triglav's summit. Tomo had checked the forecast in the morning and learned it was going to be zero degrees on the peak; fortunately, that was Celsius. While the mountain was going to be socked in all day, rain wasn't expected. We met at a gas station and he drove us in his Škoda station wagon—like my own car, packed full of climbing and camping gear—the 45 minutes to the national park, located not far from the Italian border, and paid the €8 entry fee for us.

Triglav is such a revered mountain that its likeness adorns the Slovenian flag—making it the only country in the world with a mountain on its flag. Getting its name from its three distinct summits, Triglav is a massive mountain composed entirely of one solid block of limestone, and is bleached white by the sun, making it look like it is covered in snow year-round.

Tomo intended for us to hike up the Luknja Route—which would mean we would do a complete loop over all three summits—rather than the safer up-and-back Prag Route outlined in my guidebook. This we could do, he said, if the weather held. It looked fine, so we headed up the northern flank of the mountain, and eventually reached a small saddle called The Window. Here, the wind rushed through a gap in the rocks as it forced its way over the Julian Alps toward the Adriatic Sea about 40 miles to our west.

This was where the real fun began. This was where he told me not to fall. This was where I probably would not have continued had I been alone. The "trail" immediately climbed up a steep ridgeline with exposure on both sides, and only pegs protruding from the rocks to hold on to. Most of these steel pegs had been painstakingly hammered into the solid rock many decades ago, it appeared.

Soon, we traversed a 1-foot-wide ledge, holding onto cable that was bolted to the rock face.

Normally, climbers are supposed to use via ferrata equipment here, donning harnesses with short ropes and clipping themselves to the cable. But we simply free-climbed it. Nothing to worry about. I just didn't look down, and even if I had, all I would have seen was gray nothingness, as we could not see the dizzying drops below us because of the day's thick cloud cover.

We climbed this way for nearly an hour, overtaking a solo climber on the cliff face who looked like he shouldn't have been there; certainly not alone, anyway. The climbing was exuberant as we clawed and scratched our way up the mountainside. Eventually, we reached the "plateau," as Tomo called it, between Triglav's northernmost peak and the main massif, which loomed directly in front of us darting in and out of the clouds. Here, Tomo said it was easy to lose the trail if the clouds were any thicker, and it wasn't a place to go wandering around looking for cairns, as one of the sheerest cliff faces in Europe loomed unseen just to our left; he said a party of three men had done just that not more than a week before.

Those hikers had called for help on their cell phone instead. The Triglavski Dom hut on the other side of the summit had been contacted, Tomo said, and the caretaker asked the hikers gathered there if anyone dared venture out in the bad weather to rescue their fellow climbers. Everyone just shrugged their shoulders and went back to eating their hot soup. But a 14-year-old girl took up the challenge, scaled the peak, found the missing hikers, and led them back to the safety of the hut. Each week, a local Slovenian radio station has its listeners call in to vote for the "national person of the week," and the previous week this heroic girl had been the winner.

There was still one more challenging section of via ferrata to negotiate as we climbed the main summit of Triglav, then we were on top, where the weather showed a little promise of clearing—enough so that I put on my sunglasses for the first time all day. There is a conical building, called the Aljažev Stolp, about 4 feet in diameter and maybe 7 feet tall directly on the summit with a metal flag sticking out of the top that acts as a weather vane. Built in 1895 by Jakob Aljaž, the so-called "father of Slovenian climbing," the building looked more like a phone booth or portable toilet, but obviously had withstood the elements for the past 115 years. Tomo showed me a picture on his cell phone of a winter hike he had done a year or two before when only the building's flag was sticking out of the snow.

Inside the building, someone had meticulously painted a 360-degree panorama of the surrounding mountains, but that was my only view of them. The weather quickly changed, and I had to put my sunglasses away after only a minute or so. The register book at the summit had been replaced just that day, and I was the third person to sign into the new one.

Then we headed down via the standard route, which meant continuing over the ridgeline toward the Triglavski Dom hut, located at 8,251 feet, by way of Mali Triglav—Little Triglav—a sharp spine that narrowed to just a few feet wide in some spots, with sheer dropoffs on both sides. A cable ran down the middle of this spine, but, of course, we had no gear to clip ourselves safely in. In fact, on several occasions we had to maneuver around other groups of hikers that we were overtaking, some on their way down or some still headed up. As Tomo pointed out often during the climb, "Our speed is our safety." If the weather turned, he said, we had the physical ability to hightail it off the mountain in time.

Soon thereafter, Tomo stopped at a particularly narrow place to tell me about an incident that had happened a few years before in that exact spot. He had met an Italian climber on the trail and they had been standing there talking when Tomo said goodbye and turned to head to the summit. He took no more than a single step when he heard a shout of *"Mamma mia!"* and turned to watch the Italian plummet 1,200 feet to his death.

After a quick respite at the Triglavski Dom hut, we reached another area where via ferrata cable ran along a narrow ledge above a steep drop. Tomo said he had fallen here in the winter a few years before, slipping on the ice and rocketing toward a cliff less than 200 feet away. He had his ice ax handy and was able to self-arrest in time, or he wouldn't have been telling me the story. The very next day, however, another climber had slipped at the exact same spot and was not so lucky, plummeting to his death.

Many have lost their lives on Triglav. Plaques bolted to the rock all over the mountain pay tribute to fallen climbers. Some were just teenagers.

We passed several more climbing parties, including a large group from Bulgaria, then we were finally off the mountain and headed back to the car. It had been my tenth international highpoint. And, more important, it had cemented a bond between Tomo and me that I hoped would endure. I would not see him again until 2014, when he and his daughter visited us in Colorado and he and I climbed Pikes Peak together.

But he said I should come back to Slovenia sometime so he can show me more of his country's high peaks. And just maybe, next time we'll get some views.

When we returned from Europe, I set about getting ready to leave on my Rocky Mountain tour with *Ride the Divide*. One added benefit of starting the extended promotional tour in Idaho that October was that I would get to knock off another state highpoint. I had never been to Idaho before that late September day when I pulled into the parking lot at Borah Peak, located just over Trail Creek Pass from Sun Valley, where I had a show scheduled in a couple of days. At 12,667 feet high, the peak rises nearly a mile above the surrounding plain in the Challis National Forest, and was nameless until 1934 when it was discovered to be higher than Hyndman Peak, which until then had been considered the state's highest point (in reality, it ranks only ninth). The peak was named for an outspoken U.S. senator from Idaho named William Borah, known as the "Lion of Idaho," who unsuccessfully sought the Republican nomination for president in 1936.

The sun was setting in the trailhead parking lot when I arrived. I'd intended to camp there and climb the next morning, but then I got to talking to a pair of women who were waiting for their husbands to return from the summit. One of them commented that the night before, the full moon had been as bright as daylight, and it occurred to me that I didn't need to wait till morning. I decided to make the climb one to remember by attempting it under the full moon.

I packed up my daypack, purposely leaving out my headlamp, as there were no clouds in the sky, and the moon, I figured, would provide all the light I would need. Thanks to some advice I got in the parking lot from another climber, I did bring a pair of gloves—not because of the cold, but because the rock, formed from uplifted ocean sediments millions of years old, is so sharp that it would tear bare fingers to shreds.

The peak's steep trail rises 5,262 feet in its 3.5-mile ascent, making it perhaps the steepest standard route on any of the fifty state highpoints. Many members of the Highpointers Club save Borah for one of their final peaks, and not just because of its inaccessibility. The trail is steep right from the get-go, climbing steadily to the ridgeline just before reaching a place aptly named Chickenout Ridge, which is the crux of the climb.

As I approached the ridge, which extends from roughly 11,300 feet to 11,700 feet, I could see why the novice climber might find it a bit daunting. More than one climber has turned back after seeing this exposed, razor-thin, nerve-racking arête. I, however, did not find Chickenout Ridge to be as tough as it looked. Essentially, it's little more than a Class 3 scramble over a subsidiary summit that, once cleared, provides direct access to Borah's main summit. Just don't look down on either side. I stayed on the trail and climbed directly over the top of the ridge. Even in the waning daylight, I could see that if I had dropped down on either side of the ridge, there was so much loose shale that I could easily have slid off into the abyss. It was a dizzying drop on either side, and I knew I would have to be cautious here on my descent in the moonlight.

Beyond this hurdle, the remainder of the climb was over a long, flat saddle to Borah's main peak and then another scramble of several hundred feet on sharp, pointy rocks to what my guidebook said were grand views over the entire Lost River Range. The twenty-four highest peaks in Idaho are within the confines of this range, but with darkness encroaching, I could barely even pick out Leatherman Peak, the state's second-highest mountain at 12,228 feet, which lies just to the southwest of Borah's summit.

After having enjoyed the immaculate summit registers in Europe earlier that summer, it was a bit disconcerting to again find an old Army footlocker with several wet and withered notebooks inside that were all completely filled. I had to scribble my name on a loose piece of paper and toss it back in to announce Borah Peak as my forty-fourth state highpoint.

The moon soon rose above the jagged peaks of the Bitterroots to the east, but almost immediately disappeared again. I had not noticed that clouds had rolled in during my ascent, blotting out the moon and all the reflective light I had been counting on. Suddenly, I was plunged into darkness without a headlamp. Not to worry, I thought. The trail had pretty much followed the ridgeline the entire way from Chickenout Ridge to the summit, so I figured I could easily retrace my steps by just staying on the highest ground. In the darkness, however, that proved impossible.

I soon found myself off the ridgeline on the south side of the mountain, where I had seen all the loose shale. Slowly, I picked my way along the edge of the ridge, each step creating a small rock slide that cascaded off the mountain, each crash sounding like a stack of dishes being dropped in a restaurant. I held tightly to the rocks to keep from sliding off myself.

I traversed about a dozen of these steep, little ravines before I successfully regained the ridgeline and relative safety. Still, in the pitch black, it was difficult to stay on the trail as I carefully negotiated my way off Chickenout Ridge and then down the steep trail to the parking lot. It was nearly 2 A.M. when I arrived at my car, having taken me as long to descend (3 hours 15 minutes) as it had to ascend, and I still had to find a place to put up my tent for the remainder of the night. At least I now had my headlamp to see by.

My show of Ride the Divide *at Sun Valley a couple of days later went about as well* as my climb. Only a handful of people turned out, and I lost money on the show. That pattern repeated itself just about every night until about a week later when I rolled into Flagstaff, Arizona. I arrived expecting another bust, especially considering that I had booked the film into the Orpheum Theater on the night before a four-day mountain film festival was set to begin. What had I been thinking?

An hour before the show, however, there was a line of people waiting to get in that stretched down the street and around the corner for two blocks. I could barely contain myself. More than 300 people turned out that night and I made back all the money I had lost the week before and then some. I had turned the corner. Word was getting out about this amazing little film.

The trip had been a success, and I quickly scheduled more shows around the country. In fact, I left for Hartford, Connecticut, the day after I got back to Colorado, missing Nancy by only an hour at O'Hare in Chicago, as she was returning from a race in Syracuse, New York. It was just one of many times that we would miss each other when one or both of us was coming or going.

During that tour of the Northeast, which included a stop in Lake Placid, New York, I was able to climb my first 46ers in the Adirondacks—the forty-six peaks above 4,000 feet in the range—though I didn't get to bag Mount Marcy, one of the remaining state highpoints I needed. While there, I stayed at a place called "The Bivy," which was a barn owned by local rock-climbing legend Joe Szot in the town of Keene Valley. He had converted the barn into a bunkhouse for his climbing buddies, who would show up every weekend. I had stayed there once before, but Joe had been off climbing in Chamonix at the time, so it was great to finally meet him. We hit it off immediately, as we were both about the same age and still very active in our sports. He was known as one of the area's top rock climbers, having pioneered many routes in the region. Unfortunately, in 2012, Joe was climbing in the Gunks, a popular rock-climbing destination in the Catskills, and suffered a fatal heart attack. His death hit the local climbing community hard.

On that same trip, I also returned to Rhode Island and officially "climbed" Jerimoth Hill, the state highpoint. When I was first there in 1993, the actual summit was off-limits, as access was through private land, and highpoint-ers simply had to pull to the side of RI 101 to officially "bag" Jerimoth Hill. Since then, the land has changed hands to more amenable owners and a short trail now leads a few hundred feet into the woods to the actual highpoint, which is marked by a small cairn on top of a large erratic boulder sticking out of the ground.

The plot of land encompassing the actual summit was donated in the 1930s to Brown University, which has an astronomical observation area nearby. Dave Targan—the Monadnock park ranger—is also the associate dean of the College of Science at Brown and said he was once doing some site work on Jerimoth Hill with a backhoe when he thought he had accidentally excavated the actual sum-mit. He was much relieved, he said, to realize he had not, in fact, taken a few feet off the top of the state highpoint.

After nearly seventy shows that winter, the tour was dubbed a success. Since the release of the film, interest in this underground race has exploded, with more than one hundred riders now entered annually. Its success would also lead to two more cycling films by Mike Dion and Hunter Weeks, both of which I later promoted.

Days after we had returned from Europe and while I was preparing to leave for Idaho, Nancy had flown to Pennsylvania to see her father, James, who had been diagnosed with inoperable brain cancer six months before. Tragically, he died just days later. It was a very difficult time for Nancy. She had lost her brother, David—her only sibling—years before. With no children of her own, Nancy had only her mother, Peggy, left. In October, I broke away from my tour to fly to her childhood home of Bethlehem to join her for her dad's memorial service.

That December, Nancy and I took her mother with us on a trip to Hawaii, where we spent a week exploring the island of Kauai. It was great therapy for both of them. I planned to make the trip do double duty, and flew out ahead of them to attempt Mauna Kea on the Big Island, the highpoint of Hawaii.

A lot of fifty-state highpointers save Hawaii for last, treating themselves to a vacation to celebrate their success. While Mauna Kea wouldn't be my final state highpoint, I did want the trip to be unique. So, I dreamed up the idea of doing a sea-to-summit expedition, a 60-mile ultramarathon-style trip from the Waikoloa Beach Resort to the snow-covered summit of the 13,803-foot dormant volcano. Fifty-three miles of that would be on paved road, with only the final 7 miles—from the visitor center to the observatory on the summit—on trails and dirt roads.

Measured from the ocean floor, Mauna Kea is the tallest mountain on Earth; it stands more than 33,000 feet from base to summit, higher even than Everest. Perfect atmospheric conditions at its summit make it one of the best places on Earth for astrological observation.

I spent weeks beforehand working out the logistics of my quest. The first problem I had to solve was how to get from the airport in Kailua-Kona to my starting point on the beach about 18 miles north. A Facebook friend put me in touch with Franz, a German who had moved to Kona in 1992, who agreed to pick me up at the airport and deliver me to the beach in Waikoloa. He was an interesting guy. A cyclist, Franz sported a long, gray ponytail, and was often seen riding the roads around the island. In fact, when we met, he had just completed a three-day circumnavigation of the Big Island the week before. With the sun setting behind me, he took some pictures of me with one foot in the Pacific as I started what I anticipated would be about an 18-hour ordeal.

My second problem, I had surmised, would be the weather. Days before my arrival, a winter storm had dumped a couple feet of fresh snow on the summit of Mauna Kea—the first snow of the season—and I had called the visitor center to make sure I could still hike beyond the end of the road. The ranger informed me that the mountain was closed and that I would be turned away. When I told him that I still planned to come, he responded, "Well, we can't stop you from climbing the mountain. But we can call someone who can." Not encouraging news, but I was determined. I figured if I was able to keep to my schedule, I would pass the visitor center in the wee hours of the morning and could be successfully up and down the mountain before anyone even knew I was there.

After just 5 miles of walking in the dark on the hard pavement of the Waikoloa Road, however, my feet were already hurting. My plantar fasciitis was flaring up—it had been quiet in recent weeks after coming on with a vengeance after I ran my second Massanutten 100 earlier in the year—and the ferocious winds and whipping rain were blowing me right off the road. It was barely dark, and I was already miserable, and soon realized that I had bitten off far more than I could chew with this crazy idea. So, I did the only thing I could think of—I stuck out my thumb.

Before long, a guy driving an SUV picked me up and gave me a ride as far as the turn for the Saddle Road—the 53-mile, two-lane road that bisects the island, connecting Waimea to Hilo, and goes over the saddle between the two towering volcanoes on the island, Mauna Kea and its sister to the south, Mauna Loa.

Between the thick cloud cover and the new moon, it was very dark, and with it already raining, this guy told me he didn't think I'd get another ride until morning. Fortunately, he was wrong. The second car to pass me stopped, even though the couple really didn't have room in their pickup truck for me. I crammed myself in behind the passenger seat, pushing out of the way piles of quilt batting they had bought in Kona that day. They were returning home to Hilo and dropped me off at the bottom of the Mauna Kea Observatory Road, which climbs about 6 miles to the visitor center, or so the sign there indicated.

It was noticeably cooler there, at 6,000 feet, than it had been at the beach, but at least it was no longer raining. I changed into long pants for the hike up the road, but the pain in my left foot was becoming excruciating. After close to 5 miles, and with the visitor center still nowhere in sight, the pain became unbearable, the worst I had experienced during my eighteen-month bout with plantar. I was near tears when I accepted that I was not going to summit. I turned around and started back down the steep road, not knowing where I was heading. I didn't get very far. I discovered that walking downhill was even more painful than going uphill. I was in a quandary.

Peering over the guardrail, I spotted some tall grass under a tree that was out of the wind. Even though the grass was still damp, it was the only suitable place to bivouac for the night. Fortunately, I had carried my Heatsheets bivy sack with me, given to me by the company's owner, Dave Deigan, a friend of Nancy's whom I had met at the Outdoor Retailer exposition in Salt Lake City the previous August. He had given me a sample of his product to test for him; I just didn't realize it was going to happen in Hawaii, where temperatures that night must have dipped close to freezing.

I put on all the clothes I had carried with me—three shirts and three jackets, including a down parka, plus my wind pants—and spent a relatively comfortable night in what I dubbed my "oven roaster bag." I woke up shivering several times, perhaps because I was too warm and condensation was forming on the inside of the bag, soaking my clothes. I considered turning it inside out so the silver lining would be facing away from me, but that seemed like too much work.

In the morning, I climbed back over the guardrail and discovered that my foot was feeling considerably better; I could walk on it, at least. After a couple of miles hiking back down the road, I had dropped enough elevation that I was now getting too warm again. So, I climbed into the bushes and changed back into shorts and a T-shirt. Returning to the road, the first car that passed stopped and gave me a ride the final 2 miles back to Saddle Road. They were a young couple from Hilo who had made the trip in hopes of being able to drive their four-wheel-drive SUV all the way to the summit. They had been turned back, probably by the same surly park ranger I had spoken to on the phone.

If things hadn't been interesting enough already, they were about to get downright crazy. After what seemed like an hour or more of waiting on Saddle Road, a car finally stopped to pick me up. The driver and passenger were Michael and Wayne, but they could easily have passed for Cheech and Chong.

They were driving a beat-up late-model Ford pickup that was a veritable heap; it had no door handles, no ignition—Michael used a screwdriver to turn the car on and off—and no horn, as he flicked a switch under the dashboard to honk at just about every car we passed. Whenever he stopped—which was three times in 35 miles, as they kept pulling over to go pee—Michael pointed the truck downhill so he could pop-start the clutch to restart it. In the back was a load of wood—a special variety that was very expensive, they explained, and the reason for their trip to Hilo the day before—along with a cooler full of Milwaukee's Best Ice beer, which I later learned is a potent 5.9 percent alcohol by volume.

Actually, the cooler was only half full. Although it was only about 8 A.M., they were already halfway through a case and kept tossing empties through the rear window into the back of the truck. It was the reason they had to stop every few minutes to relieve themselves.

Wayne said he was part Hawaiian, and was the quiet one of the two, though it really didn't matter, because I found it almost impossible to understand what either of them said. They spoke some dialect of English that I couldn't follow very well, sort of like when I was on Utila and couldn't understand the pirate English of Captain Hal.

Michael, who said he was 57, soon pulled a pipe out from under the seat, nearly driving off the road as he fumbled for it. After lighting the bowl, he and Wayne, who was about the same age, each took several hits, though I passed, even though sitting between them in the front seat, I was the unfortunate benefactor of most of the smoke.

Michael said it was "some good shit" that he had grown himself. He then handed me two cans of beer and said that if I wasn't going to smoke, I certainly was going to drink. While most of the vehicle's accessories didn't work, the heater did, and was blowing hot air full blast on my bare, contorted legs, giving me what felt like an instant sunburn on my shins. Since both windows were down, and likely didn't work anyway, I'm not sure why the heater was on, but I didn't dare ask. The CD player also worked, though it emitted only a tinny, metallic sound, but that didn't keep Michael from cranking Creedence Clearwater Revival, to which he was singing loudly.

When we got to Waikoloa Village, Michael pulled into the first gas station we came to in order to get water for the radiator, as the engine was overheating. He said it was a regular occurrence.

Minutes later they dropped me off at the intersection with HI 19, the main road back to Kona, and just like that, the bizarre and rather comical ordeal was over.

The very next car picked me up and, to my good fortune, was actually driven by a normal-looking guy. His name was Terry, and he said he installed satellite TV systems for rich beachfront owners. He got a big kick out of my story about my previous ride. He dropped me off right in front of the hostel in Kona where I had planned to stay that night, before I was to fly to Kauai the next day to meet Nancy and her mother.

Then things got weird again. The guy who ran the hostel had hair that stood up in a row of spikes and he said his name was Zero, which soon made sense. He said I couldn't check in until 5 P.M., and it was only 11 A.M. at the time. When I told him I needed sleep and a shower, he retorted, "How much clearer do I need to be about the check-in time?" Not a very personable fellow. He eventually relented and let me nap on one of the chaise lounges on the patio for the afternoon.

That evening I went down to the beach, where a Christmas parade was going on, which again seemed comically out of place in a tropical paradise, and then sat on the seawall and watched the sun set over the Pacific. It had been a long day and a half, and one I couldn't forget if I had tried.

By coincidence, my grandson, Cameron, was due in mid-April 2011, when I already had planned to be back in New England to run my first Boston Marathon. If you had told me twenty years ago that I would become a grandfather before I would run my first Boston Marathon, I would have said you were crazy; I would have expected to have run a dozen Bostons by then. But that did not turn out to be the case: my grandson entered the world before I toed the line in Hopkinton by a margin of about 12 hours. I ran the race with him in my prayers, as he spent the first few weeks of his life in the hospital with complications. But he is now a healthy 5-year-old, excited for his first climb of Monadnock.

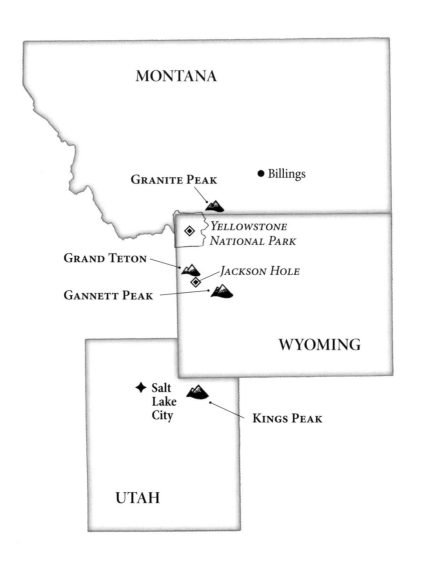

MONTANA

GRANITE PEAK

● Billings

◈ *Yellowstone*
National Park

GRAND TETON

Jackson Hole

GANNETT PEAK

WYOMING

✦ Salt
Lake
City

KINGS PEAK

UTAH

A GRAND ADVENTURE

WHEN JIM GRACE BECAME OBSESSED WITH HIGHPOINTING, HE WASN'T OUT TO get his name into *Guinness World Records*. But that all changed one day in the late '80s. "[My wife Betty and I] had done thirty-some highpoints, and when we got to Kings Peak in Utah, we saw a note in the summit register from a guy named Dennis Stewart, who was also doing the state highpoints and was from Higginsville, Missouri, only about a hundred miles from where we live [in Albany, Missouri]," Jim told me when we met in Wyoming more than twenty years later, when I was out west pursuing my own list of peaks. "When we got home, I made an effort to contact him."

Dennis suggested that he and Jim should team up for the trip of a lifetime: all the state highpoints in the contiguous United States in the shortest possible time. The current record, Dennis discovered, had been set some years before by a Brit who had done it in "like fifty-six days," Jim recalled. "Dennis put together a plan to do them all in less than a month," he said.

The trip was two years in the planning, and they invited three other climbers to join the adventure—Pete Allard, who taught at the same high school as Dennis; Shaun Lacher, who had been a student of theirs; and David Sandway, a climber from New York whom Dennis knew. Meanwhile, Dennis spent 1988 through 1990 completing all of the Lower 48 state highpoints to gain a personal knowledge of every climb.

Before they set out, a filmmaker from Massachusetts named Ken Bell contacted Dennis about filming much of the trip for a documentary about geography Ken hoped to produce. The crew planned to join the highpointers at several points throughout the trip.

"Dennis was meticulous, planning everything down to a 15-minute interval for each day and night," Jim said. The whole trip was planned for the month of July 1991. "We started on Rainier so the climb up wouldn't count; the clock started when we reached the summit," Jim noted. "And, we [planned to finish] on Gannett so we wouldn't have to include the long hike out."

In all, they drove more than 19,000 miles, sharing time at the wheel of Dennis's Chevy Crew Cab pickup. They slept in the truck's capped bed and towed a trailer of their gear behind them. "We had some car trouble when we left Missouri [to head for Rainier], but nothing during the actual expedition," Jim said of their good fortune.

They did, however, have a few mishaps along the way. In Oklahoma, when they climbed Black Mesa during a moonless night, they lost their way on the return to their vehicle, and spent a couple of hours looking for it. "We couldn't understand how we had gotten lost," Jim said. Maybe it was because they were preoccupied with all the local fauna. "Rattlesnakes were all over the place," he said, "even though it was the middle of the night. We would hear them rattle, and jump out of the way. David was about at the end of his rope."

In Florida, they were driving into Lakewood Park when a mountain lion jumped across the road in front of them. "That caused a little bit of concern," Jim said. A couple of days later, they arrived at Great Smoky Mountains National Park and found the road to the summit of Clingmans Dome closed, just as I would in 2009. "It was closed indefinitely because of some insect infestation or something," Jim, who is a wildlife biologist, remembered. "We had to go back at night and sneak past all the barriers to get that one." Later in the trip, in Ohio, they arrived at the state highpoint, located on the campus of a vocational center, to find the front gate locked, since it was after dark. Jim called his wife, and Betty contacted someone who came and unlocked the gate.

In Rhode Island, they nearly got arrested for trespassing; the owner of Jerimoth Hill must have called the police when their car pulled off RI 101 next to his home, as he frequently did. After a quick traipse into the woods to locate the highpoint, Jim said a policeman pulled in behind them just as they were returning to their vehicle.

"He put us up against the truck and made us spread our legs" for a patdown, Jim said. "We tried to explain to him what we were doing, but it was the middle of the night, and he thought we were all crazy."

Luckily, Ken's film crew happened to be there that night, and filmed the incident. Jim said their presence "lent an air of authenticity to what we were doing there. Otherwise, we all probably would have gotten arrested."

Their clock had started on the summit of Washington's Mount Rainier at midnight on July 1, 1991. "Going into it, I had thought the probability of success was very low to do it in the month of July," Jim said. "I figured we would have weather issues, or someone would twist an ankle or something, or we'd have car trouble. But none of that happened, and somehow we got all five of us to the top of all forty-eight peaks." They reached the summit of Gannett Peak in Wyoming on July 31. *Guinness World Records* confirmed their time as the new record: 30 days 10 hours 52 minutes.

The documentary never materialized, but Dennis apparently still has all the footage that Ken shot.

Since then, their speed record has been broken at least twice—official records are not kept by the Highpointers Club, of which Dennis was a charter member—but Jim noted that subsequent record holders have used more than one vehicle and were supported by a crew. In 2005, Ben Jones—a 20-year-old from Washington—completed the Lower 48 state highpoints in 29 days, and then the next year, Jake Meyer, a 23-year-old Brit, accomplished it in 23 days, 19 hours, and 13 minutes. Jim said he heard that Meyer had a crew of six people with him to do most of the driving.

"I think we still hold the unsupported record where all the people summited every peak and everyone shared the driving," Jim said. "Nobody has done it in the style that we did."

In 2000, Jim and Dennis teamed up again to climb Denali in Alaska; Jim became the ninety-third person to complete the fifty state highpoints. Dennis finished a month later, as he still needed Mauna Kea in Hawaii.

Perhaps they might team up again to recreate their epic adventure, although, since most of them are now in their 60s, their unsupported speed record is probably safe.

By mid-2011, my own state-highpoint quest had taken on a sense of urgency. After having climbed Borah Peak in Idaho the year before, I had only four more to go to complete the contiguous United States. One of those, Mount Marcy in New York, had somehow escaped my attention during all those years I had lived in New England, and the other three—the highpoints of Utah, Wyoming, and Montana—had all been too snowbound to attempt during my cross-country highpointing adventure in 2009. It was time for another road trip.

On August 1, I loaded up my '99 Jetta, which I had bought that spring— replacing the '96 Passat that had treated me so well during that cross-country trip in 2009—and headed for Kings Peak, the 13,528-foot summit located in the High Uintas Wilderness of northeastern Utah. The only road leading to Kings Peak comes in from Wyoming and includes a drive of many miles on a dirt road that would have been unplowed had I attempted it in March 2009. A wall of other 13ers hides Kings Peak, and even from the trailhead, bagging the highpoint takes a round-trip hike of roughly 29 miles through some rugged terrain. Kings Peak also includes more than 5,300 feet of elevation gain, putting it in the "strenuous" category, according to my *Highpoints of the United States* guidebook. Most people take between two and five days to climb Kings Peak; not many do it in a single day, as I planned to.

Ironically, it's named for Clarence King, the same guy who claimed to have been the first to climb Mount Whitney in California, but had mistakenly climbed the wrong peak. Besides his work with the California Geological Survey, King had been the director of a survey of mineral resources along the route of the Union Pacific Railroad that opened up the West in the late 1860s, much of that work done in Utah.

The 29 miles of gravel road to Kings Peak trailhead was smooth as a tabletop, the most meticulously maintained dirt road that I have ever driven, quite unlike the usual washboard terrain. I found the Henrys Fork Campground parking lot to be almost full, though no one was around. Everyone else, it appeared, was on-trail somewhere.

In the morning, I hit the trail early for what I knew was going to be a long, arduous day. Just 5 miles in, I came to a fast-running stream at Elkhorn Crossing. I had read online that the log bridge across this raging creek had washed out that spring, but I arrived at the crossing to discover that a new bridge had been built just two weeks before, enabling me to avoid a dangerous and unpleasant fording.

From there, the trail climbed its way into a box canyon, via a thicket of willows that soaked me with morning dew. It was also quite muddy here because of a lot of horse traffic tearing up the trail. It was the first time since that day on Mount Bierstadt—my first 14er in 2006—that I had had a lengthy battle with such a snarling mass of willows.

The only way out of this canyon was over Gunsight Pass, which loomed in front of me as a climb of about a thousand feet or so. As I began the climb up to the rim, I spotted a lone, gray coyote sauntering down the trail in my direction, by far the largest I had ever seen. It slipped silently into the scrub brush, and, like a ghost, was quickly gone. Afterward, I questioned whether it might have been a wolf, as they have indeed been spotted that far south of Yellowstone, I later learned.

Topping Gunsight Pass, I avoided a downclimb to the beautiful, green valley on the other side by traversing along the contours of Gunsight Peak, which was to my right. From there, it was a steep climb up a slabby ridge to the airy, rocky summit of Kings Peak. I made the ascent in 5 hours 5 minutes, gaining more than a mile of elevation over about 14 miles.

Leaving the summit, I ran into a guy from Long Island, who said he, too, was a highpointer, and mentioned that he had just summited Gannett Peak

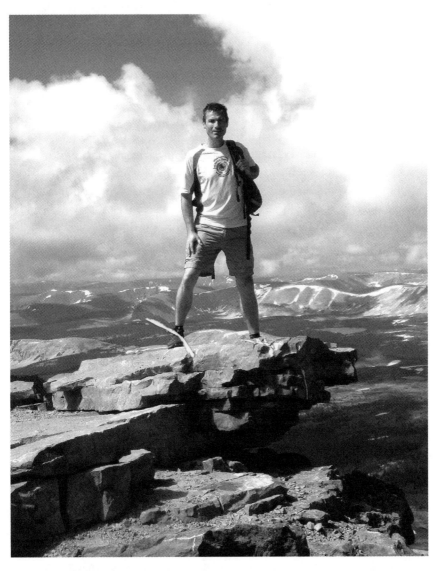

I feel as if I could step off into the clouds from the summit of Kings Peak, the highpoint of Utah.

in Wyoming a few days before. He had been guided on that trip, he said, and had used the southern route into Titcomb Basin, which was the same route I planned to use in a few days. When he told me he had endured a grueling 14-hour summit day, I decided a change of plans was in order. I would instead come in from the northern end and avoid the time-consuming climb over Bonney Pass and the hike over one of the two glaciers I would have to cross to gain Gannett's summit.

I then ran into another party that I had passed earlier in the day, and they told me about a shortcut I could take down "The Chute," a steep, scree-filled ravine. One of them told me that it would "take 2 hours" off my return trip, avoiding the descent into the broad valley and the reclimbing of Gunsight Pass. It was some fun boot-skiing down this scree slope, and I was quickly at the bottom, and able to contour along the backside of Gunsight Peak to rejoin my original trail. The shortcut did not save me 2 hours, since I completed the return trip in 4 hours 35 minutes. But my plantar fasciitis was flaring up again, slowing me down.

The shortcut did keep me dry, it turned out. The very instant I set my backpack on the picnic table next to my tent at the trailhead, a crash of thunder boomed directly over my head and I dived into my tent just moments before a torrential rainstorm pounded the valley. Later, I counted forty other cars in the parking lot, and every one of their occupants, I surmised, was currently out on the trail getting drenched. One of them soon arrived at the trailhead, looking like a drowned rat, and said he had nearly been struck by lightning several times. He was still visibly shaking, or maybe just shivering from near hypothermia.

In the morning, I broke camp and drove to Salt Lake City, where Nancy was attending the Outdoor Retailer exposition starting the following day. I picked her up at the airport and spent the next couple of days "helping" at her American Trail Running Association table. The expo, for me, was like being a kid in a candy store: just about every outdoor gear manufacturer in the world was there with all their latest gadgets on display. I spent my time mostly wandering around and picking up free samples of everything from energy gels to running socks.

The following day, I packed up for a solo drive to Wyoming to climb Gannett Peak—and, hopefully, Grand Teton—and then on to Montana to climb Granite Peak, considered by many to be the toughest of all the state highpoints. I happened to mention to Nancy that I had left home without my ice ax, and, of course, she immediately became concerned. Gannett was, after all, glacier-capped, and ice axes are essential safety gear for that terrain. I told her I would be all right without it, though I knew that was not really the truth. Sure, I had never needed to use my ice ax on any previous expedition, but that didn't mean I felt I should be up there without one. My reluctance was mostly in that I always hate to buy a piece of gear that I already own. But she insisted that I go buy one, so I relented and promised to stop at the Black Diamond outlet store—the only one in the world—on my way out of Salt Lake City to pick up another one. I got a good deal and Nancy got her peace of mind.

The only other essential item I needed to pick up was a can of bear spray at the ranger station in Big Piney, Wyoming, where I fortunately arrived at exactly 4:30 P.M., just as it was about to close. The canister of bear spray cost $50, but

I considered it a life insurance premium and gladly paid it. The Glacier Trail trailhead is not far as the crow flies from Yellowstone National Park, and the Wind River Range in which Gannett Peak lies is considered grizzly country.

The next day was going to be a long one: I planned to hike 23 miles into the high valley east of Gannett Peak to set up camp, leaving me a much shorter summit day the following morning than an ascent from Titcomb Basin would have required. I got to the trailhead for Glacier Trail with just enough daylight left to set up camp, as the 9-mile drive in from Dubois was on a very rough dirt road, not like the one that had led in to Kings Peak. That night, the heavens opened and a massive thunderstorm inundated the valley. It was so ferocious that a family with young children from Nebraska camping next to me must've packed up and left in the middle of the night, as there was no sign of them in the morning.

My 23-mile trek took a solid 12 hours the next day, as I was slowed considerably by the weight of my pack. The main culprit, I later discerned, was my antiquated cooking gear, more suitable for car camping than for backpacking; but until I got back to civilization, the situation couldn't be rectified.

The trail began with a moderate 3-mile hike in to Bomber Basin, where I met several groups on horseback on their way out. This was followed by a 2,000-foot climb up twenty-eight switchbacks to a beautiful high-alpine meadow in a small pass. Starting down the other side, I entered an eerie section of trail through an area recently denuded by wildfire. Soon, I met two bedraggled hikers; it was apparent, based on the size of their overstuffed backpacks, that they were returning from a summit bid of Gannett.

Asking if they had summited, one of them said with chagrin, "We had hoped to, but we were a little underprepared." Looking at their bulging packs, I asked what gear they possibly could have been missing, and the other one immediately responded, "Ice axes."

A lump rose in my throat knowing I had almost ignored Nancy's advice and not stopped to buy one. As usual, she had been right.

I soon came to the first of three lakes that marked the roughly halfway point, and from there, the trail quickly descended another series of switchbacks into Dinwoody Creek Basin, which would prove to be one of the most beautiful valleys I had ever seen. The fast-rushing water was glacial green, and had it not been for millions of mosquitoes swarming around my head, I might have considered never leaving this Shangri-la.

Though what happened next might have changed my mind. About halfway down the switchbacks, I stopped to take a rest and get my heavy pack off my aching back for a few minutes. Looking out at the small lake below, something interesting caught my eye. There was a spit of land sticking out into the lake from the rocky shoreline, and at the end of this little peninsula was what looked to me to be a man fishing. But, as I watched, there was no movement, and besides, I quickly realized it was much too tall to be a man—at least 9 feet—and was uniform in color—a dark brown, not the usual color of clothing. I decided after 5 or 6 minutes of watching the unmoving figure that it must be a tree, but I thought that was a very unlikely place for a tree to be growing. Giving it no more thought, I turned to grab my pack and got ready to continue hiking. Turning around, I took one last look in the direction of the lake. The hair on my arms stood on end.

The "tree" was mysteriously gone.

Now, I'm not going to claim I saw Bigfoot, but if I didn't, I have no explanation for what I saw. It was certainly not a bear; I have seen many bears over the years, and they don't stand on their hind legs for several minutes like that, and even if they did, their bodies are rounded in shape. This one was tapered, like that of a man.

Unnerved, I continued down the trail, not sure if I hoped the trail would lead me to this lake or not. At the bottom of the switchbacks, the trail turned away from the lake and followed its drainage down to its convergence with Dinwoody Creek, and I never looked back.

The creek was nearly overflowing its banks because of the runoff from snowmelt following a huge winter snowpack. I became very proficient in the art of log crossings, as there were countless creeks coming in from the side that I had to get across. Not to mention a major crossing of Dinwoody Creek itself over a wooden-plank bridge that was an inch or so below the surface of the water. I heard noise coming from a campsite somewhere off to my right and even smelled the smoke of a campfire and heard horses whinnying. It gave me comfort, if for no other reason than I told myself grizzlies don't like to be around horses. I wasn't sure about sasquatches, though.

Finally, in late afternoon, Gannett Peak came into view, and it was spectacular—a snow-covered pinnacle shining in the brilliant sunshine. I hiked underneath the entire length of the mountain; my northern approach would meet the trail from Bonney Pass somewhere south of my position and higher in the basin, but I wouldn't reach it that day. I had long since wanted to quit hiking and set up camp, but I resisted the temptation because the mosquitoes were as thick as thieves in this forested valley. I climbed higher into the basin and stopped at the last small stand of fir trees that marked treeline. The trees would protect my camp from the wind during the night, and serve for hanging my food bag to keep it out of the reach of any bears. I knew, though, that they were probably smarter than I was and would get my food anyway if they wanted to. Mostly, I just wanted my backpack off my back.

In the morning, I hit the trail early, eating breakfast on my feet as I continued to follow the diminishing creek upstream. The path soon became hard to follow as it entered a boulder field and curved around a small, emerald-green tarn. Patches of snow still held the faint tracks of previous climbers, so I just followed those, as I wasn't quite sure where I was going; all of my reconnaissance had been for the Bonney Pass route.

Facing the mountain, I climbed the first snow slope angling to my left— the south—from where I surmised the trail from Bonney Pass came in to meet it, and then turned back the other way along the top of a bergschrund, where the top of the glacier had melted away from the warmer rock it was attached to, creating a crevasse. I crossed a short rock band to stay to the right of Gooseneck Pinnacle, the sharp, pointy peak directly in front of me (or so I correctly guessed). Crossing two more snowfields and another rock band as I continued to climb steadily, two things gave me confidence that I was on the right trail: First, I saw the gaping crevasse stretching across my path a few hundred yards in front of me, with its tiny snow bridge that I would have to cross to get onto the upper glacier. Also, I noticed two other climbers not far behind me who had likely come over Bonney Pass.

The snow bridge was much sturdier than it appeared, and I was quickly across the 8-foot gap and onto the steep, 60-degree slope of the main glacier. It was so steep that I had to plant my ice ax into the snow in front of me and then pull myself up one step at a time. I repeated this maneuver over and over until I was finally on the ridge, an easy scramble of a few hundred feet away from the glorious summit.

I felt I could see all of Wyoming from the peak, including Grand Teton to the west, which I was hoping to climb in a few days. There are thirty-three peaks in Wyoming rising more than 13,000 feet, and very few of them ever see any climbers. In every direction, I saw nothing but towering peaks stretching all the way to the horizon. I was about as far from civilization as I imagined I could get in the Lower 48.

On the descent, the snow was quite a bit softer than on the way up. I was able to glissade part of the way off the glacier, twice falling and having to self-arrest, which was no problem in the slushy snow, thanks to my new ice ax.

I expected to meet the two climbers I had seen earlier, but I discovered by their tracks that they had apparently turned back and retreated over Bonney Pass without success—confirmation to me that I made the right choice by not taking that route myself. My day had been a 6-hour round-trip, as I got back to my campsite a little before noon.

Still, I was tired from the long hike in the day before, and I dived into my tent for a nap and some relief from the already annoying mosquitoes. I knew I would have to pack up soon and begin the hike out to get some miles behind me before dark; I wouldn't have the energy for another 23-mile day if I camped in the basin again. Even though it would be mostly downhill, the return trip would also include 10,800 feet of climbing. I fastidiously packed up and started out at 2:15 P.M., planning to get as far as the switchbacks leading out of Dinwoody Creek Basin, since I knew I would be too tired to climb those today.

The mosquitoes were downright relentless and murderous, despite the fact that I'd slathered on an entire bottle of bug spray. They were as bad as anywhere I had ever hiked, and that includes Maine, where the mosquito might as well be the state bird. It was a constant and unwinnable battle to keep them off. I would have gladly traded a grizzly encounter to get rid of them.

I reached the switchbacks at 6:20 P.M.—too early, I thought, to stop for the night—and pondered what to do next. I decided to keep going, so I started up, but I got only a few hundred yards before I realized I was too tired and going so slowly that the mosquitoes had me absolutely at their mercy. I stopped just ahead at a nice campsite next to a stream and the first thing I did was throw up my tent and dive inside to get away from the onslaught. But so many mosquitoes came in with me that I was immediately swatting at them like a madman; when I was done, I counted at least forty mosquito "carcasses" on the floor of my tent. But I had gotten them all, and, satisfied with my efforts, lay back and enjoyed 40 minutes of solitude as I watched thousands more buzz outside my tent, all wanting to come to the funeral of their fallen comrades.

My sanctuary was soon compromised: I still had to finish setting up camp and cook some dinner. I filled a pot with water from the stream and set up my stove just outside the front flap of the tent, unzipping it again only when the water was boiling to pour it into the pouch of my freeze-dried meal. Very few of the attackers foiled this ingenious plan, and those that did were quickly dispatched by the raving lunatic occupying a small tent in the wilderness. I vacated my asylum only once more that night when I got out to brush my teeth and go pee before bed.

I thought it would be too cold in the morning for mosquitoes to be on the prowl, but I was wrong. Though vastly reduced in ranks from the night before, legions still greeted me as I cooked breakfast and broke camp.

I still had a long, 14-mile day ahead of me, but rejuvenated by a night's sleep, I didn't find the switchbacks as hard as I had feared and I was soon back at the three lakes near the top of the pass. It seemed like an especially long hike out and the final miles were incredibly draining. I did not reach my car until 3:24 P.M., much later than I had expected, but not late enough to warrant camping at the trailhead, as I had done three nights before.

When I reached the town of Dubois, I got a bit of a scare when I stopped at a convenience store to buy some ice for my cooler and to use the restroom. When I got into the bathroom, I discovered I was peeing blood.

My kidneys apparently had been taxed to their limit by the arduous hike, which I had done in half the typical time. In my haste to get out of there, I had unwittingly failed to drink enough water on the hike out. I immediately started flushing myself by drinking lots of water. By the time I got to the American Alpine Club's Grand Teton Climbers Ranch in Moose Junction, about 12 miles north of Jackson Hole, and had taken a shower, thankfully my urine was no longer red.

It was afterward, at dinner, when I met Jim Grace, the former *Guinness* record holder for climbing the Lower 48 highpoints the fastest. That's when Jim told me the story of their adventure that was chronicled at the beginning of this chapter. Seems everywhere I go, I meet interesting people doing great things in the mountains.

After a rest day, I awoke at 1:30 A.M. on Tuesday and drove to the office of Exum Guides to begin what I anticipated might be my greatest and most dangerous adventure yet: climbing Grand Teton. Even the easiest route up the mountain is an exposed, Class 5 climb requiring ropes and climbing skills I really didn't possess.

Most people think Grand Teton is the highest peak in Wyoming, but, at 13,775 feet, it's a full 34 feet shorter than Gannett. It was going to be a one-on-one guided climb with Mark Falender, the same guide with whom I'd summited Rainier two years before.

Mark had me fill out a couple of forms—signing my life away—and after he fit me with a pair of climbing shoes, we were off. We hit the trail at 2:15 A.M. and reached the Lower Saddle between Grand Teton and Middle Teton just as the sun was coming up, as he had planned.

Mark then surprised me by announcing that we were going to climb the more challenging Exum Ridge route rather than the slightly easier, but perhaps more exposed, Owen-Spalding route. One advantage to this was that we would be in the sun more; the Exum route goes up the southwest ridge, while the Owen-Spalding route is on the west side, which would be in shadows until the afternoon. The Exum route begins by climbing a section called Wall Street, a narrow ledge that runs diagonally up the cliff face. But the ledge proved plenty wide and was not the least bit scary, and my nerves were calmed for the remainder of the day.

We then roped up for a series of pitches on which Mark led and I nimbly scrambled up behind him. It was so exhilarating to be able to climb so well on vertical rock, even if it was only 5.4 to 5.7 on the rock-climbing scale. I was amazed, and frankly so was Mark, that I climbed so well given that I had climbed on rope only two days in my life, when Nancy's friend Jamie Pierce, a certified guide, had taken me to Eleven Mile Canyon outside Colorado Springs the summer before. There was not a single pitch I had any difficulty surmounting, and after what did not seem a very long time, we were within sight of the summit.

Mark had one more treat in store first, however, before we topped out. Rather than complete the short scramble in front of us to the summit, we traversed to the west side of the ridge and then climbed a short, exposed section that deposited us on "The Horse," a narrow knife's edge that was so-named because we had to sit on the ridge with one foot on either side like it was a saddle. Then we completed the short scramble to the summit. With a deep sense of accomplishment, I finally relaxed and began to wonder why I had ever doubted my climbing abilities.

After about twenty glorious minutes on the summit, where we enjoyed incredible views of the entire Teton Range, we started down the Owen-Spalding route, and almost immediately had to put on another layer as we were suddenly plunged into the shadows and greeted by a brisk, chilling wind. We also found ourselves behind several other parties, but we were able to get past them all, with Mark having to do me the "indignity," he said, of belaying me down an icy chute in order to get around one slow-moving group.

Later, we avoided an exposed area—the one I had worried about had we taken this route on the way up—by doing a 120-foot rappel off a cliff. Peering down this cliff face—and the long drop just beyond it—as a lump rose in my throat. Mark set up the ropes for the rappel. My knees knocked as he connected me to the rope using a rappel device. I cautiously leaned back over the abyss and tried not to look down as I began to lower myself down the cliff face. But, again, my fears proved meritless, and my feet were soon on flat ground again. I had done it perfectly, remembering everything Jamie had taught me.

Soon we were back at the Lower Saddle, left with just the 7-mile hike back to the valley floor. It was interesting to discover how steep the trail was going down, and how many obstacles we had to go around, as I had remembered none of these boulders from the way up in the dark. We reached the parking lot at 2 p.m.; we had completed the round-trip in less than 12 hours, which Mark said was very impressive considering my inexperience on rope.

It was tough to leave the American Alpine Club's lodge the next morning. Initially, I had joined the club only so I could stay at the lodge, which charges members just $14 a night for a bunk, compared with $25 for nonmembers. In addition, the yearly membership fee provides climbers with insurance in case they need to be rescued on a climb, even outside the country. It was a bargain that no climber should pass up.

After stopping in Moose Junction to buy a new camp stove—a Jetboil system that weighed mere ounces as opposed to my antiquated gear—I drove north into Yellowstone Park, which I had never visited before. As I often discovered in our national parks, the place was virtually overrun with tourists. With a speed limit of just 45 mph, it took me half the day to get through the park. But first, I stopped at Old Faithful to learn that the next eruption was due in about 40 minutes.

Old Faithful blew right on schedule, sending steaming water up about a hundred feet in a constant belching that must've lasted for a couple of minutes or more. Then, it died down, and everyone got up and headed for the parking lot or the gift shop. I imagine this routine repeats itself at least a dozen times a day, with the ebb and flow of activity at this tourist attraction dictated solely by the Earth's plumbing.

It took another couple of hours for me to get to the park's northeast entrance, which lies just over the border in Montana, marking the forty-ninth state I had visited; only Alaska remained. After driving briefly back into Wyoming, I turned north and headed over Beartooth Pass, which was nothing short of spectacular. The road twisted and turned for miles as it climbed past numerous flowering meadows and stunning glacial lakes before topping out at the border at 10,947 feet.

The descent down the other side of the pass into the town of Red Lodge was just as beautiful. Montana certainly is the Big Sky State; even on tiny MT 78 it seemed like a vast expanse. On a washboard dirt road out of the town of Fishkill, it took nearly 45 minutes to drive the 14 miles to Emerald Lake Campground, located about a mile from the trailhead for Granite Peak at the Mystic Lake Hydroelectric Dam.

But the road dead-ended prematurely at a barricade at the entrance to the campground. The road beyond had recently washed out, meaning I would have an extra mile and a half to hike in the morning. I picked a site close to the raging West Rosebud Creek, as I figured it would help drown out the loud noises being made by some other campers at a nearby site. Plus, there was a large tree in the middle of the site, under which was the only dry patch of ground I could see, as it had rained earlier in the afternoon.

In the morning, I walked up the road to the power station at the dam, where the trail for the 11-mile hike to the ridge below Granite Peak began. Signs at the campground had warned campers about leaving food out to entice the bears, but no one had bothered to come empty the two large Dumpsters near the parking lot where I had left my car for the hike in. Both were so jam-packed with garbage that the lids couldn't close, so if any bears had been around, they could have had a smörgåsbord. But another hiker in the parking lot said he'd climbed Granite

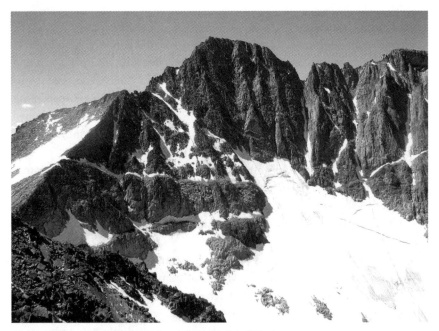

The South Face of Granite Peak, the state highpoint of Montana.

Peak six times, and had never seen a bear.

After passing the power station, the path followed West Rosebud Creek for 3 miles to the dam at Mystic Lake, gaining 1,200 feet along the way and providing great views of the long, narrow valley. At the lake, the real climbing began. I turned left onto the Phantom Creek Trail, which climbed another 3,000 feet over the next 3 miles. My guidebook called this the "Twenty-Six Switchbacks from Hell," but I found this to be a remarkably and intelligently constructed trail, perhaps the best-contoured series of switchbacks I had ever seen. I could tell by the reinforced rock walls built into the turns that a lot of care and thought had gone into the building and maintenance of this trail.

But once I got to the top of the pass and reached an open expanse, all bets were off. Known as the Froze-to-Death Plateau, the 5-mile segment passed through boulder fields, patches of snow, and wet, grassy meadows to reach a high saddle just below the summit of Tempest Mountain, overlooking the sheer south face of Granite Peak. Five miles, that is, if you took the most direct route. Good luck with that. There was no defined trail on this wide-open, wind-swept plateau, and while cairns supposedly marked the way, the book said not to trust them, because there were so many that they all seemed to lead in different directions. Turned out, if I had followed the series of large cairns that seemed to head off to my left, I would have found the shortest route. But then I would have missed out on yet another serendipitous meeting.

Unable to see Granite Peak behind the hillocks surrounding me, I wandered too far to my right and ended up at the top of a sheer cliff face. Looking to my left, I spotted two hikers coming in my direction and I headed to meet them. Not only did they provide me with trail information about the climb up Granite Peak, which they had completed that morning, they also turned out to be fellow Vermonters, and both had just finished their forty-seventh state highpoint. Granite Peak would be my forty-seventh as well.

The man's name was Bill Bender, and he was climbing with his stepdaughter, Kristen Kelliher. They lived in Norwich on the Vermont side of the Connecticut River, but she attended Hanover High on the New Hampshire side, where she was going to be a senior. Bill still had Rainier left on his list of the lower 48 states, having been turned back by a storm at the crater rim within sight of the summit when he and Kristen tried to climb it the month before. The outfitter they had used handed out certificates after that climb signifying that they had all "summited," but Kristen knew they hadn't stood atop Columbia Crest and therefore couldn't check off the Washington highpoint. So she contacted some other outfitters and found one that had a cancelation, and while her family returned to Vermont, she stayed and officially summited Rainier a couple of days later.

A week after I met her, Kristen would climb Mount Mansfield in her home state of Vermont to become the youngest woman, at 17 years old, to summit all the lower 48 state highpoints—and she didn't stop there.

While her classmates were finishing up their final year of high school, Kristen, a three-sport athlete at Hanover High, graduated a semester early and went to Hawaii to climb Mauna Kea that February. Then, that May, she got Denali in Alaska, making her the youngest female fifty-state highpointer ever. At the time of her completion, she was just the fifteenth woman to climb the highpoints of all fifty states, and the youngest by two full years. She was subsequently named one of ESPN's 18 Under 18. She summited Rainier again with Bill in June 2013, when he completed the lower 48.

I thanked Bill and Kristen for the trail info and headed for the saddle of Tempest and my soon-to-be campsite. Reaching this saddle, I found three rock walls that had been erected to protect campers from the ferocious winds that routinely whipped through there, forced back by Granite's blank south face.

Just after I finished setting up camp, the first of three vicious, back-to-back thunderstorms rolled across the plateau, each a little closer and more intense than the one before. As I lay huddled in my tent, I realized that I had left my trekking poles leaning up against the rock wall just a foot behind my tent;

I was afraid they would act as lightning rods, but I was too scared to go outside and retrieve them. I was so worried that I even put on my climbing helmet inside the tent, in case the howling wind blew a stone off the top of the wall onto my head.

It was snowing, too; not flakes of snow, like in winter, but graupel—popcorn snow. It continuously pelted the back of my tent until it sounded like I was inside a popcorn popper. By the time it stopped, more than an inch of BB-sized snowballs covered the ground. The lull between the second and third rounds was just long enough for me to get out my new Jetboil stove and boil some water for a tasty dinner of freeze-dried lasagna. I couldn't believe the extra weight I had been carrying around needlessly in my pack with my old stove.

Afterward, the weather cleared, and I was treated to one of the most beautiful sunsets I have ever seen. But the night turned out to be one of the longest I've ever endured. While it certainly dipped below freezing that night, I was snug in my sleeping bag and slept pretty well. The problem was that dawn never seemed to arrive; I awoke several times during the night expecting to see the first faint rays of daylight, but each time, it was still pitch black out.

When morning finally did arrive, I decided I'd better wait until the sun could warm Granite Peak up a bit before I ventured out on an ice-covered trail, considering the snow from the night before. At 8 A.M., voices passed my tent, and I jumped out. Brett and Janine, both from nearby Red Lodge, were headed for the summit. They were both brand new to climbing and were attempting their first state highpoint, they informed me. They did have a rope and seemed otherwise prepared, but I cautioned them about attempting perhaps the hardest of all the state highpoints first.

A third climber, Brian from Missoula, arrived at the same moment and dropped his pack near my tent and headed for the summit of Tempest Mountain, just a short scramble up the ridge from the campsite. He later caught us near the top of the first snowfield just before the famed "snow bridge," which really isn't a snow bridge, but rather an overhanging cornice at the top of a narrow couloir that gives climbers firmer footing than is found after the snow melts out later in the summer. Since he seemed experienced and said he was climbing Granite for the fourth time, I left the other two behind and continued on with Brian.

When we got to the other side of the snow bridge, however, he started to descend in order to go around a large buttress. I quickly stopped him and pointed to the narrow chute above us that I could see had protection in the form of rock-climbing gear attached to the rocks. Then, I showed him a picture in the guidebook, which showed that this was the way to go. He agreed, and led us up through these Class 4 chutes that I knew I was going to have to downclimb later on my descent.

At the top of this chimney, the well-marked trail beyond was easy to follow, until we got to the final 200 feet below the summit, where the real challenges began. The climbing was exposed and pretty scary, with no defined route. We chose the path of least resistance, which sometimes lead me into places I don't want to be. Such as the South Face. Falling behind Brian, I followed one route around to that side of the mountain and suddenly was staring at a thousand-foot drop below me. I tried the next chute, but backed off when I saw I would have to make a bold move directly over this expanse. I ultimately took a less-risky chute, which brought me back to the north side of the mountain and safer climbing.

From there, I was directly under the summit, which Brian had somehow already attained. He told me to traverse to my left to a keyhole, and from there it was just a 50-foot scramble to the summit block, where he was sitting with the register book in his lap. Gaining the lofty summit, I knew firsthand why Granite Peak was the last of the state highpoints to be conquered; it wasn't until 1923 that anyone stood atop Montana.

After we both signed in and snapped a few pictures of each other, I nearly choked on the apple I was eating when he told me he was continuing over the summit and going out another way. He was attempting a complete traverse of all the mountains surrounding Granite, and there were many: twenty-five peaks over 13,000 feet dot the Absaroka–Beartooth Range. He departed, and I contemplated my future. I wasn't sure if I should try to climb down on my own—facing the sheer drops below the chute solo—or wait for Brett and Janine to arrive so I could take advantage of their rope if it was needed.

I decided to start down and, once past the keyhole, found the route pretty much laid out before me. I reached the top of the chute above the snow bridge as Brett and Janine were exiting it, having taken an inordinately long time ascending this narrow chimney. They continued on to the summit; I don't know if they reached it, because I continued on, working my way down with careful steadiness through the "no-fall zone." The hand- and footholds, however, were well spaced and I found the descent to be anything but difficult. Soon, I was back at the snow bridge, and after dropping another 800 feet to the col, climbed back up to my tentsite to find that some visitors had stopped in while I was away.

Six mountain goats were checking out my campsite, and I promptly remembered pictures I'd seen in one online trip report in which mountain goats had ripped a tent to shreds trying to get at the food that had been left inside. Fortunately, my tent was still intact, but they hung around me like a swarm of mosquitoes while I broke camp, looking for any handout I might give them. They got so close, I had to shoo them away several times, and one of them—

the billy of the group—kept climbing up on the rock wall behind my tent to watch my progress, with the inquisitive, blank stare of a Tibetan monk.

Now don't get me wrong. I liked having the goats around. Considering it had taken three expeditions through Colorado's 14ers to see my first—and even then not until my fifty-fourth and final mountain and at some distance—this was a real treat, if a slightly inconvenient one. After I packed up and started hiking out, I looked back and saw them all standing there on the hilltop looking forlorn. A moment later, four ascending climbers passed me, headed for the campsite, so these goats weren't lonely for long.

I could have spent another night at Emerald Lake Campground, but I had only $2 on me and the nightly fee was $9, so I got in the car and headed for Billings, about 2 hours away. There were free campsites along the road—and several were empty when I passed them—but I really wanted a shower, a comfortable bed, and a good steak dinner. As it turned out, I went only 1-for-3.

At 7:45 that night, virtually every hotel and motel room in Billings was booked. Turned out it was a Friday, unbeknownst to me, since I wasn't keeping track of the days. Not only that, but the area was hosting the Montana State Fair, a blues festival, several crews on site to clean up an oil spill on the Yellowstone River, and the Little League state playoffs. In addition, some of the 100,000 bikers who had been at Bike Week in Sturgis, South Dakota, were on their way home. The cheapest room still available in town that night was for $230. Not on my budget.

They couldn't keep me from eating, however. I dragged my smelly carcass to an Applebee's and enjoyed a juicy steak and a cold beer. There, I was told that I probably could find a room about 40 miles down I-90 in the town of Harden, so I got back on the highway. I stopped at a rest area about halfway there and contemplated pitching my tent somewhere in the darkness. But between the lights, the nearly full moon, the cloudless night, and the lack of trees, there was no place dark enough or sheltered enough to spend the night. I couldn't win.

A "No Vacancy" sign greeted me when I pulled into Harden's Super 8. Inquiring inside, I was told every room in Harden was sold out, too, but I could find a room in Sheridan, Wyoming, or pitch my tent at a nearby campground. I was far too tired to drive another 90 miles that night, so I spent $19 to toss and turn in my tent, listening to teenagers hot-rod up and down the main street. I was so tired, I even waited until morning to take a shower, and it sure felt good after a fitful night's sleep.

Clean and refreshed, I got back on I-90 and headed for home, stopping only for food and gas and to visit Little Bighorn National Battlefield, where I was warned to be careful wandering around, since the place was crawling with rattlesnakes. Or so the park ranger said. Fortunately, I didn't cross paths with any.

It was another 8 hours before I pulled into Colorado Springs. Nancy, who had been home a few days from Outdoor Retailer, was glad to see me. So were the dog and the horse, as best as I could tell. The cat, of course, couldn't have cared less.

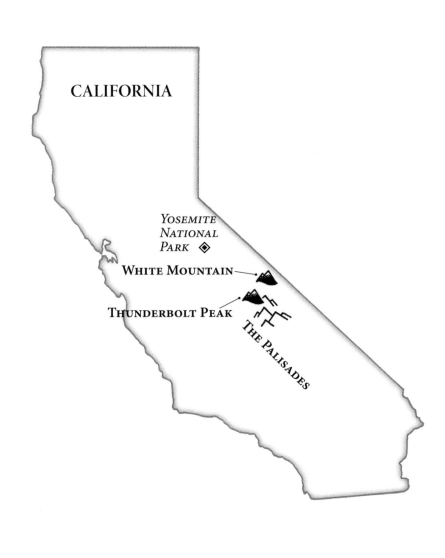

CALIFORNIA

Yosemite National Park ◈

White Mountain ⟶

Thunderbolt Peak ⟶

The Palisades

Chapter 13
September 2011

YOSEMITE AND THE PALISADES

THREE WEEKS AFTER CLIMBING GRANITE PEAK IN MONTANA, I PACKED UP AGAIN and headed for California to begin knocking off the state's remaining 14ers— so far I had climbed only Whitney—and to join Charles and Zac Bookman and their friends on a five-day camping trip in Yosemite National Park. Nancy would be traveling, too: the 2011 World Mountain Running Championships were being held in Albania, of all places. We were both due home in a couple weeks.

Leaving on a Monday morning in late August, I made good time as I drove the hour north to Denver and turned west on I-70, one of the prettiest interstate highways in the country. The road crests the Rockies of Colorado, then descends along the Colorado River through narrow Glenwood Canyon. The landscape gets even more remarkable once I-70 crosses into Utah and climbs the San Rafael Swell. The construction of the freeway through these sheer canyons is listed as one of the great engineering marvels of the Interstate Highway System, with one engineer stating that this section was "one of the most significant highway construction feats of its time." The area is also home to the system's longest stretch between service stations: I gassed up at Green River, as the next services were 110 miles away.

Then, while climbing the San Rafael Swell, my car started to sputter and the "check engine" light came on. I wasn't too concerned. It had done that often, and was usually related to a problem with the oxygen intake sensor. A few hours later, however, after I had entered Nevada on lonely US 50, the "check oil" light suddenly came on and a warning buzzer sounded. This, I could not ignore.

As has happened so many times when I've had car trouble, I was approaching the only "town" for many miles. This time it was the desolate way station of Major's Junction, a tiny outpost marking the junction of US 6, US 50, and US 93, where there was a single building—a general store, bar, and rest stop all rolled into one. I bought two quarts of oil and needed both of them in order to get anything to register on the Jetta's dipstick. Considering I had changed the oil after I'd gotten back from Montana, I couldn't figure out where it had gone. But I had no further problems, and headed over the hill and dropped into Ely, where I gassed up again for the long haul across Nevada the next day.

I pulled into almost-deserted Ward Mountain Campground, just up the hill from Ely, beneath an incredible sunset. In the morning, I awoke early and crossed Nevada on US 6. Five hours, plus a 9-mile drive on a dirt road later, I arrived at White Mountain Peak's trailhead in California.

White Mountain Peak is the most distinctive of California's fifteen mountains over 14,000 feet. Unlike the Sierra Nevada range looming across the Owens River Valley—marked by their steep, jagged spires jutting skyward—the broad, barren, desertlike mountain more resembles Colorado 14ers such as Culebra. Its biology is as unusual as its geology, as there are more than 200 species of plants found on White Mountain Peak that occur nowhere else in California. Chief among them is the Great Basin bristlecone pine, one of the longest-lived species on Earth. The oldest specimen is more than 5,000 years old and is the world's oldest individual plant; many of the other bristlecone pines found on White Mountain are more than 4,000 years old.

The road ended at a gate at 12,000 feet, and I left the car, following a four-wheel-drive track for 7 more miles to an abandoned government high-altitude research facility on the summit. The square, cement building had long since been boarded up. I went around to the backside and found a way to climb onto its flat roof to get better views of the Owens River Valley below and of the Sierras on the other side.

Running down the winding road from the summit, I passed a woman running up, then spotted a familiar-looking dog and another person, both coming up behind her.

Suddenly, this person blurted out, "Garry?"

What a surprise. It was my friend Steve Till and his dog, Pepper, with whom I had climbed Humphreys Peak in Arizona two years before and a couple of Colorado 14ers before that. I had not seen or heard from him since screening *Ride the Divide* in Flagstaff the previous October, when I had stayed with him. What an amazing coincidence, meeting him again on a remote 14er in California. The woman ahead of him was his on-again, off-again girlfriend,

Bonney. Steve said he was leaving to return to Arizona the next day, as he had a rafting trip through the Grand Canyon planned—a "work" trip, he reminded me—and then was heading to Utah for a month-long hike on the Hayduke Trail, a newly created route through 800 miles of publically protected land from Moab to Zion National Park, though to date the route is merely an unsigned suggestion. If not for the fact that I had to return to work at UPS in October, I would have asked to join him.

Entering Yosemite the next day, I headed straight for Crane Flat Campground, where I rented two adjacent sites and waited for the Bookmans and their friends to arrive for our planned five-day hike. The name was a misnomer: the campground lacked any flat ground whatsoever. I noticed that most of the tents there were set up at an angle, but I found the lone semiflat spot at our site, cut out of a sidehill with a shovel, and grabbed it, the perk for arriving first.

Then I drove into the valley, where just about everything of interest in Yosemite is found. Coming out of a tunnel, I got my first views—and they were stunning. I passed El Capitan, as well as Yosemite Falls and Bridalveil Fall, then entered the Village, where I got my first real look at Half Dome, gleaming in the midday sun. We planned to conclude our trek by climbing the backside of Half Dome, which requires a permit that was included in our hiking pass.

Looking at Half Dome, I could not fathom how rock climber Alex Honnold had free-soloed this sheer, featureless face without a rope in just a couple of hours in 2008. I had heard that some guy had committed suicide a couple of weeks before by jumping from Half Dome, and not long before, a California woman slipped from a ladder while descending in the rain on the Cable Route that we would be climbing, falling 600 feet to her death. I was later told that body recovery is one of the first jobs designated to new park rangers at Yosemite, to make sure they can stomach what is an all-too-frequent occurrence.

Indeed. People die all the time in Yosemite. Just while I was there, a 69-year-old man was found dead in his sleeping bag, bringing the death toll for the year to eighteen, the highest in Yosemite history. And it was still only Labor Day Weekend. I read somewhere that there have been as many as 900 recorded deaths in Yosemite since it was designated a national park in 1890. Even the more recent incidents hadn't affected the number of park visitors; nearly three-quarters of a million people entered Yosemite just during the month of July that year.

I spent my afternoon hiking the Mist Trail to view both Vernal and Nevada falls, two of the park's signature waterfalls. The first part of the trail was fairly steep, but it was paved all the way to a bridge crossing over the raging Merced

River. Farther up, the rugged, rocky footpath with steep switchbacks led to great views back down the valley. Many international tourists—a lot of them Germans, from what I could tell—were not discouraged by the strenuous hike, talking comfortably in their native tongues. Conversely, on my way out, I was met by dozens of huffing and puffing Americans asking in shortened breath how far it was to the bridge. To the bridge! That's barely a half-mile up the trail, and Vernal Fall, the lower of the two, isn't even visible from there. I pray that I hadn't been similarly that out of shape before I started climbing Monadnock regularly all those years ago.

Back in the valley, I found no cell service, and thus was unable to call Zac Bookman to let them know where we were camping that night. I later found a Wi-Fi hot spot and emailed them, learning that they were just leaving San Francisco. Zac, Charles, and Zac's older brother Ty arrived in Ty's '99 Audi about 9:15 P.M., along with Ty's friend Aaron, who had flown in for the adventure from Arkansas, where he worked at Walmart's headquarters in Bentonville.

Zac's friend Greg was waiting for us at the Mono Meadow trailhead when we arrived at ten the next morning, and we hiked the rest of the day, stopping only for lunch on a large, flat rock next to a fast-running stream. Everyone except Greg and I skinny-dipped in the ice-cold, 2-foot-deep creek. I decided not to embarrass myself by joining them.

Our intended destination that day was Lower Merced Lake, but somehow we hiked right past it without seeing it. We turned left at a trail junction and started toward Ottoway Lake, still more than 3 miles away. Charles, who had recently turned 64, was exhausted after hiking all day, so we decided to camp at the next stream we came to. But when we got to it, there was no flat ground nearby, and we continued on to the next one. When we reached it, Zac and I traipsed into the woods, where we found a decent tentsite high above the trail. We all enjoyed a gorgeous sunset and a rice-and-beans dinner ahead of a chilly night spent at 8,900 feet.

We reached Ottoway Lake very early the next morning and discovered several amazing-looking campsites, but we had made the right choice by stopping; Charles hadn't been the only one who was whipped after a long, taxing first day on the trail. Of course, Ottoway Lake gave the Bookmans another opportunity to skinny-dip, despite the water being near-glacial cold, as we were now at 9,700 feet. The trail from the lake to Red Peak Pass at 11,180 feet was as immaculately constructed as the inlaid rock stairs leading to the waterfalls I had visited two days before, and I marveled at the stonework as the trail switchbacked its way to the pass.

Our original plan was to climb nearby Red Peak, but, because we still had 10 more miles to hike that day, only Zac still wanted to climb the thousand feet or

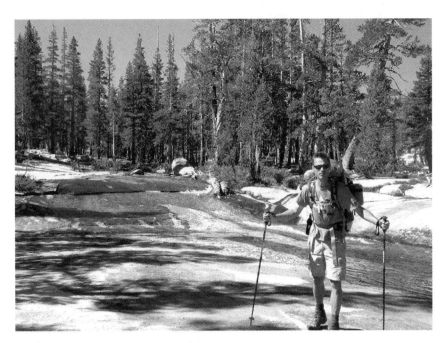

Hiking along the Merced River in Yosemite National Park.

so to the 11,704-foot summit. He finally talked Ty and me into joining him, but Ty turned back when we reached a near-vertical wall that, while not particularly exposed, required some low Class 5 climbing. It proved to be quite exhilarating, but not overly dangerous, though Zac said he would not have continued had I not been with him. I was surprised to find a register book on the summit of such an inconsequential peak, but we signed it anyway, and then descended by what must have been the standard route, as it was marked by cairns.

Picking up our packs at the small lake at which we had left them, we continued down from the pass and had gone only a couple of miles when we heard someone yelling up at us. Looking down, we spied four naked men sitting on a flat rock next to another glistening lake. Apparently, the others had decided not to hike another 10 miles after all. We joined them at Small Lake shortly thereafter, and despite it being only 3:30, they had already decided this campsite was more than sufficient for the night.

There was a 20-foot-high cliff on the far side of this lake and Ty dared Zac and me to jump from it. Feeling more comfortable among friends after two days on the trail, I finally got naked myself and swam across the lake and climbed to the top of the cliff. Though we were at nearly 10,000 feet, the water was not as cold as I would have imagined. But the 20-foot drop sure seemed higher than I had expected. Zac soon joined me, and we both jumped into the water with a hard smack. I was not aware until then how much protection swim trunks can provide to one's otherwise-exposed private parts when jumping from a cliff. It was a painful swim back across the lake to our campsite.

Dropping into the Merced River drainage the next day, we stopped to eat lunch at the first deep hole we came to. The others all went swimming again, except Charles, who left ahead of us and said he would wait for us at Washburn Lake, a few miles downstream. We followed not long after, but got sidetracked by one amazing swimming hole after another. At one of them, I stood under a small waterfall upstream and enjoyed a refreshing shower for the first time in days.

We met up with Charles at a trail junction a few miles past Washburn Lake, where he'd stopped to chat with some other hikers, and continued on to Merced Lake. The lake's campground was surprisingly uncrowded for a Saturday night on Labor Day Weekend. We marched past, and Greg recounted a story of an airplane full of marijuana that had crashed in this lake in the '70s. I thought the story dubious, but I later confirmed that it had happened—in Lower Merced Pass Lake, several miles away from Merced Lake, in the park's Clark Range.

In December 1976, a twin-engine Lockheed Lodestar stuffed with six tons of marijuana—apparently from Mexico—crashed into Lower Merced Pass Lake. Authorities mounted a well-publicized rescue expedition, retrieving several bales of the drug, but divers could not find the bodies of the plane's pilot or any passengers, so they called off the search until after the spring melt. They didn't think anyone would try to fish the remaining ton of pot out of the icy water. But they were wrong. Their oversight led to what became known as the Yosemite Gold Rush.

"Somehow, people got wind of this, and it was like the Klondike gold rush," said John Dill, a longtime Yosemite park ranger. "You couldn't find an ice ax anywhere."

It began when three members of the Valley Rats—rock-climbing bums living in vans, working as guides in summer, and scrounging for nickel-deposit cans in winter—were tipped off about the unrecovered weed and hiked the 14 miles in to the remote lake. Chopping through the 2-foot-thick ice with their axes was cold and wet work. Just before giving up, one opened a hole, and a large black plastic bag filled with marijuana floated to the surface. Smoking some of it, they found that it was the highest-quality pot they had ever tried. They immediately named it "Airplane." They were going to be rich. Or at least high for a while.

They loaded up all they could carry and headed out, only to be met by two others who had had the same idea. "There's plenty more for the taking," they told the two newcomers.

Back in the Valley, the three Valley Rats stopped at a friend's cabin and showed off the 200 pounds of marijuana they had carried out. In the morning, their friend was gone; he had called in sick and hit the trail for his share.

The news spread like wildfire. The next day, virtually every working transient in the Yosemite Valley failed to show up for work. Hikers with chainsaws and scuba gear were soon seen on the Illilouette and Mono Meadow trails. The Yosemite Gold Rush was on.

When the three original scavengers returned to the crash site ten days later, they couldn't believe what they saw: campsites ringed the western end of the lake, and at least thirty people were out on the lake chopping away with ice axes. "It was insane," one of the men, named Craig, said later. People would haul a bale out of the water, divvy it up, and immediately start hiking out on a trail that was now as well trodden as if it were summer.

A week later, the Valley regulars had become convinced that a bust must be imminent. Everyone knew about the pot. Craig was riding the shuttle bus one day when two hikers reeking of pot boarded with bulging backpacks. People no longer bothered hiding their stashes. The following Monday, the same ranger who had tipped off the Valley Rats to the contents of the plane told them that Wednesday might not be a good day to be on the Mono Meadow trail.

The feds nabbed only a couple of people on the trail, but the gold rush was over; the park service stationed two rangers at the lake to guard the crash site until spring.

For the next several weeks, things were different in Yosemite Valley. The same people who had been scrounging for food in the cafeterias were buying steak dinners and leaving big tips in the finest restaurants. They were all now drinking Beck's instead of Budweiser. Almost overnight, they had become "Airplane millionaires."

In all, a reported half million dollars worth of marijuana was carted out of the woods during the gold rush, selling for more than $400 a pound in San Francisco and Los Angeles. Many of the Valley Rats returned to Yosemite showing off thick wads of cash. A cocaine market soon blossomed in the Valley, as before, no one had been able to afford it. Months later, when asked what they had done with all their money, many of the Valley Rats simply put a finger to their nose and sniffed.

But new vans and motorcycles were bought, as well, and the local mountaineering shops quickly sold out of all the latest gear.

The Rats' makeshift camp also changed. The media kept the crash story alive well into the summer, encouraging a flood of new arrivals and hangers-on. "It became too much of a zoo," Craig later lamented; the communal lifestyle they had all enjoyed before had been swallowed up. Most of those who had profited from the rush left for places such as the Dolomites and the Himalaya. Craig was one of the few who stayed, but spent most of his time that summer in the high country, avoiding the annual influx of contemptible tourists. The bodies from the crash were finally recovered and the plane and the rest of its cargo removed. And just like that, the Yosemite Gold Rush was over.

A mile past Merced Lake, we found a great campsite right next to the trail and another glorious swimming hole. That night, Charles cooked some of his famous "mystery meat," which I didn't quite dare to ask about—it did not taste like chicken, but was a bit spicy, like it might once have been sausage. We were not as cold as previous nights, as we had descended to just over 7,000 feet; it was the first night on the trip that I had not secretly wished I had brought a down parka with me.

In the morning, we parted ways with Greg at the first trail junction we came to, as he was hiking out early to return to Los Angeles on a Sunday to avoid all the holiday traffic. The rest of us headed to Half Dome on the Echo Valley Trail. The path climbed more than a thousand feet and then leveled off at a burn scar from a fairly recent wildfire. New growth was creeping in on the trail, and we probably should have paid a little more attention to all this low-lying vegetation.

We were all walking single file, pushing through new growth creeping in on the trail, Charles in the lead. Suddenly, we heard the unmistakable sound of a rattle in the bushes. Charles screamed, wheeled around, and turned back toward us in a panicked rush. Ty turned, screamed, and sidestepped Aaron, crashing instead into Zac, who in turn backpedaled into me. I tumbled off the trail into the bushes. Charles knocked Aaron to the ground, and ran him over. When he fell, Aaron landed on a sharp rock, scraping a large portion of skin off his palm. The ordeal had been like watching an old rerun of the *Keystone Cops*, or, better yet, the episode of *Seinfeld* in which George knocks over a bunch of kids at a birthday party trying to escape when a fire breaks out in the apartment's kitchen.

The whole episode would have been quite comical had Aaron not been in-jured. Our trekking poles were strewn all over the trail, like a pile of pickup sticks. While Zac and Ty tended to Aaron's hand, Charles and I started back along the trail—cautiously—to make sure the snake was gone. It had apparently made as hasty a retreat as we'd attempted. Once we'd regained our composure, we continued on, using our poles as minesweeping devises until we were satis-fied that it had been a one-time occurrence. We were soon on the more-traveled trail leading to the backside of Half Dome and no longer had to worry.

The iconic granite Half Dome rises nearly 5,000 feet above the valley floor and is probably Yosemite's most familiar rock formation. It adorns the California state quarter that was issued in 2005, and now is also pictured on some California license plates.

We showed our climbing permits to the ranger stationed at the bottom, then started up. Steep switchbacks beat an exposed path to the rounded summit of a smaller dome that flanks the much-larger main dome; even this climbing was not for everyone. Beyond, a cable ladder led 400 feet straight up what appeared to be a near-vertical wall. Dozens of tourists moved up and down the rungs, passing each other with only the utmost of care. It boggled my imagination and stretched the boundaries of what I would have expected to be legally permissible in an American national park. I wasn't even sure something like this would have been allowed in Guatemala, where I had stood face to face with erupting volcanoes. It was insane, and we were about to join the madness.

About 50,000 tourists a year scale this harrowing Cable Route, yet fewer than ten people have died from a fall here, the most recent being the previously mentioned woman from California, who fell only the month before my visit. Fortunately, the direct path to the Cable Route is an 8.2-mile hike past Vernal Fall; the demanding trail must deter most of those out-of-breath tourists that I had seen only a few days earlier. With easier access, the body count would certainly rise dramatically.

The cables' angle of steepness probably did not exceed 60 degrees, but that was still enough exposure that many of the people above us were freaking out. Some moved very slowly or not at all. It was difficult enough to get past these climbers, but we also had to contend with those who were on their way down. The cables were held in place by metal posts hammered directly into the rock, with boards stretched along the rock face every few feet serving as footholds. Most people wore gloves available at the bottom to protect their hands from metal splinters, but I found I got a better grip on the cables without them.

About halfway up, someone above me dropped a water bottle, and it rocketed down the slope, barely missing me and other climbers before disappearing over the edge of a cliff and out of sight. I could only imagine how many people might be swept off the ladder by a falling body.

Near the top, the steepness lessened dramatically until I could stand upright and walk normally. I explored the large summit, which covers about 3 or 4 acres, I guessed. The views were beyond stunning. I edged out onto an overhang called The Visor and someone took my picture, but I didn't dare dangle my legs over the lip like my friend Howie Stern said he had done. A large, fat marmot, however, was sunning itself on the warm rocks just inches from the edge of the cliff, perfectly oblivious to the 5,000-foot drop it would have experienced had it rolled over. I have no idea how he got up there.

Descending felt like it took forever; there was still a conga line of people climbing up. But we eventually made it down and called it a day. We spent our final night together at the Little Yosemite Valley backpackers' campground, easily our least favorite campsite of the trip. This campground was crowded, and quite a distance from the river, and even Zac and Ty weren't able to skinny-dip here. In the morning, we passed Nevada Fall—which I had visited the week before—and turned left onto the John Muir Trail, which led us back to the Mono Meadow trailhead, where we had started five days before.

It was tough to say goodbye after such an incredible trip. They all headed west back to San Francisco, while I returned all of our rented bear canisters to the ranger station and headed east through beautiful Tuolomne Meadows. Getting back to CA 395 in the town of Lee Vining, I put one adventure behind me and headed for the next.

I began reading about California's Palisade Range when I had started planning my trip to bag the state's remaining 14ers. My knees went weak at the route descriptions. The pictures alone took my breath away. The range is steep, jagged, and extremely exposed, protected by the Sierra's largest glacier, and summiting them would require rock-climbing skills that I had only begun to acquire. Only veteran rock climbers, with the expertise and the equipment to scale these steep, jagged spires, should step foot in the Palisades, and I certainly was not among them. The Palisades were far more technical than even what I had experienced on Grand Teton, where I had had the luxury of a paid guide to get me through. It would be the most challenging and physically demanding mountaineering I had yet undertaken. My chances of winning the lottery were likely higher than successfully solo climbing any of the peaks in the Palisades range.

I needed a guide, but I couldn't afford a professional one. And I did not want to be shepherded to the summits; I wanted to experience them in a more personal way. I reached out to my friend Doug Seitz, with whom I had climbed Mount Hood two years before, and I offered him a deal. If he would guide me through the Palisades, I would pay for everything, including his plane ticket from Seattle to Reno. Doug immediately said yes. The deal was fair: he got a free trip to the remote, rugged peaks he'd always wanted to climb, and I got the security of a guide without the irritation, hassle, or price tag of hiring a pro.

Doug did the research and thought that we would be able to climb all five 14ers in the Palisades in one day, traversing from Thunderbolt and Starlight peaks, over to North Palisade and Polemonium, then on to Mount Sill at the far end of the ridge. Polemonium, at 14,080 feet, is often overlooked by mountaineers as not being a true 14er, due to its proximity to higher North Pal, but it's a favorite of many climbers and it didn't make sense not to bag it on the way to Mount Sill. We knew our plan was a bit on the ambitious side, but looking at the map, the distance between the peaks was marginal—at least as the crow flies.

While waiting in Reno for him to arrive, I stopped at REI and dropped $320, picking up the down parka that I had desperately wished I'd had in Yosemite, and a water filtration system, among other things. All too often, I am too cheap to purchase gear I might need only a handful of times, resigning myself to the inconvenience of being without it over the inconvenience of a thinner wallet. But with the financial tradeoffs I'd made—all in order to be in the mountains with regularity—I could afford to equip myself properly.

Doug's plane arrived at 1 P.M., and we drove the 4 hours south to Bishop and spent the night at the Willow Campground on the road to South Lake trailhead. We hiked 8 miles the next morning, from the parking lot to the top of Bishop Pass, passing several beautiful lakes along the way. The last of these was Bishop Lake, from where the trail switchbacks wonderfully right up the cliff face to Bishop Pass at an elevation of 11,972 feet.

Traversing under the west faces of Agassiz and Winchell, a pair of high 13ers that mark the northern end of the Palisades, we crossed Dusy Basin and angled toward Thunderbolt Pass, where we found several appealing campsites and set up camp on a mostly flat, sandy bench. To lighten our packs, we did not bring a tent, as the weather forecast did not call for rain over the next two days. A 20-foot-high granite block to our right would protect us from the wind whipping over Thunderbolt Pass.

Our Palisades itinerary was not for the faint of heart. We decided to start on one of the range's toughest summits: Thunderbolt Peak. Not only is the approach steep and exposed, but the summit block, like the one on neighboring Starlight, requires some serious rock-climbing moves to ascend.

The description in *Climbing California's 14ers*—the guidebook I was using by climbers Stephen Porcella and Cameron Burns—was daunting enough. "For many years, due to its illusory guise of arêtes and gullies, Thunderbolt Peak remained untouched by mountaineers," Porcella and Burns wrote. "Thunderbolt was the last 14,000-foot peak to be climbed in California, and yet it is one of the most spectacular. A straightforward route to the summit is not apparent from any direction. Even after you've gained the main Palisade Crest at the 13,800-foot level, the difficulties are still ahead of you. The final obstacle is a triangular monolith lacking any noticeable features. Of all the 14,000-foot peaks in California, Thunderbolt's summit monolith is the most difficult to surmount."

Thunderbolt was named and conquered in August 1931. That summer, Francis Farquhar, editor of the *Sierra Club Bulletin* newsletter, invited Harvard philosophy professor Robert Underhill, who edited the Appalachian Mountain Club's *Appalachia*, to come to the Sierras. Farquhar wanted Underhill to instruct climbers there on the new techniques Underhill had unveiled in a still-famous article entitled "Of the Use and Management of the Rope in Rock Work," which first outlined the techniques of belaying and rappelling that are still the staple of rock climbing today.

While there, Farquhar and Underhill headed to the Palisades, teaming up with legendary mountaineer Norman Clyde, who had put up more first routes in the Sierras than any other climber. The three were among seven climbers who had completed the first-ever traverse from North Palisade to Starlight Peak, which Clyde had been the first to climb the year before. A week later, the seven set their sights on the unclimbed and unnamed 14,003-foot peak next to Starlight.

On August 13, 1931, despite threatening clouds that were coming over the ridge from the west, the party ascended a chute on the east side of the mountain that would later become known as the Underhill Couloir. Once reaching the ridge, they decided to scramble over a precarious knife's edge despite the onset of the storm.

When they arrived at the summit block—a large pyramidal block of smooth, solid granite—the men created a human ladder, enabling two members of the party, longtime climbing partners Glen Dawson and Jules Eichorn, to scramble to the top. But blue sparks were dancing and flickering about the summit and they all scrambled for safety. Dawson descended, and Eichorn began to follow when a sudden burst of light flashed, followed by a deafening clap of thunder. A bolt of lightning had struck the summit block. When Eichorn caught up to the others, he informed them that "a thunderbolt just whizzed past my right ear!" It had been a narrow escape, and had given the mountain a name.

The other five had to forgo a summit bid on this expedition, but Clyde returned two years later and succeeded, establishing a new route from the west side. Nearly eighty years later, Doug and I started up the same route, entering the chute directly behind our camp the morning after our arrival. We climbed steadily and had little difficulty ascending the 1,700 vertical feet to a small notch in the ridgeline. From there, we carefully worked our way along the same narrow knife's edge that the Underhill party had negotiated in 1931, and soon we, too, were standing in front of the huge summit monolith.

Looking at its smooth, featureless contours, I didn't think there was any way I was going to be able to get to the top. The block is rated as a 5.9 climb on the rock-climbing scale, more difficult than the Milk Bottle atop Starlight, which we could now see little more than a quarter-mile to our south, and harder than anything I had even contemplated before. Doug had his doubts, too.

Climbing up on the edge of the triangular block, Doug said he found no solid hand- or footholds. And he wasn't quite sure he wanted to commit to a bold, unprotected mantle move, where he would have to bring his feet up to where his hands clung to the smooth rock before trying to stand up. It might have gotten him past a small lip, which would deposit him onto the smooth side of the block, or he might have fallen nearly 2,000 feet. I didn't blame his uncertainty. It looked scary as hell.

Doug scratched his head. Maybe this predicament would stymie us. My heart sank. I feared that I had come all this way only to fail.

Then Doug got the idea to try to lasso the summit, which tapers to a point just a few inches in diameter. Directly on the summit were two slings and two carabiners left by previous climbers, and Doug thought he could snag one of them with his rope. Try as he might, he couldn't. He was getting frustrated, and as more time passed, I was beginning to accept our fate.

Then a miracle happened. As the rope missed the summit yet again, it snagged on the nub of a broken-off bolt, which Doug had not noticed before since it protruded only about a quarter-inch above the rock face. As he slowly reeled in the rope, it pulled tight on the bolt, and when he put some weight on the rope, it held secure.

Climbing back onto the summit block with the protection of the rope, he committed to the mantle move and got his foot over the corner of the monolith. From there, he scrambled up the smooth side of the block and seconds later was standing on the tiny summit with a big smile on his face. Coming down after securing a belay for me, Doug roped me into my harness and I repeated his moves, bringing my foot up to where my hands were and standing up, completing the difficult mantle move. From there, I got my right foot over the corner of the block and then quickly scrambled up the smooth edge until I stood on the summit, peering over a drop of a couple thousand feet.

At the time, it was perhaps the most precarious perch in which I had ever found myself, but that would be exceeded later that day once we got over to the Milk Bottle. Descending back to the safety of the ridge, I now had the permission of the mountain to sign the register book, which had once been located directly on the top of the summit block—much to the consternation of defeated climbers— but was now located down in the rocks by our feet.

While Starlight looked close enough that Doug might have been able to lasso that, too, it was, in fact, a difficult and dangerous traverse over to the neighboring peak. A sheer drop of several hundred feet separated the two peaks. We had to rappel into this notch from Thunderbolt's summit ridge, then scramble along an exposed ledge to regain the ridgeline on the other side. From there, however, we still had some serious climbing along the ridge crest to ascend Starlight.

Norman Clyde had been the first to successfully climb the Milk Bottle, making a solo attempt on July 9, 1930, arriving at the summit just as a thunderstorm

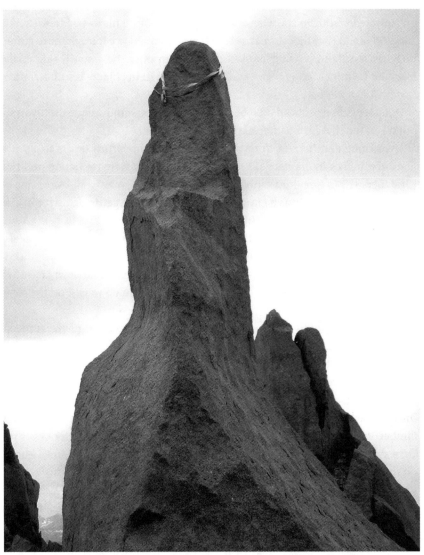

The infamous Milk Bottle sticks straight up on the summit of Starlight Peak like a middle finger thrust in the air to defy all who attempt to climb it.

was racing in across Dusy Basin below. After attempting to lasso the 30-foot-high tower unsuccessfully, he swung the rope around the spire and, tying both ends to his waist, he shimmied up the monolith like a lumberjack climbing a redwood tree. A famous photograph, taken the following year during the Underhill expedition, shows Clyde sitting atop the Milk Bottle.

The climbing was quite sketchy for me and Doug kept a keen eye on my progress as we slowly descended into a narrow chute, which led to the summit.

Once in the chute, the climbing was less exposed and quite safe, and I arrived first at the infamous Milk Bottle, which has turned away many a summit bid.

The 30-foot-high monolithic slab of smooth granite sticks up like a middle finger thrust into the air, defying anyone who might attempt to climb it. The column tapers to a square platform less than 2 feet wide, constituting the entire summit of what many consider the toughest 14er to climb in the continental United States. The apex overlooks a sheer drop of several thousand feet to the valley floor, testing the resolve of even the most seasoned climber.

"The summit of Starlight Peak offers the bold mountaineer the most exciting summit of all the peaks in the Palisades," the guidebook read. "In fact, it would be difficult to find an apex more worthy of this distinction anywhere in the Sierra Nevada. Upon reaching this diminutive point, the climber's senses are besieged by vertigo as well as euphoria. The ridge below, much like one's stomach, seems to drop out from beneath. The view, like the exposure, is nothing less than exhilarating." Just reading those words had been intimidating enough for me.

Standing beneath the Milk Bottle, with its rating of 5.7—meaning it was nearly vertical with few holds—I was unsure I could climb it. I quickly noticed how exposed the Milk Bottle was on its east side, as well, and I didn't see how Doug was going to get up this one, either. But he made the first move quickly, getting past the protruding edge near the bottom, and then, holding the opposite corners of the spire with his hands, walked his feet up the smooth, vertical wall. Once at the top, he looped his rope around the iron bolt that some unknown climber had drilled into the 2-foot-square summit sometime in the '50s, and I was able to belay him from there.

We didn't have much time. Like in 1931, during Clyde's first ascent, we too could see a storm coming in from the west over the expanse of the John Muir Wilderness, even though the forecast had not called for rain. It was already snowing lightly. Thousands of feet of descent separated us from the safety of our camp on the valley floor. Doug said we might have to bail off Starlight without me tagging the summit if I wasn't successful on my first attempt. My heart sank. I was only going to get one shot at this.

Hooking into the rope, I was a bit hesitant. I could find no purchase for my left foot on the smooth granite slab. Finally, I found a nubbin. I lifted myself up. My hands gripped the edges of the narrowing spire, more tightly than I had the crucifix atop Gerlach štít in Slovakia two years before.

Two crisp moves later, I was peering over the top, surprising myself and perhaps Doug, too. But while touching the summit with my right hand might constitute conquering the mountain among peakbagging circles, I knew that what I really needed to conquer here was my own fear. My knees were knocking as I tried to work up the courage to do what I had told myself I probably would not have the *cojones* to do—stand up on this tiny, airy platform like a high-diver 2,000 feet above the ground. But, gulping hard, I very methodically brought one foot up to the top of the pillar and then with a bit of a wobble, slowly stood up, and even raised my hands high into the thin air. I felt like Leonardo DiCaprio in *Titanic*. "I'm the king of the world!"

With one hand holding the rope, Doug grabbed his camera with his other hand and snapped a couple of pictures of me. Cautiously, I lowered myself back to the rock, grabbing it tightly with both hands, just as I'd seen Doug do, and descended back to the relative safety of the mountaintop by Doug's side.

A smile burst onto my face. I had never been so scared or so exhilarated in my life. I *was* king of the world—if even for a brief instant.

After signing the register book, I took my first look at the summit of North Palisade, which, too, was little more than a quarter-mile away. But North Pal would have to wait.

The day's climbing had proven harder than we had anticipated, and with all the lost time atop Thunderbolt and the encroaching storm, we had to get back to the safety of the valley as soon as possible. This we had not anticipated, having expected—albeit perhaps unreasonably—that we would complete the entire traverse in one day. Fortunately, we had built in a buffer, as Doug's flight home wasn't until the day after tomorrow.

Starting down the chute we had ascended, we soon found the descent too steep. We ended up rappelling down eight pitches, including one on an over-hanging ledge that momentarily left me dangling in midair. At camp, the snow had changed to rain. Using our trekking poles and a rope, we fashioned a tent out of our tarp—using the overhang of a rock—and found ourselves quite cozy despite the storm.

At 14,275 feet, North Palisade is the highest peak in the Palisade range, and also the third-highest mountain in the Sierras. Ever since early climbers first laid eyes on the jagged spires of this range, North Palisade has enchanted them.

"There is no more spectacular peak in the Sierra Nevada," wrote Norman Clyde, who put up several new routes on the peak in the 1930s, "none more alluring to the mountaineer than North Palisade."

Clyde was not the first to climb it; a party of three men, led by Joseph N. Le Conte, had conquered the mountain in 1904. They had at first turned back after reaching the distinctive U-Notch that separates North Palisade from neighboring Polemonium, but found another route to the summit two days later. Clyde, however, did pioneer the route above the U-Notch, which was our destination the following morning.

Hiking along the base of North Palisades' west side, we looked up the first gully and saw that it went nowhere. Moving on, we guessed the second would lead to the U-Notch and started climbing. The solid Class 3 chute brought us to a notch between the two peaks, but we were unsure that we were in the right place. While we contemplated this, four other climbers arrived in the notch having climbed up from the east side, which was chock-full of snow. Telling us they were all engineers from Alaska, they confirmed for us what we had suspected: we were in the U-Notch, just below the summit.

While the Alaskans roped up and climbed straight out of the U-Notch on very exposed terrain, Doug and I climbed a slightly more protected Class 4 chute, which dropped us into a little bowl.

Upon reaching it, Doug announced that he had a massive headache and thought he was going to throw up, the obvious signs of altitude sickness. He said he had a bad feeling about continuing in that condition. A jumble of blocks and spires beyond denied easy access to the summit, the same blockade that nearly turned back Le Conte's party in 1904. I had not planned to climb these large blocks—with dizzying drops on all sides—without Doug's assistance. Again, I deflated at the prospect of failure.

I asked if we should descend immediately, but Doug said he thought he would be all right, though he didn't feel well enough to continue ascending. He said I could make it to the summit on my own, since it was only a couple of hundred yards away. But I wasn't as confident as he was.

Carefully working my way around a spire that blocked my path, I scoped out a trail along the narrow ridge that mostly followed the path of least resistance. Twice, I thought I had dead-ended at a cliff face. The first time, I swung out around a boulder that was sitting atop a vertiginous drop. The next time, I climbed over a narrow fin onto the ledge above. There, I stood on a small block that led to a large, flat rock that appeared to be the summit. But gaining access to this bench required a veritable leap of faith: I lifted my foot off a little pinnacle and swung it out over thin air until it reached the top of the block, which was at shoulder level. I got up on the first attempt.

Sitting atop the summit block, which was about the size of a typical dinner table, I once again marveled at what I'd achieved, at reaching what had seemed unreachable just moments before. I blew the whistle on my backpack to let Doug know I was there, and he snapped some long-range photos from his vantage point. I was so caught up in the moment that I forgot to look for the summit register, and never did sign in.

Getting off the summit was harder than attaining it. I hung off the edge of the exposed rock and blindly searched with my foot for the tiny pinnacle. I found it, then carefully lowered myself down. I retraced my steps along the ridgeline, passing the four Alaskans as they made their way to the summit. When I got back to Doug's location, he said he didn't feel any better, and needed to descend back to the U-Notch immediately. I didn't dare ask what we were going to do once we got there, since the summit of Polemonium, the next 14er in the range, had to be reached from the other side of the notch and looked to be rather easily ascended. I suspected we were going to bail, which made the most sense given Doug's incapacitated condition.

He had already set up a rappel over the same airy pitch the Alaskans had ascended, and a lump rose in my throat as I looked at the exposure below us. It took us three raps to get back to the U-Notch—we could have done it in two, but the rope was 7 feet too short on the second one.

I was a bit surprised when Doug said he felt good enough to continue to Polemonium, despite the fact that it was already afternoon and we could see another storm brewing, just like the one the day before. I certainly was grateful to keep going; I couldn't imagine heading back there on my own. From the U-Notch, we climbed a diagonal traverse over two pitches that Doug free-climbed before belaying me from above. From there, we faced a climb straight up the exposed west face.

Doug said he was quite impressed with my climbing ability, but I chalked it up more to survival instincts; I knew if I fell, I would probably die. That's a great motivator. But in all the climbing we had done over the previous two days, not once had I faltered on the rope, with no slips or falls that would have put all of my weight on the rope and caused Doug to have to brake me. Even I was impressed by this.

While he coiled the rope, I made for the summit just a few yards away. The Class 5 moves that this short distance required now seemed like a cakewalk after Thunderbolt and Starlight peaks. True 14er or not, many climbers find the airy exposure of the ascent exhilarating, ourselves included.

By then, it was nearly 4 p.m., and snow had begun falling, even before we'd reached the summit of Polemonium. There was no chance that we were going to be able to continue along the ridge and bag Mount Sill. Plus, we still had to get off the mountain, break down camp, and complete the long hike out, not to mention the 4-hour drive back to Reno, since Doug's flight was the next morning. We figured it would be at least midnight before we reached our motel.

Doug said it would take two rappels to get us down into the V-Notch, which was the next gully southeast of Polemonium's summit. The first one went without incident, but the second had an overhanging ledge, which Doug negotiated by kneeling against the lip of the ledge and lowering himself gracefully under it. Since my knee was very swollen from having knelt on all the rocks while climbing North Palisade earlier in the day, I attempted to get past this overhang by putting my feet against it, and then letting out enough rope that I could safely swing under the ledge. It almost worked. I failed to let out enough rope and came crashing into the ledge, pinching my hand between the rock and the rope, smashing my middle finger. When I reached Doug, I was bleeding profusely and it looked like I might need a stitch or two.

We were not carrying an emergency kit, but I remembered I had finished a roll of toilet paper that morning. I pulled out the empty, flattened cardboard tube and Doug cut a small strip off it. I also had wrapped some duct tape around a Nalgene bottle prior to the Yosemite hike, and Doug used both to fashion a pseudo tourniquet to stop the bleeding. When he was done, there was a considerable amount of blood in the snow at our feet. I joked that the next climber was probably going to think someone had butchered a marmot.

Descending into the V-Notch, we could have done a series of rappels straight down the couloir to the basin below, and then had a short hike back to our camp. But instead we continued over the ridgeline, which had eased considerably and looked like it might be faster. We stayed on the ridge too long, however, and mistakenly dropped down into the large, glaciated basin underneath Mount Sill, leaving us on the wrong side of Potluck Pass. We had to regain about 500 or 600 feet of elevation to get back into Palisade Basin—and from there spent a seeming eternity hopping from boulder to boulder to cross it. We arrived at our campsite at 7:30 P.M., a 12.5-hour round-trip to climb just two peaks. It had been only an 11-hour excursion the day before.

Quickly breaking camp and crossing Dusy Basin, Doug used his altimeter to keep us at or near the 12,000-foot level of Bishop Pass, which we reached at 9:50 P.M., well after dark. We still had an 8-mile hike back to the car. And it was insufferable: my back and shoulders were in misery by the time we reached the car at 12:40 A.M., making it nearly an 18-hour day. And, of course, we still had a 4-hour drive to Reno.

In Bishop, we made a quick stop at McDonald's for our only real meal of the day—if we could call it that—then drove north until I couldn't keep my eyes open any longer. We pulled off on a turnout at 3:30 A.M. and slept in the car until first light. We checked into the motel at 8:30 A.M., as they had thankfully held the room. While Doug showered and got ready for his flight, I went down to the lobby and enjoyed a continental breakfast. I am sure I looked quite a sight, not having showered or shaved in four days and sporting a bloody finger with a toilet paper roll duct-taped around it.

I planned to drop Doug off at the airport and then go back to the motel and sleep until checkout time. Instead, after thanking him for such a tremendous job helping me get those four summits, I headed for home across the expanse of US 50, designated as the "The Loneliest Road in America."

I much preferred US 50 to I-80, as I could drive just as fast on this desolate highway and it enters Utah in the middle of the state, not in the northern part near Salt Lake City, which enabled me to enter Colorado on I-70 instead of going through Wyoming on I-80, which would have taken several hours longer. Most people think it makes more sense to stay on the interstate as much as possible, but that isn't always the best option. At least not out West.

In the middle of Nevada lies Austin, a tiny old mining town in the Toiyabe Range at the bottom of some switchbacks. The town—named after Austin, Texas—was founded in 1862 as part of a silver rush reportedly triggered by a Pony Express horse kicking over a rock. Though it is now a shadow of its heyday, when 10,000 residents lived there, the town still retains much of its Old West charm.

Stopping at the Toiyabe Café for lunch and still feeling the effects of my sore knee and lack of sleep, I looked forward to my return home the next day. A sign on the café wall kind of summed things up for me: "Midlife: When your mind makes promises your body can't keep."

Touché.

Despite the high notes of the Ride the Divide *tour, I thought my "career" as a film* promoter was over, a one-time deal. But then Stephen Auerbach, the producer of *Bicycle Dreams*, the amazing film about Race Across America, contacted me out of the blue. He said he had seen what I had done for *Ride the Divide* and wanted me to do the same for his film.

Our nationwide tour for *Bicycle Dreams* during the winter of 2011–2012 was even more successful than the one with *Ride the Divide*, and suddenly I had producers of other adventure documentaries contacting me to promote their films. I had created a niche industry for myself. While my new career as a film promoter enabled me to make some additional money in the winter months— when I was not able to umpire softball or drive for UPS—it did take me away from Nancy more often than I wished. But she seemed to understand how my unconventional work schedule allowed me to continue maintaining a flexible lifestyle.

Since then, I have worked with several more films, including another mountain-bike film by Mike Dion called *Reveal the Path* and a fly-fishing film made by Hunter Weeks entitled *Where the Yellowstone Goes*. I have worked with other cycling films, as well as some running films and a rock-climbing film festival. In 2015, Mike Dion came out with another cycling film, *Inspired to Ride*, for which I also scheduled about a dozen shows.

I have my Facebook buddy Andy Garza to thank for it all, and, later, when I went to Bozeman in the summer of 2012 to run the Bridger Ridge Run, a grueling 20-mile trail race in the mountains outside of town that tore up my quads, I bought him a big steak dinner as I had promised. I'm sure glad his roommate hadn't made a porn film.

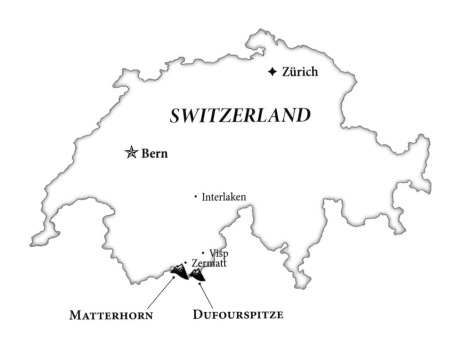

✦ Zürich

SWITZERLAND

☆ Bern

· Interlaken

· Visp
Zermatt

MATTERHORN   **DUFOURSPITZE**

THE MATTERHORN: CULMINATION OF A DREAM

I'M NOT SURE WHEN I FIRST BECAME ENTHRALLED WITH THE MONOLITHIC PYRAMID of the Matterhorn, which juts impossibly straight into the sky like a giant, stone arrowhead. But I imagine it was in the third grade, when books first opened the world to me, and I first saw the mountain in pictures. At this impressionable age, I became a voracious reader, devouring books like they were Halloween candy. My teacher, Mrs. Hemenway, had instituted a reading program in which students could attain "Moon explorer" status by reading a certain number of books during the school year. A handful of other students and I reached this level; however, I alone went on to become a Mercury, Venus, and Mars explorer, as well. Already I was determined to tick off accomplishments and lists.

Of all the mountains in the world, the Matterhorn, to me, stands out as the single most definitive example of what a mountain should look like—chiseled and worn as if it had been sculpted by the hands of man, rather than the ancient glaciers that carved out its smooth, featureless faces. While most would-be mountaineers covet standing on top of the world, climbing Everest has never had such a powerful draw on my psyche as has the Matterhorn.

I imagine that Edward Whymper—then a 20-year-old British illustrator who had never seen a mountain in his life before being hired to go to the Alps to sketch alpine scenes for a soon-to-be-released book on mountaineering—felt the same way when he first laid eyes on the Matterhorn in the summer of 1860. He arrived in the Zermatt Valley that July already enraptured by the mountains he had seen along the way, but the Matterhorn grabbed his attention like a face full of ice water.

The iconic view of the Matterhorn from the town of Zermatt has been photographed, sketched, and painted perhaps more than any mountain in the world, its massive presence looming over the entire valley with more magnificence than the great pyramids of Giza. It was this view that ignited in Whymper an urgent desire to be the first to stand atop this last, great unclimbed peak in the then-known modern world.

Whymper returned to England that September, already determined to climb this "unassailable summit," the so-called "impossible mountain." The locals believed that any climber reckless enough to challenge its dominion would never return, but Whymper was determined to prove them wrong, even though to that point his only climbing experience had been ascending the seven flights of stairs in his Paris hotel.

The Golden Age of Mountaineering had begun a few years before in 1854 with Alfred Wills's ascension of the Wetterhorn. Over the next decade, prominent British climbers—many of them the same ones who formed the Alpine Club in London in 1857—conquered the remaining unclimbed peaks of the Alps. Any number of those adventurers could have been the first to climb the Matterhorn—and some of them tried—but none of them became as obsessed with this last great prize as did Whymper.

For the next four summers, Whymper returned to the respectively Swiss and Italian valleys at the foot of the Matterhorn in hopes of being the first to summit. Whymper and his on-again, off-again guide, Jean-Antoine Carrel—an Italian climber out of the town of Brueil who himself aspired to be the first atop this last great prize in the Alps—climbed a thousand feet shy of the summit during various attempts between 1861 and 1864. Meanwhile, Whymper honed his limited mountaineering skills on lesser peaks in the French Alps.

Unbeknownst to Whymper, the recently formed Italian Alpine Club had secret plans to climb the Matterhorn in 1865. By the time Whymper arrived in Breuil that July, plans were well under way for their assault on the peak. Carrel, of course, was part of those plans, but had not let on about them. The competing interests were about to square off in the most fateful and exciting real-time race in the history of mountaineering. In the annals of exploration, this rivalry would be matched only by the race to the South Pole in 1911 between Roald Amundsen and Robert Falcon Scott, and perhaps by the space race between the Americans and Soviets in the 1960s.

When Whymper arrived in Breuil on July 6, he learned that Carrel was already on the mountain with a team of Italians who had departed for their attempt. A thick fog drove the Italian team back into the valley. Whymper met with Carrel, who agreed to climb with Whymper in three days' time. So Whymper crossed back over the Theodul Pass to Zermatt. When he returned two days later to check on a sick British climber in Breuil, Carrel said he would not be available for "a couple more days." Whymper thus was shocked to learn upon waking the next morning that he had been double-crossed: Carrel and the large Italian team had left early that morning for the summit.

Whymper was mortified as he watched their progress through a telescope. But he knew that a party that large would climb slowly. As luck would have it, a British climber named Lord Francis Douglas arrived in Breuil that morning, fresh off a first ascent of nearby Ober Gabelhorn. Douglas told Whymper that his Zermatt guide, Peter Taugwalder, had remarked that he had recently climbed above the Hörnli Pic high on the ridge of the Matterhorn and had said he felt

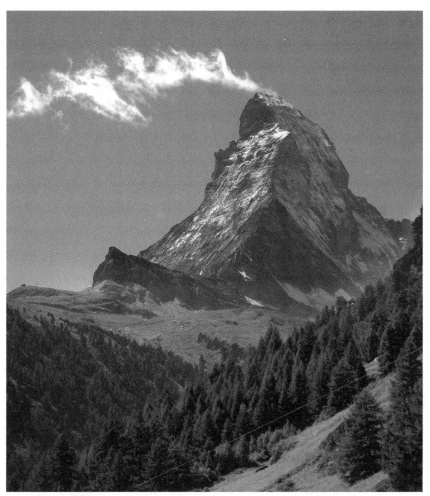

The iconic rooster tail of clouds streams off the summit of the Matterhorn as seen from the Swiss village of Zermatt.

the mountain could indeed be scaled from the Swiss side, heretofore deemed impossible. That was great news, Whymper thought, and he and Douglas returned to Zermatt on July 12 intent on seeking out Taugwalder.

More good luck greeted Whymper in Zermatt. Michel Croz, an accomplished guide with whom Whymper had climbed many times in the French Alps, had arrived in town along with his British clients, Reverend Charles Hudson and 18-year-old Douglas Hadow. Hudson and Hadow had climbed Mount Blanc the week before, and Hudson also had it in mind to climb the Matterhorn the following day. They decided to join forces and sought out Peter Taugwalder, who agreed to guide them, along with his son, "Young Peter."

Starting out the next morning up the Hörnli Ridge—the most popular climbing route today—they climbed steadily to about 12,000 feet and set up camp. Croz and the elder Taugwalder then scouted ahead, returning 3 hours later to report that they had found the climbing not difficult at all and that they could have summited themselves, had it not been so late in the day. All were excited.

By ten o'clock the next morning, they were at about 14,000 feet, where the ridge turns vertical and some difficult climbing begins. Several times they thought they heard voices coming from the summit, but each time decided it was just the wind. Gaining the top of these cliffs took some doing—Hadow's inexperience slowed them down considerably—but once above them, they were elated to discover only a 200-foot snow slope between them and the summit. "The Matterhorn is ours!" they exclaimed, as Whymper and Croz unroped and raced to the summit, arriving in a dead heat to find nothing but untrammeled snow; there was no sign of the Italians. They were overjoyed.

Crossing over to the slightly lower Italian summit, Whymper looked down and spotted the Italian party about 1,200 feet below them. They yelled and threw rocks, but could not get their attention; finally they created a small rock slide that caused the Italians to look up. You can imagine the expression on their faces when they spotted Whymper on the summit. Shocked and completely deflated, the Italians turned around and returned to Breuil with their tails between their legs.

When Croz used a tent pole and his shirt to erect a flag on the summit, the people in Breuil celebrated the sight, mistakenly thinking it signified the success of the Italian team. Meanwhile, those on the Zermatt side celebrated as well, correctly guessing that their climbers had reached the summit first. They quickly went about preparing a heroes' welcome for the seven conquerors.

But there would be no celebration. Disaster struck on the descent, turning what would have been perhaps the greatest mountaineering achievement in history into an unmitigated tragedy, forever tarnishing Whymper's reputation.

Slowly descending the steep cliff section that they had previously surmounted, Hadow slipped and fell onto Croz. The two started to slide. The rope connecting the seven climbers quickly snatched Hudson and Douglas from their perches above. The rope came taut with such a force that it snapped between Douglas and the elder Taugwalder, who, along with his son and Whymper, were helpless as they watched their companions plummet more than 4,000 feet to the glacier below.

The three survivors were unprepared for the shock of what they had just witnessed. Looking at the rope, Whymper was surprised to see that it was the weakest and thinnest of the ropes they had carried, and not the one they should have used to rope together. After much effort, the three made it back to Zermatt, where news of the deaths completely overshadowed their great accomplishment. The disaster captured the public's attention like no mountaineering story before. Rather than be exalted in triumph, Whymper would be haunted by tragedy the rest of his life.

Whymper led the recovery efforts to retrieve the bodies off the Matterhorn Glacier and, when found, they were mangled almost beyond identification. Douglas's body, in fact, could not be located, and has never been recovered. In the midst of the horrific scene, Whymper was heard to mutter, "I will never step foot on a mountain again." He was only 25 at the time. He might have gone on to become the most famous climber ever, had it not been for the tragedy.

Carrel, incredibly, returned to Breuil and put together another party and headed back up from the Italian side, knowing nothing of the events that had unfolded on Whymper's descent. He reached the summit just three days after spotting Whymper on the ridge above him, coming within 72 hours of achieving his personal dream of recording the first ascent. The mountain was not summited again until Carrel did it a second time two years later. It would not be until 1868 that another party successfully climbed from the Swiss side.

The Swiss government promptly convened an inquest, though only Whymper and the elder Taugwalder testified. Authorities quickly concluded that the accident was caused by Hadow's inexperience, but the court of public opinion just as quickly found fodder for the rumor mill. The rope soon came under scrutiny. People asked why Taugwalder had placed the most inferior rope between himself and Douglas. Even Whymper had considered this suspect. But, it was later determined, this was the same style of rope that Taugwalder had used during his ascent of Ober Gabelhorn with Douglas the week before, when the two had nearly fallen to their deaths from the summit, saved only by their rope. So it was thought that Taugwalder would have considered this rope sufficient for the task.

Then another rumor circulated that Taugwalder had cut the rope to save his own life—and that of his son—but Whymper dismissed this instantly. He stated that the incident happened so quickly that no one would have had time to reach for a knife and cut the rope. Indeed, the rope is still on display in the mountaineering museum in Zermatt, showing no signs of having been cut. Still, Taugwalder defended himself against the charge in the streets of Zermatt, telling anyone who would listen of the burn marks on his fingers caused when the rope slipped through his hands.

Old Peter never shook the speculation about the rope and rarely guided again, though Young Peter would go on to be a successful guide in his own right, climbing the Matterhorn again in 1872 and opening up new opportunities for other guides on the mountain. By then, the Matterhorn was and continues to be as much a staple of the economy of Zermatt as working on Everest is to the many Sherpa villages in Nepal.

Since that fateful day in 1865, nearly 500 climbers have died on the Matterhorn, making it one of the deadliest mountains in the world; to put that in perspective, it is also the most-climbed 4,000-meter peak. It should be noted that all but one of those deaths were of climbers who weren't using a guide.

A sullen Whymper returned to London trying to avoid notoriety, but the British press besieged and excoriated him. The public outcry was so severe that Queen Victoria even considered banning all British subjects from mountain climbing. Finally, Whymper answered their charges with a 3,000-word letter to the editor in hopes of putting the matter to rest, but, as he later wrote, mention of the word Matterhorn became "hateful" to him, its conquest nothing but "bitterness and ashes."

Though Whymper returned the following year to Zermatt, he never really climbed again in the Alps. Later, he became interested in the study of the effects of high altitude on climbers, and did much research in the Andes. In fact, he and Carrel repaired what could have been a fragmented relationship and climbed together in Ecuador, achieving some notable first ascents, including 20,702-foot Chimborazo in 1880, when they became the first Europeans to summit a 20,000-foot peak.

Ironically, Carrel died during a climb of the Matterhorn in 1890, most likely from a heart attack. Whymper died a lonely death in 1911 while visiting Chamonix, France, under the shadows of some of the great mountains he had once been the first to climb. The Golden Age of Alpinism had concluded the day Whymper stepped foot on the summit of the Matterhorn, and with his death, so closed the chapter on what was perhaps the greatest achievement in mountaineering history.

Jamie Pierce's career as a mountain guide essentially got started with a lie to his parents. The winter after he graduated from high school in Illinois, he told them he was flying to Colorado for a ski vacation. What he didn't tell them was that he had bought a one-way plane ticket. Once in the Rockies, he called his parents and informed them he wasn't coming home.

Armed with little more than a book on beginning rock climbing, Pierce spent the next few years living the so-called dirtbag lifestyle of a climber: skiing and climbing in the Rockies by day and cooking dinner at a Colorado guest ranch by night. Eventually, he became an apprentice guide, then spent four summers working in Antarctica at a scientific research center and cut his teeth by guiding in the nearby mountains along the Weddell Sea. He eventually got his guiding license and with it a job with Alpine Ascents, traveling all over the globe to guide in places such as Alaska, the Andes, and Africa.

Jamie went on to become certified as an international mountain guide with the International Association of Mountain Guide Associations (IFMGA) and started the Pikes Peak Alpine School out of his home in Colorado Springs.

I first met Jamie in the summer of 2011, when Nancy suggested I contact him to learn how to rock climb, in anticipation of my climbs of Grand Teton and the Palisades. She had met Jamie a few years before when they had worked together on a climbing and hiking project on Pikes Peak sponsored by Chick-fil-A, which had brought several of its employees to the region as part of a health and wellness program.

Jamie took me on climbs in the Red Rocks Canyon Open Space in Colorado Springs and to Eleven Mile Canyon in nearby Lake George, giving me a great introduction to rock climbing. We spent the day climbing pitches from 5.7 to 5.9, relatively moderate on the rock climbing scale, but totally exhilarating to me. Jamie said I was a natural rock climber and encouraged me to climb more often, but other than those subsequent trips to Grand Teton and the Palisades, I had not been able to do that.

But then the opportunity that I had seemingly been waiting a lifetime for started to come together. Jamie said he was available in the summer of 2012 to guide me up the Matterhorn. He was getting married that July and would be spending his honeymoon in Europe, and had a two-week window in August to climb if I wanted. Sure, I could have hired a local guide in Zermatt for much less, but I had confidence in Jamie. Plus, he said we would attempt some other nearby peaks—most notably Dufourspitze, the highpoint of Switzerland, located across the valley from its more famous neighbor.

I flew into Zürich on a Thursday morning, unable to sleep on my overnight flight from Dulles. I made my way to the train station, lugging an overstuffed backpack with everything I would need for the climb except an ice ax, which I would rent in Zermatt. I purchased a Swiss Rail Pass for $198 and boarded a train for the 3.5-hour trip to Visp, located at the base of the Zermatt Valley. I spent the entire time glued to the window, staring out at staggering scenery that was around every bend in the track. I could have gotten off in Interlaken and easily spent the rest of my life there.

After a group of young revelers, who had disembarked with me in Visp, boarded another train headed to Sierre to attend a Woodstock-like music festival, I was about the only one left at the station and sat eating an apple in a light rain as I waited for the train to Zermatt. Once aboard, the scenery became even more breathtaking as we climbed up the narrow valley to the end of the line in Zermatt, where I got out and immediately started looking around for views of the Matterhorn.

Unfortunately, you can't see the mountain from the village square, so I walked up the narrow streets—cars are not allowed in Zermatt—to find my room at the Arben, the guesthouse Jamie had booked for me. I will only describe my room as "cozy." I was hoping that Jamie was not also staying in such a tiny room, since Adrienne, his bride of just two weeks, was with him.

Jamie had told me not to go to sleep upon arrival, hoping to avoid any effects of jet lag, so instead I went for a run through town toward the trail that I knew headed in the direction of the Matterhorn. Suddenly, it came into view, and it was every bit as magnificent as I had imagined. The east face was cloaked head to toe in clouds, but the north face was completely exposed. I almost soiled my pants when I got my first look at the insanely steep northeast ridge, which we would be climbing.

For a moment, I could not formulate any coherent thoughts; I simply stared at the mountain with my mouth agape. I then remembered Whymper's words about first laying eyes on the Matterhorn: "Men who ordinarily spoke or wrote like rational beings, when they came under its power seemed to quit their senses, and ranted and rhapsodized, losing for a time all common forms of speech."

I, too, was speechless. I watched the clouds dance upon the sheer walls of the mountain, with the iconic rooster tail streaming from the summit. I, at least, had the reassurance that the route was safe—it is now climbed thousands of times a year—but I can only imagine the trepidation that must have addled the mind of the 20-year-old Whymper.

After my run, I got some dinner, washed it down with a beer, and went to bed, waiting for Jamie and Adrienne to call on me in the morning. They collected me at 7:45, and after a quick breakfast, we headed for the tramway, where we boarded the Gornergrat Bahn train for a short ride up into a high valley, where we disembarked for our planned climb of the Riffelhorn, a sharp, pointy pinnacle with views of more than a score of 4,000-meter peaks from its rocky summit. The three of us would be rock-climbing on its backside, where several solid, spectacular routes awaited. I mistakenly paid for the train ride, not knowing that my Swiss Rail Pass already covered it. Sorry, no refunds, I was told later.

Getting off the train, the three of us traversed along a rocky path looking directly at the Gornergletscher a few hundred feet below us—the same glacier that descends from the upper reaches of Dufourspitze off to our left. It was hard to believe that Dufourspitze, the highpoint of Switzerland also known as Monte Rosa, was several hundred feet taller than the Matterhorn, which, too, was staring at us directly across the valley. The two mountains were about equidistant from us, but the Matterhorn looked impossibly higher.

Our destination was The Egg, a route rated "4b" on the European scale, according to the metal plate attached to the rock. Jamie said this corresponded to about a 5.8 or 5.9 on the Yosemite Decimal Scale; it was not significantly harder than what we had climbed in Colorado the year before, he promised. Still, the route took five pitches and was difficult for a novice like me. On one steep, featureless section that lacked adequate holds, I hesitated slightly, which did not go unnoticed. Jamie, who was belaying me from above, said he could not only see my tentativeness, but could feel it in the rope, as well. I was certainly not climbing as surely as I had when I was in the Palisades with my friend Doug the year before.

Too many times he spied me searching high above my head for handholds. He admonished me to climb more with my legs and to worry more about securing my footholds than my handholds. He said if I climbed like that on the Matterhorn, I would be trashed after about 4 hours. But this was why he had taken me to the Riffelhorn, so there would be no surprises on the real climb in a couple of days. It was a hard climb for me, made all the more so by the nearly new boots I was wearing.

After summiting, and a quick lunch, it was time to descend, which, Jamie said, would require rappelling. I had not been aware that we did not have a hikable trail off the front side of the Riffelhorn, and as Jamie had not mentioned that I would need a belay device until now, I had not brought one. As a result, he had to lower me down three or four rappels before we could hike off the mountain and return to the train station. I felt Jamie had become a little annoyed with me.

A high-pressure system had come up from the Sahara and had been parked over Europe since I had arrived, giving us a window of warm, clear weather. Because of this, we decided to climb the Matterhorn on a Sunday—typically a busier day on the mountain—as the weather was expected to change by the following day.

I didn't sleep particularly well that final night at the Arben, and awoke from a fitful sleep a bit anxious in the morning. After a quick breakfast, I met Jamie and Adrienne at a local climbing store and rented an ice ax, and we all headed for the cable car and the 12-minute ride up to Schwarzee, the starting point for ascents of the Matterhorn. The gondola terminus is located at the edge of a small lake along with a hotel and a tiny chapel—undoubtedly the same one at which Whymper stopped to pray during his recovery mission to retrieve the bodies of his companions off the Matterhorn Glacier. Today, many successful climbers stop at the chapel on their way down to give thanks for a safe climb.

From there, it was a 2-hour hike up to the Hörnli Hut, situated at 10,695 feet. I arrived far enough in advance of Jamie and Adrienne that I had already finished my packed-in lunch by the time they arrived. Many others crowded about the deck of the large stone building, eating at the restaurant and enjoying a brilliant, sunny afternoon. Jamie later remarked that the day was the hottest he had ever experienced in Zermatt, perhaps as warm as 75 degrees Fahrenheit. About 3 P.M., most of the others headed back down the trail to catch the final gondola of the day at 4:50 P.M.; only climbers and those waiting for their return, including Adrienne, remained at the hut overnight.

Soon, a steady stream of descending climbers arrived, having summited earlier in the day. They all looked in good condition, and I hoped I would look as good the next afternoon upon my return.

One of Jamie's friends, a guide from Idaho named Daniel, was also at the hut with his client from New York, so they spent some time catching up. Meanwhile, I hiked up the sharp rise behind the hut to the edge of the northeast ridge and took a long, hard look at the route above. I could see that the bottom third and the top third of the route were not as steep as they had appeared from the valley floor, but the middle third looked to be nearly vertical. Back at the hut, Jamie then went through my pack and arranged everything, with the items I'd need first on top.

The Hörnli Hut sleeps about 120, with the bunks little more than large wooden shelves stacked one above the other. I'm sure I had not slept much before we awoke at 4 A.M. for our breakfast of bread, cheese, and marmalade. Then we suited up and headed for the route. It was immediately apparent that we were about the last client-and-guide tandem to leave the hut; I could sense Jamie was a bit perturbed, and I wasn't sure if it was because of this unexpected tardiness or something I had done. Or maybe both. I didn't want any personal issues getting in the way of a safe and successful climb.

The Hörnli Route starts just above the hut at the base of the mountain, with an immediate technical climb up a short wall fitted with fixed ropes. Despite this first pitch seeming rather benign to me, Jamie belayed me anyway and kept me on rope the entire time we were on the mountain. I felt as if I was on-leash, and I was. We climbed in the dark for the first couple of hours, which was probably a good thing since I was unable to see any of the exposure. But even as it got light, the climbing as yet had not been very difficult or very exposed; I could easily have free-climbed it without reservation.

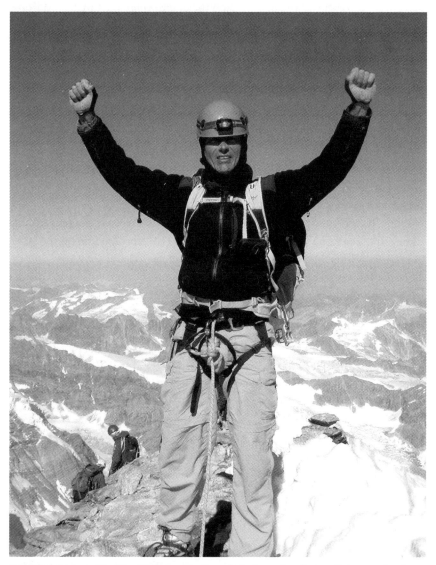

Reaching the summit of the Matterhorn is the culmination of a climb well done and a dream come true.

That changed soon after daylight, when we reached an especially steep pitch just below the Solvay Hut, a tiny refuge perched on a small ledge at 13,130 feet. We had a similar climb directly above the hut and then, for the remainder of the ascent, we were on some serious steeps. We climbed straight up the razor-thin northeast ridge, with the near-vertical north face directly to our right and the nearly-as-steep east wall to our left. The climbing was very precise, with zero margin for error. It was the first time on the climb where I felt that a fall would definitely kill me. One benefit of our late start was that no other parties were trying to scoot past us, as most everyone else was already higher on the mountain. Of course, because of this, we were always wary of falling rocks.

Soon, we reached a shoulder where the slope leveled before shooting skyward directly toward the summit. This was the transition area between the bottom two-thirds of the route and the top third, and where we stopped to put on our crampons for the first time. There was much ice and snow here, though the weather was relatively calm, since it was not particularly windy on this day.

Jamie sat me down on a rock that was perched precariously close to the edge of the north face and I tried not to peer down its sheer expanse while I strapped on my crampons. To do anything else would have been to invite terror and paralyze me on the spot. Normally, I am especially clumsy in crampons, but I knew there were no missteps allowed here. We continued climbing the steep, narrow ridgeline, with Jamie going up each pitch first and then belaying me as I climbed up to him. We repeated this procedure over and over until we were above the long section of fixed ropes, as well as one that had sported a chain-link ladder.

Though the summit appeared close and though the slope lessened to about 75 degrees, this was no place to relax. We still had a lot of dangerous footwork ahead. With the risk of sliding off the north face looming below us, our every step was precise and purposeful. I found it hard to believe that Swiss climber Ueli Steck soloed the north face in less than 2 hours in 2009. It seemed pure suicide to me.

Gaining the summit ridge, I was unnerved to discover how incredibly razor-thin it was—barely a foot wide—and I am not sure why this seemed to surprise me, since there had been dozens of photos of the summit hanging on the walls of the Hörnli Hut. Any slip, in either direction, would result in a free fall of several thousand feet. But what really unnerved me was the two-way traffic on this ridge; climbers on their way down after having reached the summit passed us in the other direction, and we had to step cautiously to our right as we passed them. Imagine two gymnasts trying to pass each other on a balance beam 4,000 feet above the ground. I concentrated solely on proper placement of my feet and tried not to look over either edge as we made it the final few yards to the summit—the culmination of a lifelong dream.

I could not believe that I was standing on the summit of what I considered the most famous mountain in the world. I cannot describe the euphoria I felt at that very moment. My whirling thoughts were interrupted by Jamie's voice.

"I suppose you need to touch the other summit, too," he said, peering over to the Italian side.

The Italian summit was about 50 yards away on the other side of a short little dip along the ridge and, at least from our perspective, appeared to be slightly higher than where we were currently standing.

"That's why we're here," I replied. But, looking across this expanse, I wasn't so sure.

Between us and the Italian summit—the border runs directly through the saddle—was an even more exposed ridgeline, with a sidehill snow climb past a 6-foot-tall wrought-iron crucifix, where a number of other climbers were congregated, blocking the way. Beyond that, the ridge widened to 4 or 5 feet and even more climbers were sitting about enjoying what for them must have been as rewarding an experience as it was for me.

Not until we had reached the other summit and turned around did we realize that the first summit was actually the higher of the two, by about a meter or so. But the Italian side was more dramatic, with long views down into Italy—surely the same view Whymper had had when he peered over the edge and saw Carrel and his party still several hundred feet below him.

It was a beautiful, sunny day and unseasonably warm on the summit, with little wind. In fact, I needed only a pair of cycling gloves on my hands— the kind with no fingertips—rather than the pair of ski gloves that I had mistakenly left in the bag I'd locked up at the Zermatt train station, much to Jamie's consternation.

Matterhorn's descent is far more treacherous than its ascent, for obvious reasons borne out by the Whymper tragedy. For one thing, climbers are facing away from the mountain on the descent, making any fall more potentially perilous; plus they are tired, dehydrated, and not as mentally focused after the euphoria of the summit. Most mistakes happen on the way down.

Jamie had kept asking me if my hands were getting cold, since I had on just the fingerless gloves, but except for when we had stopped to put on our crampons, they had been plenty warm. But, as we began the descent, I noticed that I had not strapped my crampons on properly. The toe plates were constantly sliding off the tips of my boots, meaning I didn't have any front points to rely on. The crampons were, in fact, slopping around on my feet. This was a serious problem, given the importance of each individual step as we slowly made our way off the summit. I tried to stop and cinch them tighter, but my hands were a little too cold to work the straps. I ended up just kicking the toe plates back into place against the rocks that were protruding from the snow. Of course, this gave me less stability as we clung to the 75-degree slope directly above the north face.

A series of large bolts attached to the rocks coming down from the summit gives climbers something to tie into for extra protection, a safety precaution that Whymper's party had not had, though they had discussed tying off to the rocks on their descent, which they ultimately neglected to do. Had they done that, it might have prevented the tragedy entirely and changed Whymper's legacy forever.

We were working our way quite deliberately from one bolt to the next when several groups of climbers came barreling down behind us at an alarming rate, kicking up bits of snow and ice on us as they raced past. Jamie instantly became agitated and yelled at some of them, but they kept rappelling past us. At least one group was downclimbing without using the bolts at all, each a slip away from cartwheeling down the north face into the next day's headlines. We were just hoping they didn't take us with them.

An ironic thing happened next. As safety-conscious as Jamie had been the entire time, he accidentally lost his grip on his ice ax as he was yelling at the other climbers. We could only watch as it slid off the east face and plummeted to an icy grave on the Matterhorn Glacier 4,000 feet below—the same route taken by Whymper's four unfortunate companions.

Jamie was beside himself with his gaffe. "I have *never* dropped something like that on a mountain before!" he exclaimed. Fortunately, the climbing route was not directly below us at the time, so no one had been in immediate danger. Not to undo the gravity of the situation, but later on the descent, Jamie miraculously found another ice ax wedged under a rock near the bottom of the mountain, likely dropped from above by another climber. I laughed and told him that he had played the mountain even par for the day, but he was not amused.

It was many long rappels before we got off the mountain, and, as I have said, I have never been a big fan of rappelling. It is disconcerting, to say the least, to lean back into thin air with nothing below me but a certain-death drop and to trust a rope and a piece of metal that has been anchored into the rock for untold moons. But it was by far the quickest and easiest way down—and certainly the safest—despite my trepidation.

It seemed like forever before we arrived at the Solvay Hut, which marks the relative halfway point, but the lower half of the route seemed to take even longer than it had coming up in the morning, when we had been in darkness. Jamie kept me on a short leash the entire way down, and we had at least a dozen more belays, mostly because Jamie kept losing the way on the convoluted trail and we all too often descended trails that would dead-end above another pitch off of which we would have to rappel.

It was well past 6 P.M. when we returned to the Hörnli Hut, with a concerned Adrienne waiting for us. Whereas it had taken us about 5 hours to summit, the descent had astonishingly taken us an additional 9 hours. We had not expected it to take 14 hours for the climb, and while Jamie said it was due to all the crazy climbers trying to pass us near the top and the tough route-finding on the lower half, I wondered whether part of it might have been Jamie losing confidence in my climbing ability due to the crampon problem. He certainly did seem irritated, but I wasn't sure if it was directed at me or at himself for dropping his ice ax.

Once back at the hut, however, I had tears in my eyes as I thanked Jamie for helping me complete a dream come true. As I stood there in the waning afternoon sunlight, I stared back at the magnificent mountain, with its impossibly steep walls jutting directly overhead, and savored a moment that would be forever etched in my soul. "I just climbed the freaking Matterhorn!" would soon be the status posted on my Facebook page.

After dinner, we went straight to bed—I was exhausted both physically and mentally—and I almost overslept breakfast in the morning. Only a few crumbs of bread and hunks of cheese were left by the time I rolled off my bunk about 7:30 A.M. As I finished these scraps, Jamie and Adrienne began the hike back to the gondola. I packed quickly, headed out, and soon overtook them on the trail. My throat felt a bit sore on the way down, but I otherwise was in tolerable shape after the previous day. I waited for them at the Schwarzee Hotel. Then we took the cable car back to Zermatt, retrieved our bags from the train station, and crossed the street to the Hotel Bahnhof, where I had rented a bunk in a dorm room for CHF40 a night—more than twice the rate of my favorite Leadville Hostel. I had the next two days to rest up before Jamie, Adrienne, and I would begin our attempt on Dufourspitze, the highest point in Switzerland.

Dufourspitze, the main summit of Monte Rosa, is the second-highest peak in the Alps after Mont Blanc. Standing 15,203 feet, Monte Rosa is a massive mountain—a massif, in fact, in that it is connected to several other high peaks around it, unlike the freestanding Matterhorn directly across the valley. After climbing the Matterhorn, Dufourspitze might seem a lark, since it has only a few, short technical sections just below the summit. The danger on Dufourspitze, however, is in the massive glaciers that adorn its upper slopes and in the many crevasses hidden under its perpetual blanket of snow.

On Tuesday, I had wandered around town, which didn't take long since it's quite small, and visited the Matterhorn Museum, mainly because it was free with my Swiss Pass card. Most of the descriptions of the items there were in German, so I wasn't sure what I was looking at, but I did see Whymper's famous rope. There was another exhibit about a local guide who had summited the Matterhorn a record 370 times, the last time at the age of 90.

By that night, however, the sore throat I had experienced hiking out from the Hörnli Hut two days before was now a full-blown cold, and my nose ran constantly. In the morning, I took the Gornergrat train up to the Rotenboden station—remembering to use my Swiss Rail Pass this time—and waited for Jamie and Adrienne, who arrived two trains later. Unlike on the Matterhorn, Adrienne would be joining us for the summit bid of Dufourspitze. I sat in the sun to ward off the chill of the 9,236-foot elevation and listened as a guide addressed his large group of eighteen climbers, who were on some sort of company retreat, about the hike up to the Monte Rosa Hut.

After Jamie and Adrienne arrived, we began our trek to the hut by traversing a single-track trail underneath the summit of Gornergrat, where the train ends at a hotel and observation area far above us. Below us was the Gornergletscher, a huge glacier running down from the slopes of Dufourspitze, now directly in front of us. Our trail ended at a sheer 20-foot cliff descending onto another smaller glacier that was coming in from our left. Jamie remarked that this cliff had not been there the last time he made this hike; the glacier had receded hundreds of feet in the interim and no longer reached the main glacier running down the center of the valley. Whereas before, climbers had been able to step directly out onto ice, a new pair of steel ladders descended down this cliff to a metal footbridge, under which rushed a torrent of glacier melt.

Here, also, we found ourselves jammed in a bottleneck behind the group of eighteen hikers, who stacked up like lemmings at the top of the ladders waiting to be belayed onto the glacier below. When our turn came, Jamie belayed us down the ladder, and we walked across the tiny bridge onto the glacier. We stood in a pile of sawdust deposited for better footing and put on our crampons for the crossing. The glacier was not particularly wide, and it wasn't long before we were back on rocks and dirt and were able to remove our crampons. But the spikes went on again moments later when we reached the edge of the much larger Gornergletscher, which was streaked with gaping crevasses everywhere, like they had been carved into the ice by a giant steak knife.

Scattered along this glacier were tiny red flags on wooden tripods to mark the way through, but it was obvious that these flags were being repositioned almost daily due to shifting ice. Crossing this minefield was serious business, but we made it safely through and soon reunited with terra firma. Glistening on a cliff face about a thousand feet above us was the Monte Rosa Hut, which we arrived at about an hour later.

The Monte Rosa Hut is an architectural marvel. The space-age, high-tech building looks more like it belongs on the surface of the moon than atop a cliff face surrounded by glaciers in the Swiss Alps. Built by the Swiss Alpine Club, the hut is a solar-powered, self-sustaining building that was completed in 2009 at a cost of $18 million. The five-story, crystal-shaped building, which sleeps 120, is covered on the outside by a silver aluminum shell and is designed to obtain 90 percent of its energy requirements from the sun. Melting glaciers above provide a water source. It took more than 3,000 helicopter trips to transport all the materials and workers to the construction site. The distinctive spiral interior captures radiant heat from the sun. It might have been the most energy-efficient building I had ever seen, and perhaps the most remote as well.

The full-service restaurant on the main floor of the hut prepared a fantastic roast beef dinner that night—complete with real mashed potatoes and gravy— before we retired to our little cubicle of a room on an upper floor to catch a few hours' sleep. I hardly slept a wink, waking up several times in a start because I felt as if I was choking on my own phlegm. I felt gurgling coming up from my lungs—sort of like a burp—and I was concerned that what had started out as a cold suddenly had transformed itself into high-altitude pulmonary edema (HAPE). I had never had even so much as a headache at altitude before, but I also had not been this high with a cold before, either. Well, there was that time in Colorado when I was wheezing from a head cold and some guy from Seattle helped me change a flat tire, but that had been long forgotten.

Alarms rang at 2 A.M. ahead of the day's assault of Dufourspitze. I informed Jamie of my concerns at breakfast, and he spent a few minutes considering our options. Then he told me we wouldn't be climbing that day and to go back to bed. He said he would not have let one of his regular clients climb in such a condition, so why should I be any different? I slept away most of the day, but was up by late afternoon when a hard, soaking rain lashed at the aluminum sides of the hut for a couple of hours. After a dinner of chipped beef and polenta that night, it was off to bed again, but I did not sleep a wink this time and was still wide awake when Jamie got us up at 2 A.M. to get the day started.

I felt considerably better than I had the day before, but certainly was not 100 percent. Unfortunately, now Jamie, too, was complaining about a sore throat and a headache, and said he felt "generally miserable." After short deliberation, we decided to give it a go anyway.

Since we had been all packed and ready to go the previous morning, we were the first climbers out the door. The trail behind the hut climbs about a thousand feet before it reaches the edge of the glacier. It was still overcast and a bit chilly, but I could see stars twinkling between the gaps in the clouds. In the darkness, we almost immediately lost the main trail among the myriad rocks and gullies, and had to pick our way upward. While the path we took got us where we wanted to go, it required Jamie to put a rope on me and Adrienne on a couple of the pitches.

It also began misting slightly, then progressed to light rain, though certainly not like the drenching we had gotten the previous afternoon. With Jamie not feeling well and my condition being less than ideal, I could sense that he was going to call off the climb. Especially after we arrived at the edge of the glacier, and we could see the headlamps of other parties—all of which had left the hut after us—now all ahead of us. As the drizzle picked up, Jamie announced it was best that we head back to the hut. He said he didn't have a good feeling about continuing.

As we turned to descend, I commented to Jamie that all the climbers above us must have lost the trail. Above us, headlamps darted in all directions as people scrambled about the ice. Whereas the trail above had previously been well worn and easily recognizable from as far away as the Riffelhorn—I had spotted the route from there during our climb on that first day in Zermatt—the heavy rains must have washed away the trail, resulting in the apparent confusion. We gave it no more thought, and retreated to the hut and went back to bed.

Soon, however, helicopters were buzzing around the hut and one even landed on the helipad outside our window. Again, I gave it little thought as I rolled over and tried to sleep. Later, we learned that a rescue had been in progress, as one of the parties ahead of us had fallen into a crevasse when a waterlogged snow bridge had collapsed. That, it was now apparent, was why I had seen headlamps flashing all over the slope. Other climbers had raced to the aid of the three who had fallen into the hidden crevasse.

Jamie said he should have realized what was happening when I remarked about the headlamps, but he hadn't put the pieces together until after more helicopters arrived. We got only a few fragments of information about the incident. While no one had been seriously injured, one of the climbers had fallen to a depth of 25 feet, necessitating a helicopter rescue to extract him.

We were extremely fortunate that it had not been us in that crevasse. Had we taken the correct route from the hut, we would have been the first group out on the glacier, and perhaps no other parties would have been close by to help rescue us. After breakfast, we packed up and headed back to Zermatt, and it was a quiet, somber hike back to the train station. Once back in town, I headed back to the Bahnhof for a few more nights, while Jamie and Adrienne prepared to leave town for the remainder of their honeymoon.

Even though the highpoint of Switzerland eluded me on this trip, it had been a tremendous week of climbing. I would not have traded my summit of the Matterhorn for anything. I was extremely grateful that Jamie had gotten me safely up and down the most incredible mountain I had ever climbed. As I stared at the wispy clouds frolicking on the summit of the Matterhorn from the tiny window on the fifth floor of the Bahnhof, it was hard to believe that just a few days before, I had stood there myself. I can't imagine that any other summit, whether it be Denali or Everest, could convey such a sense of accomplishment as that which I had experienced on the Matterhorn.

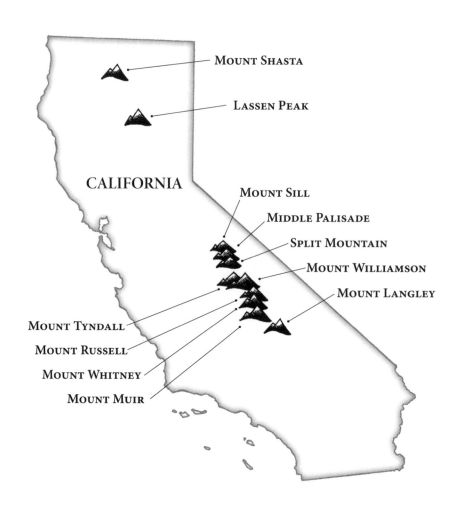

MOUNT SHASTA

LASSEN PEAK

CALIFORNIA

MOUNT SILL

MIDDLE PALISADE

SPLIT MOUNTAIN

MOUNT WILLIAMSON

MOUNT LANGLEY

MOUNT TYNDALL

MOUNT RUSSELL

MOUNT WHITNEY

MOUNT MUIR

Chapter 15
September 2012

SHASTA AND THE REMAINING SIERRAS

ALMOST EVERYTHING I KNEW ABOUT MOUNT SHASTA—THE SECOND-HIGHEST volcano in the Cascades and the fifth-highest peak in California—had come directly from the writings of John Muir. Certainly, no one in the late 1800s knew the mountainous regions of California better than Muir, who spent most of his later life campaigning for the preservation of the lands that would eventually compose Yosemite and Sequoia National Parks.

Even before my peakbagging journey, I think I had read every word ever written by Muir, but one story stands out in my memory above all others: his epic survival story on Mount Shasta.

Muir and fellow climber Jerome Fay started up Mount Shasta by starlight in the predawn hours of April 30, 1875, their objective to take barometrical observations on the summit for the U.S. Coast Survey. Another man, Army meteorologist Captain A.F. Rodgers, took simultaneous readings at the mountain's base.

Upon gaining the summit near dawn, Muir wrote that he was surprised to see several hundred square miles of cumulus clouds to the east, portending the onset of a storm. He was not particularly concerned at first, since previous knowledge had told him that these late-season wintry storms were typically not very ferocious.

The day warmed up nicely as Muir and Fay began their readings at 9 A.M. Clouds, meanwhile, continued to build, but Muir was undaunted, knowing that Rodgers was counting on him to make his final reading at 3 P.M. Soon, however, Muir realized that the storm descending upon them was not ordinary.

By the time he made his final observation and put away all their equipment, the maelstrom was upon them.

The two men scrambled to get off the summit. Fay lagged behind, and Muir had to wait for him just below some fumaroles, where hot, sulfuric gases emanated from the ground. Muir urged Fay to hurry, but his companion was not as experienced a climber and refused to continue. Instead, Fay fought his way back against the wind to the fumaroles. Knowing he could not leave Fay to an uncertain fate, Muir decided to stay. Despite the fact that neither man was properly dressed to spend a night out in wintry conditions, Fay announced he was going to lie down among the gas jets in hopes of avoiding death by freezing. Muir was left with no choice but to join his companion. But what would protect them from the acidic gases?

Lying in the bubbling mud pots, they were at once scalded on one side and frozen on the other. Snow piled up on their chests; in all, nearly 18 inches fell before it abated sometime during the night.

Still, it was well into the next morning before the sun rose high enough in the sky to ward off the chill night air, and it was 17 long hours before the two men were able to rise from their prone positions. Their muddy clothes had frozen solid, making it nearly impossible for either of them to walk as they clumsily made their way off the mountain to safety. A rescue party met them at their camp.

It must have been quite a sight to see Muir and Fay plodding their way down the upper slopes of Shasta with their clothes frozen solid by the caked mud, as stiff as the Tin Man from *The Wizard of Oz*. Very few mountaineers, I imagine, would have had the resolve to save their lives by lying down in the boiling mud of the fumaroles to keep from freezing to death. Muir wrote about that experience in an article for *Harper's New Monthly Magazine* in 1877, and the story reads as one of the most gripping tales of averted disaster in the annals of mountaineering.

I'm not sure what I might have done in a similar predicament. I certainly would not have wanted to abandon my climbing partner, but at what point did Muir's choice put his own life in peril? Perhaps it was part of the reason I preferred to climb solo. I prayed I would never have to face such a decision.

My euphoria from climbing the Matterhorn didn't last long. I returned from Switzerland on a Monday night, packed my car on Tuesday, and left on Wednesday morning for California, where I hoped to summit the remaining 14ers, including Mount Shasta. Once again, I wouldn't be going alone: my friend Van Pol planned to join me for a couple of the climbs.

It was August 29, and Nancy and I were once again two ships passing in the night. She was also leaving that afternoon for Europe and that year's WMRA Championships in Italy.

I headed back across US 50 in Nevada to pick up Van at the airport in Reno. We planned to climb Lassen Peak and Mount Shasta together before pressing on. He wanted to summit Mount Whitney, and I needed to check off the two 14ers that flanked it, so it made sense to tackle California's highpoint a second time. We also planned to visit Redwood National Park.

Though Van had arrived in Reno on time, his luggage had not. We killed the few hours' wait for its arrival on the next flight by going to Walmart to buy supplies and to REI, where I resisted the temptation to drop another $300, like I had the year before.

Despite the delay, we reached our campsite at Lassen Volcanic National Park before dark. The next morning, we set out to explore the park. Charles Bookman, who had visited the park just a few weeks prior, recommended the 1.5-mile hike to hell, one of Earth's hottest geothermal sites, Bumpass Hell. We smelled it long before we could see it. Its bubbling mud pots, sulfur vents, and boiling pools certainly conjured up images of the underworld. Boardwalks around the 16-acre site let us explore without the risk of falling in and getting burned.

That's exactly what had happened to Kendall Vanhook Bumpass, a local cowboy who first discovered the fumaroles in the 1860s. Hiking around the site, he broke through the crust and scalded his leg in a mud pot. Telling friends and townspeople about his discovery, he described it as hell. He hoped to turn the area into a tourist attraction, and invited a local newspaper reporter to visit the site with him. Bumpass again broke through the crust, but this time his leg plunged into water that was more than 200 degrees Fahrenheit. The area was certainly too dangerous for tourists. Not only did Bumpass lose his dream, he lost his leg, too, as it had to be amputated.

All this sightseeing was merely killing time before our real objective for the day: Lassen Peak itself. Also known as Mount Lassen, the peak is the southernmost active volcano in the Cascades, and rises about 2,000 feet above the surrounding terrain, making it one of the largest lava domes on the planet. It last erupted in 1915, spreading ash more than 200 miles to the east and devastating nearby areas. The only other volcano to erupt in the contiguous United States in the twentieth century was Mount St. Helens, in 1980.

The trail up Lassen had been closed for renovations the entire month of August, but was set to reopen that night, just in time for that month's blue moon. Because the path was a popular full-moon hike and because it was the Friday of Labor Day weekend, we expected to be part of an especially large crowd.

Leaving the parking lot right at dusk, we watched the sun set in the west and an enormous full moon rise in the east as we started up the Lassen Peak

Trail. We didn't need our headlamps; the moon was more than bright enough to illuminate uniform switchbacks leading up the east side of the 10,457-foot volcanic peak. Too many of our fellow hikers, however, felt the need to use their headlamps, and the descending hikers' lights were a distraction; the narrow focus of the artificial light limited our range of vision. I thought it defeated the purpose of the full-moon hike.

We found the recent trail work quite impressive; from what we saw, the trail was on its way to becoming the most manicured mountain trail anywhere (the full, five-year project was completed in fall 2014). We stumbled a few times near the summit when we crossed onto the west side and into the shadows cast by some pillars, but were soon standing on the summit next to a conical—and comical—metal structure. I can't imagine who approved the design for the 15-foot-tall phallic structure, or what possessed someone to think they could somehow disguise its appearance by painting it in camouflage. But it is part of the Lassen Volcanic Center's seismic monitoring system, so the rather obscene form may have been overshadowed by its important function.

As we made our way down, dozens of people were still heading up, even though it was now after 9 P.M. As we drove away from the parking lot and looked back at the mountain, the patches of snow near the summit glowed in the moonlight.

Mount Shasta is enormous, the most voluminous mountain in the United States—bigger at its base than even Rainier—and has a prominence of nearly 10,000 feet over the surrounding plain. Once believed to be California's highest peak (it's actually the fifth highest), an eight-man party led by Captain Elias D. Pierce climbed it in 1854, the first recorded summit by white climbers. The local Klamath people considered the "White Mountain" sacred, home to one of their gods, and were forbidden to climb it.

Others share different legends of Shasta. At the turn of the twentieth century, Frederick Spencer Oliver's posthumously published book, *A Dweller on Two Planets,* began to popularize one story. In the late 1800s, some archaeologists theorized that a continent—Lemuria—had disappeared in the Pacific, and Oliver's novel wove a tale of the land's destruction and its superhuman inhabitants' continued survival in a city built in Shasta's cone, which they named Telos. A second book, published in the 1930s, continued spreading this belief. It is also considered by many to be the site of one of the world's great "energy vortexes," similar to Sedona, Arizona, and Lake Atitlán in Guatemala.

For Van and me, Shasta was just another lofty mountain to climb. Driving into the town of Mount Shasta, we found the main street cordoned off for a custom car show and took back streets to The Fifth Season, the local outdoor store and the best source of information for climbing the mountain. While Shasta can usually be seen towering over the town, on this day views of the peak were obliterated by wildfire smoke blowing in from somewhere to the west.

After lunch, we drove the 14 miles up Everitt Memorial Highway to the trailhead at Bunny Flat, which was at one time the parking lot for the old Mount Shasta Ski Bowl. In 1959, this ski area received nearly 16 feet of snow from one storm, the most ever from a single storm, according to *Guinness World Records*. I had driven this road once before, during a scouting mission in April 2011, when I was showing *Ride the Divide* in nearby Redding; the snowbanks lining this road had been more than 10 feet high.

Bunny Flat is at an elevation of 6,950 feet, and after packing up and getting current trail conditions from a park ranger, we hiked the 1.6 miles up to Horse Camp, about a thousand feet higher. The one-story stone structure—built in 1923 and owned and operated by the Sierra Club—is considered base camp for those who climb Shasta via the Avalanche Gulch route. During my 2011 scouting mission, I had hiked to Horse Camp, only to find the snow so deep that just the chimney of the building was visible. Having been advised that the avalanche danger was too great that day to risk a solo ascent, I turned back. About 15,000 people attempt Shasta each year, and only about a third of them reach the summit.

When Van and I arrived, a caretaker was at the hut, watching some of the climbers above through her binoculars. We topped off our bottles from the nearby spring, and I thought it was just about the best-tasting water I had ever had—better even than from Falcon Spring on Mount Monadnock. Leaving the lodge, we hiked for more than a half-mile along Olberman's Causeway, a stone pathway built by the hut's first caretaker, Joseph Olberman, in the 1920s and '30s.

Two hours later, we arrived at high camp at Lake Helen at 10,400 feet, where most climbers spend the night before making a predawn summit bid the following day. Several rock walls served as windbreaks, but I could not see the lake, as Lake Helen rarely reveals itself from under its blanket of snow. Though it was still the holiday weekend and though the weather conditions were perfect, only two other parties were there when we arrived, and only a few others showed up later.

From camp, we had a clear view of an area known as the Heart, a pendant-shaped patch of dirt surrounded by a pair of snow gullies, which we would have to hike past to get to a cliff band called the "Red Banks," a 50-foot-high strip of red rock stretching across the top of the ridge. There was a narrow notch in this ridge that would lead us to the top of these cliffs, depositing us at the base of Misery Hill, just below the summit.

We awoke at three the next morning—Saturday—and were on the trail 25 minutes later, climbing in the dark past the Heart on snow so hard that our crampons had difficulty biting. We wondered when and where the notch would reveal itself, and with the onset of dawn, the notch came into view right smack in front of us, like a magical doorway.

The notch was narrow—we could touch both sides—but this only helped with our climbing, as the notch itself was chock-full of ice and snow, and contoured at a slope of about 35 degrees. The climbing was not hard, but the chute was deceptively long. We emerged from it just in time to see the sun rise to our right, always a magnificent spectacle at high elevation. Shasta's immense shadow stretched onto the western horizon, and Van stopped to snap some photos.

Then we climbed Misery Hill, which was not particularly steep, but was quite high. It got its name because many climbers mistook its top for the actual summit, which, we knew, was still a ways beyond across a glacier. The snow atop this glacier was fluted and difficult to walk on, but once across, it was just a short trudge over Shasta's sulfur-stenched crater and then a quick scamper up the far ridge to the summit.

We had made the summit from Lake Helen in just 4 hours and were back at our tents just 2.5 hours later, seeing no one else above the Red Banks. Getting back to base camp, we quickly packed up and were back at Bunny Flat by 2:15 P.M. Peering back at the peak, I wondered why it had such a reputation as a hard mountain to climb. For Van and me, it had been a relative lark.

From Mount Shasta, we headed south on I-5 to Redding and then west on CA 299 toward the coast, stopping only for a quick dip in the inviting—and frigid— Trinity River somewhere along the way. We arrived at the Redwood National and State Parks, on the northern California coast, just about dark; without a reservation, we also found all the campgrounds in Prairie Creek Redwoods State Park filled for the holiday weekend. We should have known better.

A ranger directed us to a private campground, where we forked over $29.50 to sleep in a meadow surrounded by family RVs and the noise of screaming kids. Trying to look at the bright side, Van remarked that we had slept in worse places, most notably, the cockroach-infested room we had shared in Honduras; I reminded him that that room had cost us only $4. About the only worthwhile campground amenity was the hot shower I enjoyed the next morning before we hightailed it out of there.

Redwood National Park became a reality only in 1968 after several decades of lobbying by such groups as Save the Redwoods League, the Sierra Club, and the National Geographic Society. Much of the old-growth forest of giant redwoods had long before fallen victim to the lumberjack's ax prior to President Lyndon Johnson's signing a bill to establish the park. One section of some of the tallest redwoods was set aside and named for the first lady, and we stopped to hike the 1-mile trail that looped through Lady Bird Johnson Grove. It was remarkable how big these trees were, but Van assured me they would pale in comparison with the ones we would see that afternoon.

Our original plan had been to park at the trailhead for the Redwood Creek Trail and hike the 7.5 miles to the Tall Trees Grove, where some of the tallest redwoods could be found. But when we stopped at the visitor center in Orick to pick up our hiking permit, the ranger discouraged us from the plan since there had been a rash of trailhead break-ins. He suggested starting at the Tall Trees Trail parking lot, which was 6 miles past a locked gate—to which he gave us the combination—where our car would be safe. From there, Tall Trees Grove was a short 2-mile hike away. As Van promised, the grove's trees along Redwood Creek were even taller than the ones we had seen earlier, and Van snapped lots of photos.

Crossing the creek, we pitched our tents on a sandy beach. It was an idyllic spot, with the creek flowing gently beside us. While Van went for a dip in the chilly water, I collected deadwood for a fire that I soon had roaring. When it got dark, the stars lit up the night sky, and it reminded us of the night we had spent camping on the riverbank in Batopilas with Rich in Copper Canyon.

In the morning, Van packed up before me and hiked the 7.5 miles out the Redwood Creek Trail, and I was to pick him up at the trailhead in a few hours. The first thing I had noticed when I drove in was that a car in the parking lot had its window smashed out, the victim of a break-in. That likely would have been my car had the ranger not warned us against parking there. Fifteen minutes later, Van arrived and we headed out.

We spent the rest of the day retracing our route back to Reno, where we got a room for the night. The following day, we picked up Van's rental car—we would be parting ways after climbing Whitney, so he would need his own wheels— and he followed me the 5 hours down US 395 to the town of Lone Pine, where we were to pick up our climbing permit at the ranger station just south of town.

To our good fortune, we discovered there were some unused permits to hike in that day on the Mountaineers Route—the same one Zac and I had climbed in 2009. We left Van's car in town and drove mine up to the Whitney Portal and packed for the three-day hike as a light rain began to fall. It took us about 2 hours to make the steep ascent to Upper Boy Scout Lake, where Zac and I had met the Romeros three years before.

The trail appeared much different than it had on that previous climb.

Zac and I had had a lot of snow to deal with in March, but Van and I were there in September, and the trails were clear. We followed the trail as it crisscrossed the North Fork of Lone Pine Creek and climbed several granite slabs and benches known as the Ebersbacher Ledges, which Zac and I had been able to bypass in winter conditions.

Van and I camped at Upper Boy Scout Lake, as this was where I thought I would be starting from in the morning when I attempted to summit Mount Russell, a 14er located just north of Whitney. But some guides coming down the trail informed me that the starting point for Russell was at Iceberg Lake, which was the next lake higher in the basin. From there, I would have to cross something they referred to as the "football field." But we already had our tent set up in a spot that we liked, hidden in the rocks, and there was little light left, so we stayed put.

The morning was so cold that neither of us wanted to venture out of the tent, but eventually nature called, and we had to answer. It took about an hour to hike the remaining mile or so to Iceberg Lake at about 13,000 feet. We set up camp again and I repacked for what I had hoped would be a quick scramble up Mount Russell, which, though 14,086 feet itself, is dwarfed by the stunning presence of its higher neighbor, Whitney. Heading around the eastern shore of Iceberg Lake, I climbed a broad hummock in hopes of finding the trail the guide had told me about. Instead, I quickly found myself at the top of a steep cliff that, I could plainly see, led me back into the same drainage as Upper Boy Scout Lake, where we had camped the night before. A gully on the far side led to a broad plateau that connected to Russell's summit ridge. This looked like the most apparent route, if I could get to it.

Seeing no other way off the cliff, I climbed straight down, even though it was nearly vertical and several hundred feet high. I picked my way down without incident, relying upon all of my rock-climbing skills, and crossed the drainage by hopping over some large boulders. Once in the chute at the bottom of the gully, the climbing was fairly straightforward, except when I had to negotiate around a large chock stone that blocked my path. Once around this obstacle, I quickly topped out at the edge of a broad plateau, which angled up to the saddle between Russell and its shorter neighbor, Mount Carillon.

Once on this impressive ridgeline, I turned left and started up an incredibly narrow knife's edge that had dizzying drops on both sides as I made my way over several smaller summits. While not as treacherous as the Palisades I had climbed the year before, this was not a mountain that was recommended to solo. I could see why. The exposure was staggering. Then it started to snow. I contemplated turning back, but I had summit fever; the top was only a few hundred yards above me. I just hoped the rocks would not become too slippery, or the route obscured by clouds, on the way down. I had come too far to bail now on what might have been the hardest route I had yet soloed.

The final climb to Russell's summit was over large boulders similar to those on top of Granite Peak in Montana, and, with the snow intensifying, I stayed only long enough to snap a selfie and to sign the register book. The descent seemed much easier than coming up—probably because I picked a better line through the rocks—and once back at the saddle, it was an easy hike across the open plateau back to the top of the chute I had ascended.

Rather than reclimb the cliff across the basin, I instead hiked back to Upper Boy Scout Lake and retraced the main trail back to Iceberg Lake. Van was curled up in the tent, as the snow had turned to rain at the lower elevation. All my gear was wet from the climb and I was very cold, so I quickly changed into the driest clothes I could find and dived into my sleeping bag for a nap. The rain stopped a couple of hours later, and I spread out all my wet clothes on the rocks in hopes that they would dry overnight. But I held out little hope for my soaked sneakers; they were the only pair of shoes I had brought on the climb.

We awoke at seven the next morning to sunlight filtering into our basin. All of the clothes I had put out the night before had frozen solid, with ice clinging to them. And they were the clothes I had to wear that day. Van boiled some water for breakfast and soon thereafter hit the trail ahead of me, starting up the steep, 1,500-foot gully above the lake, which would bring us to a notch just below Whitney's noble summit. I stayed behind, hoping to dry out my clothes, and eventually was able to put on a relatively dry pair of pants.

Despite the half-hour delay to my start, Van arrived at the top of the notch just minutes before I did. It was enough time for him to check out the route above us, and I could tell he was quite apprehensive. From the notch, we traversed south onto the west side of Whitney, bringing us to the top of a huge cliff, which left Van weak in the knees. Remember, he had avoided climbing any exposed routes when we had climbed the 14ers in Colorado. He was even less happy when I told him we had to scramble up the steep gully behind us, the one Zac and I had easily climbed wearing crampons. He was not convinced this was the right way, but I assured him it was the *only* way. I told Van it was no steeper than the Homestretch on Longs Peak, which he had climbed without hesitation.

Fortunately, we had reached this point just minutes after the sun had emerged over Whitney's summit, instantly warming the rocks and melting the ice that had accumulated overnight. I told Van just to stay in the sunshine, and he managed this section better than even he thought possible. In moments, we topped out on Whitney's broad summit plateau to be greeted by warm sunshine and lots of other climbers, all of whom had come up the standard route.

Our plan was to descend via this route, which would take us underneath the summit of Mount Muir, the other 14er I needed to bag on the way down. Hikers at the summit, however, told us that because of trail maintenance, a portion of the trail below Trail Crest was going to be open only from 11:30 A.M. to 12:30 P.M., and after that would be closed for several hours. That left us with only a 2-hour window to reach Mount Muir and make it below the closure, so we quickly signed the register book and began our descent.

I found the standard route to be quite wide and relatively flat; it didn't drop much elevation while winding through the many gendarmes—huge, towering spires—that line the ridge. This trail was high and airy, and very exhilarating. So much so that we accidentally passed the unmarked turnoff to Mount Muir, which is little more than the highest of these spires along Whitney's south crest. Looking up at what we thought was the summit, we dropped our packs and scrambled up together. "Easier than Mount Sherman," Van exclaimed, referring to what most consider the easiest 14er in Colorado.

But when we got to this "summit," we peered over the top and saw that Mount Muir actually rose another 200 feet and that the summit block was a steep, vertical rock face.

"See you later," Van said, and he turned and headed back down.

I told him I would catch up to him later, but knew that if I didn't hurry, I would not make the 12:30 cutoff before the trail closed ahead. I gave him my car keys just in case he had to wait.

It was a short scramble over to the cliff face, and, approaching its base, I saw that the climbing would be no worse than simple Class 4, with very pronounced footholds the entire way. I made quick work of what previously might have been some intimidating climbing and was on the summit moments later, logging into the register book. Back on the main trail, an ascending hiker told me that it was 12:20; I was still a half-mile from Trail Crest. Shouldering my pack, I ran, crossing over the crest that leads back to the east side of the mountain and passing the workers just as they were wrapping up their lunch.

I descended 1,600 feet over the next 2.2 miles down the infamous "97 Switchbacks" to reach Trail Camp, where most climbers using the standard route camp overnight on their ascent. It's still another 8 miles or so back to the Portal from there. Van, worried I hadn't made the cutoff, was much relieved to see me trudge in 5 minutes after him.

We parted ways in Lone Pine; Van planned to finish up his trip by exploring Yosemite and Lake Tahoe, and I had six 14ers to complete my list.

Back in 2010, I had run two 50K races in California and used the week in between to dabble in the Sierras, but was unable to summit any of the peaks I tried, largely because of the weather.

One of them was Split Mountain, which may be the most magnificent peak no one's ever heard of. It's often overlooked among California 14ers, as climbers are more naturally attracted to the Whitney massif to the south or to the Palisades in the north. Split is not easily seen from CA 395, as it stands behind some lesser peaks. And it's not easy to reach, either; the approach is long by vehicle or by foot. The 14,058-foot peak is named for its two summits, split in half by a gully that plummets 2,000 feet, making it one of the longest sheer walls in the Sierras. Several spectacular rock-climbing routes run up its east wall for the experienced technical climber. In 2010, I chose a pedestrian route that would require a long day of climbing; most others take two or three days to climb what I tried to tackle in one.

That day, I made it all the way to the bowl just below the saddle between Split and its neighbor to the north, Mount Prater. Wispy storm clouds raced over this saddle, and I realized I didn't have enough time to summit and retreat to safety. I probably had never put in more effort without enjoying a summit.

Mounts Williamson and Tyndall, too, turned me back. Not more than a half-mile in, I completely lost the trail in deep, drifting snow, and wisely I gave up.

But I treated these more as reconnaissance trips than summit bids, and although I had borrowed Nancy's Toyota Tundra for the trip specifically to reach these trailheads—eating the poorer gas mileage for the rest of the trip—I hadn't any real aspiration of standing on a summit.

When I returned to the Sierras in 2012, that wasn't the case. I was in official peakbagging mode when I parted ways with Van and headed back to Split Mountain. In Nancy's Toyota Tundra in 2010, I had easily navigated the network of dirt roads that connected Tinnemaha Creek Campground and the Red Mountain Creek trailhead, my starting point for the hike to Split. But in my Jetta, I had difficulty avoiding all the large rocks in the road, and bottomed out several times, peeling back the protective plastic molding from underneath the engine. I took several different roads as I tried to work my way as close to the trailhead as possible, but in the end, I abandoned the car and hiked the final 4 miles.

At what I had remembered as the trailhead, I checked out the trail info on a kiosk, then hiked past it, and started up the drainage for Red Mountain Creek. This was the same way I had gone in 2010, when I simply followed previous hikers' tracks in deep snow. But even with a couple of small cairns marking the way instead of footprints, I could tell something was amiss: the trail was far too faint, and soon disappeared entirely. I was extremely perplexed.

I looked to the other side of the creek and saw another faint trail traversing the sidehill, so I decided that must be it. But it was extremely difficult to cross this creek, since it was chock-full of willows. There is nothing less appealing than having to hike through a stand of willows. Once across, however, I discovered the trail was little more than a herd path, and I knew I was screwed. I bushwhacked up the left side of the creek and saw previous boot tracks, telling me I was not the first person to make this mistake. But after about 2 miles of this, I knew that the trail I needed must be on the other side, and I looked for a place where I could cross back over the creek. Before I found such a spot, however, the creek split into two branches, meaning I was going to have to tackle the willows twice to get across.

The first crossing wasn't too bad, but the second was awful. The willows were so thick that I had to crawl on my hands and knees to get under them. The tips of my trekking poles, which were sticking out of the top of my backpack, kept catching on the branches, forcing me to squirm out of my pack and pull it through behind me. Finally on the other side and already exhausted, I slowly climbed a steep, grassy slope to discover the correct trail exactly where I had expected. I wasn't sure how I could have missed it from the parking lot.

It was still a long climb up unending switchbacks to reach Red Lake, where three guys from Sacramento had pitched their tents. Hiking on, I came to a second, smaller lake, which also had a tent set up next to it, but no one was about.

Above treeline, I came to a talus-filled basin with a steep moraine in the middle, which led me to the bowl where I had turned around in 2010. This time, though, the weather was fine, and I continued on, scrambling up loose dirt and scree to a notch that angled to the left and climbed another long ridge on more loose rock. I slid back one step for every two I took. I found more solid rock dangerously close to the edge of a cliff, but I took the trade-off. I expected to be close to the summit when I surmounted this ridge, but was discouraged to find that I still had at least a thousand feet of climbing ahead of me, all of it on large talus blocks. Ugh.

It was a long scramble to the summit on tired, sore legs, and it was a testament to my perseverance that I made it. I topped out after 7 hours, 11 or more miles, and perhaps 9,000 feet of gain from the parking lot. This was a well-earned summit, made even more so by the additional effort from my previous attempt.

I wasted little time on the summit, as it was thundering. I overtook the three climbers from Sacramento above the saddle as it began to hail. Fortunately, as I descended back into the basin and down to the lakes, it turned to rain, though it continued the remainder of the afternoon, making for a miserable hike out.

Near the bottom of the trail, I met two hikers—a guy and a girl—coming up wearing small daypacks. I thought it strange, since it was obviously too late in the day to summit and then hike out without camping. Turned out they were the two occupants of the tent I had seen at the upper lake; they had summited in the morning and had mistakenly taken the wrong drainage off the peak, descending all the way to the bottom. Now they had a long, wet climb back up to their tent despite being exhausted. And I thought I had had a bad day.

Closer to the parking lot, the trail's true path was clearer. The lower part of the trail stayed high up on the sidehill, meaning that I never should have been down by the creek to begin with. The trail ended not at the kiosk, where I had started, but a couple of hundred yards up a side road. I had noticed a silver Ford pickup parked there that morning—it belonged to the Sacramento guys—and seeing that vehicle should have tipped me off. I was still a bit miffed that someone had once decided it was better to put the information board at some place other than the actual trailhead. As I said, I knew I was not the first person to make the mistake.

I still had a 4-mile walk on wet, wrinkled feet back to my car, and it was dark by the time I got back to the campground. I thought I would sleep like a baby after such a long, grueling day, but being at only 4,000 feet here, it was too hot in my tent. At least the sky was clear, as the rain had stopped, and the wet clothes I had hung out were dry in the morning.

After a fitful night's sleep, I considered making Sunday a rest day, but decided instead to drive to Independence and hike into Shepherd Pass, the main trail to Mounts Williamson and Tyndall. I still had a bone to pick with these two peaks, which had also turned me back on that previous trip.

Driving along US 395, the plastic molding under my car was dragging along the highway. When I turned onto Foothill Road, which leads to the trailhead, I pulled over and duct-taped the dangling material to my bumper. As I finished "MacGyvering" it back on, a four-wheel-drive Ford van pulled alongside and asked if I needed help. It was one of the local shuttle services, bringing a group of hikers to the trailhead. I said that I should be fine, but I was not sure I could drive my car all the way to the trailhead, so I told the driver that if he saw me parked alongside the road on his way out, I would pay him to drive me back in. I wasn't looking forward to another 4-mile hike to the trailhead like the day before. But, it turned out I had no trouble following them all the way to the trailhead. The road was in great shape.

My route for the day was an 8-mile hike on a trail that included a steep climb up fifty-four switchbacks, which gained 3,000 feet in less than 3 miles to reach a small pass before continuing to Anvil Camp at about 10,000 feet, where most climbers camp for the night. It was raining lightly when I arrived at camp at about 7 P.M., and I quickly set up my tent, got the rain fly attached, and threw everything inside just moments before the skies really opened up. A vicious thunderstorm lashed the area for a solid hour. It was dark by the time it stopped, and I was able to crawl out and cook dinner. But the clouds cleared to reveal an immense sky with too many stars to count. I considered this a good omen.

The next morning, the pleasant 2-mile climb from Anvil Camp to Shepherd Pass was on an astonishingly well-groomed trail; even the steep final climb to the pass was not bad, thanks to the well-laid switchbacks. But that all changed once I topped out in the pass. I crossed a broad, grassy plateau and descended into Williamson Bowl, a nasty, talus-strewn boulder field that separated Williamson and Tyndall.

I headed first to Mount Williamson, the second-highest peak in California at 14,375 feet, negotiating a mile-long section of talus blocks to reach the edge of some cliffs. I tried to locate the gully that my book said would lead me past the band of black rock that I could see above me. I chose one and started to climb, but I knew right away I was in the wrong gully, since there were not a lot of other tracks evident in the snow and dirt. But the gully went straight up, and so did I, managing to climb around a couple of chock stones that blocked my path higher up. Near the top, I angled to my right over some exposed Class 4 rock and came out on a broad shoulder stretching toward a subsidiary summit. Gaining this, it was just a short scramble over some more talus blocks to reach the summit.

On the descent, I took the correct chute down, but it was so loose and sandy that I was glad I had not followed it up. Crossing back over Williamson Bowl, I headed for Tyndall by climbing straight up a rib that protruded into the bowl off the peak's northwest flank. This rib turned out to be one of the most enjoyable climbs I had done; it was one smooth, spotless piece of granite that reminded me a lot of Huntington Ravine on Mount Washington in New Hampshire. While it was already early afternoon, the weather was clear, and I continued to climb.

Gaining the ridge, I was surprised to find the summit still a very long way off and over a somewhat exposed and narrow ridge. I could have easily descended to my right, traversed an easier slope, then regained the ridge nearer to the summit, but I didn't want to give up any elevation. I stayed on the ridge the entire way, which made for some exhilarating climbing.

Upon reaching the top of the 14,015-foot peak, I found that the actual summit was an 8-foot-tall block perched delicately on top of another larger rock. This true high point extended out a little over a 2,000-foot drop to the Williamson Bowl. It was a bit unnerving to climb, but I figured it had been there for millennia, and was not in danger of catapulting off the summit, unless an untimely earthquake suddenly occurred. But then I remembered that the second-most-powerful earthquake in recorded California history had struck not far from here in 1872; the temblor, which rocked the town of Lone Pine, was later estimated as an 8.0. Even that had not dislodged this monolith. Up I went.

It was a long hike back to Anvil Camp, and I did not arrive until 4 P.M.; too late in the day to hike out, I decided. The hikers who had been shuttled in just ahead of my car all planned to attempt Williamson and Tyndall over the next two days and were amazed that I had climbed both peaks in just 10 hours. I'd managed it only because the weather had held. I packed up in the morning and hiked out, reaching the trailhead with only one thought in mind—to find a shower. I stank horribly.

The best hot shower of my life deserves a mention.

Sitting in the parking lot of Valley Market in Independence, I noticed a sign that read, "Showers $5," and inquired within. Turned out they had a little bathroom facility in a building behind the parking lot, and for five bucks I enjoyed a steaming-hot shower without the clock running. Too often while traveling, I have found showers where you had to keep pumping quarters into a slot to keep the water running, but here there was no timer. Rinsing off a week's worth of dusty trail and shaving off a week's growth of whiskers turned me into a human again.

I dreaded the next two peaks on my agenda most—far more than I had the Maroon Bells years before. Middle Palisade and Mount Sill would undoubtedly be the steepest, scariest mountains I had yet attempted to solo. They were part of the Palisades range that included Starlight and Thunderbolt, and I would not have the luxury of someone like my friend Doug Seitz to guide me this time. I was on my own.

The rain at the Glacier Lodge trailhead only made things worse: I had a 2-hour hike in to camp, and that meant I'd be attempting Middle Palisade the next day with wet gear.

At the ranger station in Bishop, I picked up my permit, which called for me to camp at Brainerd Lake. My book said I'd have a 5-mile hike from Glacier Lodge to reach it. But I remembered that when I last ran into my friend Steve Till—and his dog, Pepper—on White Mountain the year before, he had shown me his stunning photos and told me he had camped at Finger Lake when he climbed Middle Palisade. He had also said that he had summited with Pepper, so I wondered if I might be worrying for nothing.

It was still raining slightly when I hit the trail at 4:45 P.M. I hiked up the valley to a series of switchbacks that ascended an impressive cliff face to reach Willow

Lake, where the trail faded considerably. The next body of water I came to was a tiny little cesspool of a pond, which I somehow mistook for Brainerd Lake, since I saw no other bodies of water on my map. Hiking beyond, the trail seemed to fizzle out, but there was a cairn—the first one I had seen—on my right. It seemed to very adamantly mark a little trace path going off into the woods. I followed it over a small ridge and down into the next drainage.

This "trail" went straight up the bed of a fast-running creek, crossing from side to side, and I surmised correctly that it was the outlet from Finger Lake. By the time I emerged at the edge of a long, narrow, boxed-in fjord that I recognized from Steve's photos, it was almost dark. I climbed high on the bluff on the west side to get past some cliffs, but found no indication of a campsite by the time I had reached the far end of the lake at dusk. I did, however, find a small, grassy island that I could step onto from the shore. I knew I was not supposed to camp within 200 feet of any body of water—per park restrictions and Leave No Trace ethics—but it was too late and I was too tired to do anything else. It was a beautiful spot, one I would certainly have chosen had there been no restrictions, and I ate a late dinner under a blanket of a billion stars.

I'm not sure I have ever woken up in a more beautiful setting. The morning sun illuminated Middle Palisade high above me, and its sheer eastern face seemed unclimbable from my vantage point. Leaving the lake, I climbed up alongside a waterfall, which tumbled into the lake from the glacier above before disappearing under all the talus blocks I was climbing. I reached the rocky moraine that splits Middle Palisade Glacier in half; my destination was the rocky nose that juts out into this moraine, where the two "easy" routes on Middle Palisade begin. I say "easy" because both were Class 4, rather than all the other routes, which were Class 5. As I approached this "nose," however, I could not imagine that the route that lay before me was not also a Class 5 climb.

Middle Palisade was one of the last California 14ers to be conquered, due to its nearly inaccessible summit. The first attempt came in 1919, when a party led by J. Milton Davies climbed the southwest face and wound up atop a subsidiary peak instead, staring across the expanse of an impassable ridge at the true summit. They named this point Disappointment Peak and descended by the way they had come.

Two years later, Francis Farquhar and Ansel F. Hall took a stab at the climb and wound up on top of Disappointment Peak as well. Retracing their steps, they ascended a more northerly gully, and eventually found themselves in such a precarious situation that they decided to descend. They soon realized that climbing down was impossible, and instead continued going up. They gained the summit, which revealed no evidence of any previous climbers.

Both those ascents came from the west side of the peak. In 1930, the legendary Norman Clyde, whose name adorns a subsidiary peak just north of Middle Palisade, became the first to solo the mountain, this time by the same northeast-face route that I would be attempting.

Standing in front of the buttress, I studied the first 50 feet of the route, which I knew was the crux. There seemed to be two ways to surmount the initial wall, both of them requiring vertical climbs where a fall would do some serious damage. It was not for the faint of heart. I started up and found the climbing difficult, but not overly so. The footholds were solid. Once above this 50-foot cliff, the chute above me mellowed in steepness and probably was not higher than Class 3. Steve said Pepper had climbed this chute all the way to the ridge after he had carried her up the first steep part in his backpack, like he had when we had climbed together on Wetterhorn. The gully was no longer a concern, leaving me to worry more about the narrow ridge at the top and the downclimb back to the moraine still ahead.

Still, it took quite a while to ascend this chute, which must have been a couple thousand feet in height. And at one point higher up, it calved into two gullies. I took the right path, which appeared to have had more foot traffic. (I later checked my guidebook: I should have gone left.) Topping out on the ridge, I was near what I thought was the summit, but after scrambling over some incredibly exposed blocks teetering on the ridge crest, I found that the other summit—a few hundred yards to the south—was actually higher.

It took some precise, calculated climbing over this extremely narrow and exposed ridgeline to traverse over to the real summit. I was unable to locate the register canister—I later saw other trip reports stating the same, so I wondered if there ever was one.

After a well-earned, half-hour lunch break, I carefully began my descent down what I had hoped was the proper gully. I came to a flat bench about 50 feet below the summit that was smooth and sandy; it was barely big enough to put two sleeping bags side by side, but would make for an incredibly airy camping spot for anyone who wanted to sleep at 14,000 feet. Maybe next time. I continued downclimbing; though sketchy, it was not as difficult as I had feared, and it wasn't long before I was back at the top of the 50-foot cliff that would lead me back to the moraine. There were two ways down, and I chose the one I had not ascended, mostly because it was over the edge of the glacier, and, if I fell, the "softer" ice might provide more of a cushion. But as I carefully worked my way down this face, I saw that if I fell, I would miss the glacier and tumble into the bergschrund between the rock and the snow instead. This was deep enough that I might not have been able to climb out of it if I had fallen in.

Fortunately, I did not. I leapt from the rock wall over the bergschrund onto the glacier, and made my way back to the moraine. My camp was far below, little more than a tiny orange dot on a green speck in a glacial-blue lake. For the first time all day, I relaxed.

Getting out from Finger Lake proved even harder than getting in to it, as the trail was hard to follow. I ended up bushwhacking east until I cut across the trail coming up from Willow Lake. From there, I had to locate the trail to Lake Elinore, one of the other drainages emptying into Willow Lake, which was the way to Mount Sill. The guidebook said I would find this trail at the first creek crossing after leaving Willow Lake, but it was not where I expected it to be. I hiked back and forth up and down the trail, stopped to scratch my head a few times, and then decided to sit down and read the book word by word. Then it dawned on me. The book said the "cross-country trail" to Lake Elinore began at the first creek crossing. It was not an obvious footpath, which was what I had been looking for.

I walked into the woods in the direction of the drainage and found a faint herd path, which grew stronger and stronger the farther I went, until I was certain it was the right trail. The path climbed steeply along a raging creek for about a mile to a water crossing. Here, there was an adequate campsite that appeared to have been used many times before, and I slid my heavy pack off my weary shoulders. I could see Mount Sill, so I knew how far I would have to hike in the morning to reach its base. There even was a small fire pit in the crevasse of a rock, and even though it was against regulations, I started a small fire—not for the warmth, but to fight back the tiny black flies that were swarming around me, the first bugs I had seen on the entire trip.

In the morning, the first thing I noticed was that my raging creek was now just a gurgling stream, having dropped about 8 inches overnight. I imagined that this was a daily phenomenon, the ebb and flow as the glacier above me melted from the sun, releasing its pristine water, and then refreezing at night.

The trail led me straight up the steep drainage over some flat granite slabs, over which some tiny waterfalls cascaded. Higher up, I hopped across talus blocks the size of sofas to gain the edge of Sill Glacier, located directly below Mount Sill's vertical east face. Here, things looked a bit dicey—perhaps my poor route choice on this day was the real problem.

I had intended to climb the Class 3 East Couloir route, which was considered the easiest route from the east side of the mountain. I likely should have taken the Northeast Couloir, which was also rated Class 3, but the book said that came out of the North Fork drainage—a typical ascent from Glacier Lodge—and I had hiked in along the South Fork, which led directly to Middle Palisade. So

I wrote off the Northeast Couloir route. What I hadn't realized was that both drainages converge at Glacier Notch, the saddle between Sill and Mount Gayley; I could easily have climbed to the notch from my position on the edge of the Sill Glacier had I known.

Instead, I plunged straight forward onto the glacier. I had with me only my MICROspikes, which I slipped over my running shoes, but I really needed my crampons. The incline to reach the glacier's lip exceeded 45 degrees, but I was quickly atop it. From there, I saw a wide bergschrund between the top of the glacier and the steep rock face of Mount Sill. I turned right and gingerly hiked along the top of the bergschrund, not getting too close to the lip to avoid breaking off a cornice and falling in, and not getting too far from the lip, where I risked slipping and glissading down the steep slope. Below, piles of rocks jutted out of the snow like the broken teeth of a once-smiling Cheshire Cat.

As I tiptoed along the lip of the glacier, I was unsure how to cross the gap of the bergschrund, which in spots was at least 10 feet wide. I eventually was opposite a chute where a purple fixed rope dangled down around an icy corner. A large boulder that had fallen off the peak conveniently had plugged the crevasse created by the bergschrund and made a short bridge that appeared to be my only way across. I quickly stepped across, not daring to put too much weight on the boulder, and stared at the route ahead of me. It certainly was not Class 3, so I definitely was nowhere near the East Couloir. I pulled out my guidebook. A big lump rose in my throat: I was either on the 5.7-rated East Face route or, worse, one of the two Dead Larry's Pillar routes—one of which was rated 5.9 and the other 5.10. These were not places I should have been climbing alone. And who was this Dead Larry anyway? And how did he die? I didn't want to know.

Grabbing the purple rope, I pulled myself up around the first corner, which had a long, icy tongue running down its center to the edge of the crevasse. Reaching the end of my rope—both literally and figuratively—I saw a very steep cliff face above me, but now I was committed. I had promised Nancy I would never climb anything that I didn't feel I could climb down, even after having promised myself that long before, but in my peakbagging lust, I clearly was about to break that promise. No way did I think I could downclimb what I saw above me. My only hope was that there was an easier way down from the summit.

Several times I climbed past chock stones and chimneys that tested every ounce of my meager rock-climbing skills. I'd never been so relieved in my life when I finally emerged at the ridgeline and then scrambled over some large blocks along a very narrow ridge crest to gain the summit, where the first thing I did was check to see if I had soiled myself. I wasn't sure which couloir I had climbed, but I didn't care; I was just glad I was still alive.

The view from the top of Mount Sill is said to be the best anywhere in the Sierras, and it certainly was stunning. To the northwest stood the rest of the Palisades in their striking glory—Polemonium, North Palisade, Starlight and Thunderbolt—the four peaks I had climbed the year before with Doug. They looked impossibly steep and inaccessible from this vantage point, and if I hadn't known differently, I would have sworn that there was no way I could ever have climbed them. To the south, Middle Palisade—the peak I had climbed the day before—loomed nearby, and beyond that the twin crests of Split Mountain.

Fortunately for me, there were other people on the summit. I don't know what I would have done had I been alone. And for more good luck, one of them was a guide. His name, aptly enough, was Cliff Agocs, and he was the lead alpine and rock guide for Timberline Mountain Guides in Bend, Oregon. His two clients, Frank and John, were both from Boulder, Colorado. They had climbed the Class 3 Northeast route out of the North Fork drainage—as I mentioned, a route that I had not even noticed in the book, having failed to do my homework. Cliff told me to simply follow the three of them back down. I was incredibly relieved, as I feared certain death if I had tried to go back the way I had come up. In fact, I now admitted to myself that I had taken a foolish risk climbing that route, and my only solace was that it was the final difficult mountain I had left in my quest to summit all the 14ers in the Lower 48; only Mount Langley remained, the easiest one in the Sierras.

The climb down was as easy as Cliff suggested, with only one tricky spot that he said might have been Class 4. While his clients were roped up the entire way down, it was a cinch to follow them unroped after what I had just endured. Reaching Glacier Notch, they turned left toward their campsite below Palisade Glacier and the North Fork drainage, and I turned right and descended into the South Fork drainage, not needing to traverse the steep Sill Glacier, which was now above me. It had been a piece of cake.

Hiking out from Lake Elinore, I was extremely exhausted. I'd summited eight 14ers in the past seven days—several of which had pushed the limits of my skill and mental endurance. I knew there was no way I had the energy to complete the 21-mile round-trip to the top of Mount Langley the next day and drive all the way to the outskirts of Los Angeles that same night. I didn't have a second day to spare; I was due in Riverside, California, on Saturday to umpire a weekend girls' softball tournament for Triple Crown Sports, an organization I had worked for since moving to Colorado in 2010. Finally willing to call it while I could, I chose instead to use tomorrow as a leisure travel day for the 3-hour drive south.

My destination for the night was the Whitney Portal Hostel in Lone Pine, and I was heading there at about 7 P.M. when I got a text from my friend Steve Till, the one from Flagstaff. He had seen my posts about being in the Sierras, and he and Pepper were at that moment camping only a few miles from Lone Pine in the Alabama Hills just off the Whitney Portal Road. And, he said, the beers were on him.

Steve's "free" campsite was little more than a dirt pull-off from one of the many side roads, and it was littered with broken glass and shell casings from previous partygoers. We sat and chatted for a while as we drank his free-but-warm beers and then turned in.

I hated to make the 200-mile drive to Riverside without finishing the 14ers first, but it would have to wait until the following week. I had a great time at the softball tournament, despite it being well over 100 degrees Fahrenheit both days, and must have impressed them enough that I was assigned to work home plate for the weekend's championship game for the 18-year-old division. It was quite an honor to work a game in which virtually every player on the field was headed off to play for a Pac-12 school the following year.

On Monday, I drove back up US 395 to Lone Pine and checked into the hostel, and the next day headed up Langley via the Cottonwood Lakes Trail. The road twisted back and forth for 23 miles as it climbed 6,000 feet to a campground and the trailhead. The hike itself was not particularly interesting, except for the five Cottonwood Lakes, where several people were camping and fishing. From there, I climbed one giant, sweeping switchback to the top of Old Army Pass, and then it was just a long slog up some sandy slopes to the summit plateau. Not until reaching a little rocky stretch just below the summit did I need to take my hands out of my pockets for the first time. That's how easy the climb had been.

On the summit, I found it hard to believe that Clarence King had once stood here and thought he was on the highest point in California. Mount Whitney, which stands almost 500 feet higher, and other peaks along the Sierra Crest were clearly visible and also looked higher, even from this distance. I mean, even the three fishermen had realized there was a taller peak just to the north, and became the first to climb the true Whitney the following day. And they weren't seasoned mountaineers like King was.

Returning to the Whitney Portal Hostel for one final night, I resisted the temptation to wander up the street to celebrate my success at the Double L Bar, as Zac and I had done after summiting Whitney three years before. I imagine all of the same surreal characters would have been there that night.

By climbing Langley and completing all of the California 14ers—plus the Colorado ones years before, as well as Rainier—I had now summited all the 14,000-foot peaks in the lower 48.

Or so I had thought.

When I got home from the trip, I logged my summits on the two peakbagging sites I follow—peakbaggers.com and listsofjohn.com—only to discover that, unbeknownst to me, Mount Rainier has two ranked summits. As I mentioned previously, I had not known this when I summited Rainier with the Yukmans in 2010, when our guides brought us to the highpoint of Columbia Crest. Turns out a subsidiary peak known as Liberty Cap—an hour-long slog from the main summit—is ranked in its own right, as it has a prominence of 492 feet in relation to the saddle between the two summits. Washington adheres to a prominence rule of just 400 feet.

According to Lists of John, only seven people have climbed all sixty-seven of these 14ers, including Liberty Cap, while I joined a list of five others who have climbed them all except for Liberty Cap. (Note: Another eight people completed the then-known list of 14ers in the early days of peakbagging, before the list of sixty-seven was finalized in the late '70s.) The list of completers includes Bob Packard, the legendary hiker from Oregon, whose climbing résumé is unrivaled in the history of peakbagging. Another is the only woman on the list, Teresa Gergen of Boulder, who, like Packard, has also climbed the lower 48 state highpoints. I only needed Mount Marcy to join Packard, Gergen, and Brian Kalet as the only people who have summited all the 14ers (excluding Liberty Cap, that is) and the lower 48 state highpoints. Of course, Packard and Gergen have also climbed Denali and Mauna Kea to complete the fifty state highpoints, something I had yet to do.

The Peakbaggers site included a few more names, but now adheres to a list that includes just sixty-four 14ers in the lower 48. This list of completers includes a husband-and-wife team of Victor Henney and Susan Wyman-Henney, who also have climbed the fifty state highpoints.

For some reason, I decided to contact one of the other five climbers I saw on the Peakbaggers website who also had climbed them all except for Liberty Cap. His name was Dave Hart, from Anchorage, Alaska, and he said he probably summed it up for the others on the list by stating that no sensible mountaineer would ever look at Rainier and claim it has two summits. Columbia Crest, he said, would do it for him. Of course, Dave's résumé also includes Denali and most of the remaining mountains over 14,000 feet in Alaska, of which there are twenty-one.

Then, I got another email from Dave a few days later. It seems that he was poring over my list of summits on Lists of John and discovered that, incredibly, we had both climbed North Palisade on the same day in 2011. He asked if I had been the climber suffering from altitude sickness above the U-Notch that day; no, that was my friend, Doug, I wrote back. It turns out that Dave was one of the four climbers from Alaska whom we had met at the top of the notch.

Just a couple of weeks later, Dave came to Colorado to climb some Centennial 13ers and we met up for three of those ascents. We made plans to climb again the next time he came to Colorado.

It was a bit of a mystery how Mount Marcy could have eluded me all these years. I had seen the 5,344-foot peak from the windows of my dorm during my college days in Burlington, Vermont, especially in winter, when its snow-covered summit glistened on the outstretched horizon beyond Lake Champlain. While I had climbed Vermont's Mount Mansfield several times while attending college, I had never ventured across the lake to the inviting high ridgelines of the Adirondacks with its forty-six 4,000-footers, compared with just five in Vermont.

Likewise, when I began my peakbagging quest with my first excursion to the White Mountains in 2004, I never considered the Adirondacks, although a drive from southern New Hampshire was only about 90 minutes longer to upstate New York than it was to the Whites.

Therefore, after climbing Granite Peak in Montana in 2011, the only state highpoint remaining on my list of the Lower 48 was Mount Marcy.

I had climbed in the Adirondacks only once before—in the fall of 2010 when I showed a film in Lake Placid, bagging my first four 46ers on that trip. But Marcy had not been among them, as early snows had made an excursion to the secluded highpoint prohibitive. So I returned in the spring of 2012 to finally check off the final state highpoint on my list.

Marcy is a majestic peak, standing sentinel over a great range of 4,000-foot peaks that, in fact, goes by the name of the Great Range. This range sits at the heart of the High Peaks region of 6.1-million-acre Adirondack Park, the largest state park in the United States. The area's native people called it "Tahawus," or "Cloud-Splitter," because its upper flanks would rend the clouds that would encircle its summit.

I found the summit to be nothing short of glorious on the late April day I climbed it in 2012, following in the footsteps of Teddy Roosevelt, then the vice president, who was high on the rocky ridgeline of Mount Marcy in 1901 when word came to him that President William McKinley had died of an infection caused by a would-be assassin's bullet. The country held its breath 12 long hours without a president before Roosevelt could reach Buffalo, New York, where he was sworn in as the youngest president in the nation's history at the age of 42.

Only a handful of other hikers were on hand to help commemorate my achievement, including a couple of college kids from the Washington, D.C., area. I was the 426th person to complete the lower 48 state highpoints, according to highpointers.org. On the way out, I also climbed fellow 46ers Table Top and Phelps Mountain.

The following summer, I returned to the Adirondacks and completed a "Great Range Traverse," a 25-mile circumnavigation of nine peaks in the range—seven of them 46ers—which included Marcy in the middle. The traverse consisted of 17,600 feet of climbing and is rated by *Backpacker* magazine as the third-hardest day hike in America. It was another epic day, which left me with eighteen of the 46ers in the bag, and with some newfound friends. Hopefully, a lengthy return trip to the Adirondacks in the near future will enable me to finish this list as well.

While back East in 2013, I had also gotten to hike again with Van—the first time I had seen him since we had climbed Shasta and Whitney together the year before. Van has gone on to experience many adventures of his own. He has hiked Hawaii's Nā Pali Trail; he went to Ecuador, and climbed several high volcanoes, including Chimborazo; he went to Africa and summited Kilimanjaro, perhaps the first Cambodian to climb one of the Seven Summits; recently, he went to Iceland and posted some incredible pictures in front of some massive waterfalls. At this writing, he is in China, in the mountains of Guilin Province.

He has yet to return to his native Cambodia, however. He said he nearly did so a couple of years ago, when his mother went back for the first time. He was all set to join her when an aunt warned him that his mother had an arranged marriage planned for him when he arrived. He quickly canceled. His parents still think there is something wrong with him, wanting to spend all of his time alone in the mountains, a bachelor still in his 30s.

Van and I climbed Monadnock together on Christmas Day 2013, along with our friend Karen Potter, the mountain biker from Massachusetts, who was the one who'd first set me on this peakbagging mission a decade before. In fact, this hike marked the tenth anniversary of meeting Karen on Monadnock on Christmas Day in 2003.

It is hard to fathom all the great adventures I have had since that first trip to the White Mountains in 2004, when Karen and I summited Moosilauke on a crisp winter day and I felt the rush of the wind on my face, setting me on this peakbagging expedition. I have met some amazing people along the way, people I have stayed connected to thanks to our mutual love of the mountains.

Some would say I have given up a lot; many people have questioned my decision to turn down full-time employment at UPS when it was offered again and again, telling me I should have thought about my "retirement." They call me crazy for living what they call a footloose and fancy-free lifestyle. But, to me, they are the ones who are crazy, slaving away at a 9-to-5 job and never really enjoying life. I have missed out on some things, granted. I don't see my children as often as I would like, or my new grandson, who is already excited about a promised climb of Monadnock in the summer of 2016, when he turns 5.

But I have no regrets. I could never have written this book if I hadn't dared to step out of my comfort zone and rediscover my earlier dreams. I encourage you to do the same.

Take stock of your own life, as I did mine more than a decade ago. Rediscover your own earlier dreams and the courage to take the action required to make them happen. I did, and you can, too. It's not too late.

See you on the summit.

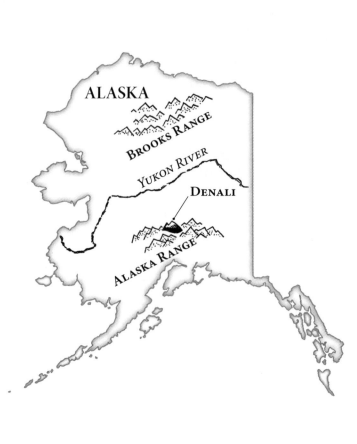

Epilogue
2013–2016

DENIED
ON
DENALI

SINCE COMPLETING THE 14ERS IN THE LOWER 48 WITH THAT CLIMB OF MOUNT Langley in 2012, I had been in a bit of a climbing funk. In 2013, I learned that I was only 800 hours shy of becoming vested in a small pension with UPS, and I could not let that pass me by, but it meant returning to New Hampshire to complete the hours. That spring, I gave some thought to climbing Denali anyway. I even set aside some money for the trip, but changed plans when my second daughter, Megan, announced she was getting married. The money went to much better use instead.

Climbing momentarily took a backseat to a job and I didn't want what began as an opportunity to become a burden. Somehow, though, I trained for and ran the inaugural Kodiak Ultra Marathon, a 100-miler in September 2013 in Big Bear Lake, California—incidentally put on by my friend, Paul Romero. I went out and surprised myself by winning the race, the greatest achievement of my running career.

My pension secured, I returned to Colorado after Christmas rush and settled back into Nancy's home, but things were no longer the same between us. Despite previously enduring all the time we spent apart, we suddenly found ourselves in what for me was all-too-familiar territory: on the verge of a breakup.

We made one last trip together to Europe in the fall of 2014; I went over in advance to climb Zugspitze, the highpoint of Germany. While there, we competed in the World Masters Mountain Running Championships in Austria, then spent several days touring Switzerland en route to that year's World Mountain Running Championships just outside Pisa, Italy.

By Christmas, when I finished up another stint at UPS—this time in Colorado Springs—it was apparent that our relationship had run its course. Hoping some more time apart might provide both of us with an opportunity to reassess, I headed to San Diego for the first few months of 2015 to stay with my brother and to umpire softball games in Southern California.

Around the same time, I was in negotiations to secure another film to promote, and I knew this one would require a commitment that far exceeded any of my previous deals. I believed *Run Free: The True Story of Caballo Blanco* would be well-received in the running world, and I wanted to see it succeed. My friend (and Caballo Blanco's once-girlfriend) Maria Walton was an executive producer on the film and put me in touch with the filmmaker, Sterling Noren. We reached an agreement for me to promote the film nationwide. I was honored by this opportunity, but also knew that to do it right—and to keep costs down— I could not fly between cities, rent cars, and stay in hotels on the tour, as I had done with other films. Instead, I decided to buy a van, convert it into a camper, and drive from city to city in one big loop around the United States.

This was not an entirely new idea for me. I had been telling Nancy for some time that I would like to buy a van to use when I traveled to races and to softball tournaments, but she hadn't taken me seriously and I never took the plunge. But with the acquisition of this film and Nancy's request that I move out as soon as possible, what had previously been mostly folly took on a sense of urgency. I located a 1998 Dodge Ram 1500 van on Craigslist a couple hours north in Greeley, Colorado, and drove with a friend to pick it up. The van was in immaculate condition considering its age and only had 114,000 miles on it. It also came equipped with some of the items I needed for the conversion, such as a power inverter, a second battery in the back, a microwave oven, and even a TV.

It took me about a month to transform the van and when I was done, I was quite impressed by how things turned out: I added a stove, a refrigerator, a bed, and a sink with running water—far more than I'd had when camping between 14ers and highpoints. It was everything I'd need to really live on the road. And then I was off.

First stop was back in Southern California, where I still had a couple more softball tournaments to umpire. After that, I spent most of the month of August parked at Ocean Beach in San Diego, working on scheduling shows for *Run Free* out of the back of the van. I had several people walk past and stop to admire the van, especially when I showed them the running water. I was told I had the coolest van on the beach, which was littered with other vagabonds living in their vehicles.

Life on the road has intrigued mankind ever since the invention of the automobile. Just consider the strength of the metaphor of putting life in the rearview mirror, for moving forward with our lives, never looking back and always wondering what lies ahead. "Nothing behind me, everything ahead of me, as is ever so on the road," were the poignant words of Jack Kerouac in *On the Road*. I settled into this life as comfortably as putting on a pair of slippers. Days and nights spent in roughly 60 square feet may not be comprehensible for some, but I found it entirely liberating. Everything I needed was in the van with me, except perhaps a place to shower, which I took care of with a membership to the YMCA.

By day, I drove from city to city, showing *Run Free* four nights a week, and at night I pulled over at truck stops or maybe a Walmart parking lot and drew down the window shades. No one knew I was inside. By morning, I would be on my way.

My tour, which eventually expanded to include 104 shows in the United States and Canada including twenty that sold out, took more than a year to complete. I made my way up the Pacific Coast into British Columbia, and then eastward across the northern United States where I arrived in New England in time to drive for UPS in New Hampshire for the final two weeks before Christmas. After the holidays, I was back on the road, heading south all the way to Florida and then back west across Texas to where the tour had begun in New Mexico fifty-four weeks before. In all, I drove more than 27,000 miles in the van, which performed remarkably well, breaking down only once—in Reno, Nevada— when a small transmission problem nearly sidelined me for a few days.

I wound down the tour in March 2016 in Silver City, New Mexico, for another sellout that included both Maria Walton and Sterling Noren in attendance. After the show, we all spent the weekend in the Gila National Forest—where Caballo Blanco had died in 2012—to celebrate his life with a memorial run that took us all to the exact spot where his body had been found four years before. It was a magical weekend among friends new and old and put a fitting climax on the tour.

One benefit of such a successful endeavor and all the work I'd put in with the film was that I'd saved enough for the Denali trip. I booked it for May 2016 with Mountain Trip, a guide service out of Telluride, Colorado. Despite my prefer- ence to avoid guided trips, Denali is the tallest mountain in North America and a 20,310-foot peak is not the place for the uninitiated. I knew it would be the harshest environment I had ever explored, and certainly more difficult than the Matterhorn, Rainier, or the Palisades. It was exciting to finally be going to Alaska—the only state I had yet to visit—but all that time on the road with the film had kept me from properly training for the expedition. I hoped my general fitness would carry me through and that I would fit in with the other climbers, who had all been training diligently, according to the emails we'd exchanged.

I arrived in Anchorage on May 1, and was picked up by Dave Hart, the engineer from Alaska whom I had first met high in the Palisades on that climb with Doug Seitz back in 2011. Dave and I became friends a year later when we corresponded online and climbed together when he came to Colorado to bag some Centennial 13ers.

Dave had previously climbed Denali and most all of the other big mountains in Alaska, and allowed me to stay with him and his family ahead of the trip. He even loaned me much of the equipment I needed for the climb. I met our guides and my fellow climbers later that week, just before packing up and being dropped off in the town of Talkeetna about two hours north of Anchorage, from where we would be flown in to the Kahiltna Glacier at 7,200 feet to begin our expedition up the standard West Buttress route.

We seemed to have a very strong team of eight climbers and we all gelled instantly. Scott, a fellow Vermonter, had previously summited Everest, but had struck out on a previous trip to Denali with Mountain Trip the year before. Brent, an attorney from Anchorage, had always wanted to climb Denali, though he still referred to the mountain by its Anglicized former name of Mount McKinley. That, too, was true of Mike, a surveyor from Anchorage who was the oldest of the group at 65.

Donn, from North Carolina, was a few days' shy of 60 when we started out and had been beaten back by Denali twenty years before: he had attempted the difficult West Rib route and was caught in a vicious storm that left him in the hospital for weeks with severe frostbite. Gustav, a Swiss native, had since relocated to the Bay Area. Grant, from Australia, had spent most of his adult life at sea, but was now making a name for himself on land, having recently summited Aconcagua in Argentina and having twice finished second in the Badwater 135 ultramarathon in Death Valley, which he was planning to run again a few weeks after our climb.

The final member of our team was Mario; at 24, he was half the age of the next youngest climber. A Nordic skier who had just gotten his masters at the University of Alaska–Anchorage the week before, Mario was headed back to his native Italy after the climb to get some good home cooking from his mom before starting a pending job in New York City in the fall. Our guides were Yoshiko, a Japanese woman with considerable alpine experience, and a pair of twenty-somethings from Colorado, Jeff and Josh.

After two days at base camp, we loaded up our packs and hauled our sleds on a 9-mile slog along the glacier to Camp 1, at 7,800 feet, where we stayed the next two nights. Then, we moved up to Camp 2, at 11,000 feet, and spent three more nights sleeping on the glacier and acclimatizing for the heights above.

At this point, we were all in great spirits, especially Mario, who had us laughing at every opportunity. Even the weather had been tame. We all thought it was a lock that we would summit. Finally, after a week on the mountain, we made our way to Camp 3, at 14,000 feet, from where the upper reaches of Denali seemed so close we could touch them. In two days' time, we figured, we would be making our bid for the summit.

But then the weather turned.

A day after our arrival at Camp 3, a storm rolled in from the Pacific. It was so severe that the Weather Service named it—Claude. It pinned us in our tents for eight nights waiting for the weather to break, but two additional storms piggybacked Claude and winds as high as 80 MPH were forecast for the mountain's upper reaches. Ominous lenticular clouds encircled the summit and the spindrift whipped off the ridge about 2,000 feet above us on the headwall, foretelling our future if we dared move higher.

We heard that others were at Camp 4, at 17,000 feet, awaiting a weather window in which to summit, but no word came from above as to whether anyone even attempted going higher, let alone succeeded. After nearly a week at Camp 3, the forecasts only seemed to get worse. Whereas we had all been "99 percent sure" we would summit once we had reached Camp 3, that number plummeted daily. By the end of the week it had shrunk to almost zero. Nightly temperatures were dropping to about 30 degrees below Fahrenheit. We were running out of food, as well as days in which to complete the trip. Finally, all any of us wanted to do was descend and get out of there.

Faced with this reality, morale continued to decline. Then, as he so often did, Mario came to our rescue. Faced with no prospects of ascending, Mario decided to have some fun. He orchestrated a pull-up contest among all the climbers in camp—of which there were upwards of fifty. Mario dug a deep hole in the snow and used some ice axes propped up on some blocks of snow for cross bars. A trekking pole served in place of a microphone as he emceed the event as if he was a game show host. He even tied with one of our guides, Josh, and another climber from Pennsylvania, for first place in the competition with twenty-two pull-ups. The winners received chunks of snow as trophies. The entire camp was in stitches even as most everyone there was accepting the fact that they probably would not summit.

Two days later we returned to Talkeetna and then to Anchorage where we parted ways after a big cookout hosted by Brent and his wife.

Had I succeeded in summiting Denali, I had planned to change my return flight by way of Hawaii, where I would have climbed Mauna Kea and completed the fifty state highpoints. But I decided to put that on hold while I contemplated whether I will return to Denali sometime in the future to try again. I don't think I will be able to afford to go guided again, but perhaps I might team up with some others—such as Grant—to try it on our own, since we now have a reasonably good idea of what it entails.

As this book goes to press, I am considering what other lists I might work on next as I continue to drive around living in my van. Sixteen years of peak-bagging and there still never seems to be a shortage of mountains to climb or lists to complete. Though Dave had previously told me that he was not interested in climbing Liberty Cap—the subsidiary summit on Rainier that represents the only ranked 14er in the lower 48 that either of us has not climbed—he has apparently changed his mind. At this writing, Dave and I have made plans to climb Rainier again and tag Liberty Cap in August 2016. While in the Pacific Northwest, I also hope to climb Mount Baker with Doug Seitz, and perhaps Washington State's Mount Adams as well.

Then, in the fall it's back East for the release of this book and, hopefully, to climb the remaining 46ers in the Adirondacks and, perhaps, that elusive Mount Fort in northern Maine, which would complete the AMC's Hundred Highest list.

If you need me, that's where you will find me.

BIBLIOGRAPHY

Adams, Jerome R. *Notable Latin American Women: Twenty-Nine Leaders, Rebels, Poets, Battlers and Spies, 1500–1900.* Jefferson, NC: McFarland, 1995.

Barcott, Bruce. "The Secret Life of Guides." *Outside,* December 1999.

Bearak, Barry. "Caballo Blanco's Last Run: The Micah True Story." *New York Times,* May 20, 2012.

Bernhardson, Wayne. *Moon Handbooks: Guatemala.* Emeryville, CA: Avalon Travel, 2001.

Blackison, A. Hooton. "Antigua—A City with a Wonderful Past." Supplement, *Scientific American*, no. 1841 (1911).

Blanc, Katherine. *The Boy Who Conquered Everest.* With Jordan Romero. Bloomington, IN: Balboa Press, 2010.

Bookman, Charles. "Incidents of Travel in Mexico." Unpublished essay. 2008.

Bookman, Zachary. "The Double L Bar." Unpublished essay. 2009.

Brain, Yossi. *Ecuador: A Climbing Guide.* Seattle: Mountaineers Books, 2000.

Brandon, Craig. *Monadnock: More Than a Mountain.* Keene, NH: Surry Cottage Books, 2007.

Elliott, Jack D., Jr. "Paving the Trace." *Journal of Mississippi History* 69, no. 3 (2007).

Farquhar, Francis P. *History of the Sierra Nevada.* Berkeley: University of California Press, 1969.

Fontana, Cyndee, and Mark Grossi. "Crashes in Sierra Have Spawned Legends, Tragedy." *Fresno Bee.* September 13, 2008.

Harrington, Bryon. *Campo: The Forgotten Gunfight*. CreateSpace, 2009.

Harrington, Garry. *Greetings from Gringotenango*. CreateSpace, 2010.

Harrington, Garry. "Cold Mountain." *Boston Globe Magazine*. March 28, 2004.

Henry, Emil. *Triumph and Tragedy: The Life of Edward Whymper*. Leicester, UK: Matador Press, 2011.

Hillsbery, Kief. "Airplane: A Modern Gold Rush." *Mountain Gazette*. December 1977/January 1978.

Hinton, Alexander Haban. *Why Did They Kill? Cambodia in the Shadow of Genocide*. Berkeley: University of California Press, 2005.

Holmes, Don W. *Highpoints of the United States*, 2nd ed. Salt Lake City: The University of Utah Press, 2000.

Howe, Nicholas. *Not Without Peril*. Tenth Anniversary Edition. Boston: Appalachian Mountain Club Books, 2009.

Huxley, Aldous. *Beyond the Mexique Bay*. New York: Vintage Books, 1934.

Kiernan, Ben. *The Pol Pot Regime: Race, Power and Genocide in Cambodia under the Khmer Rouge, 1975–1979*. New Haven, CT: Yale University Press, 1996.

Kerouac, Jack. *On the Road*. New York: Penguin, 1976.

Jenkins, Peter. *A Walk Across America*. New York: William Morrow, 1979.

Jenkins, Peter and Barbara Jenkins. *The Walk West: A Walk Across America 2*. New York: William Morrow, 1981.

Maynard, Joyce. "In Guatemala, a Torturous Drive to a Remote Eden." *New York Times*. September 12, 2012.

McDougall, Christopher. *Born to Run: A Hidden Tribe, Superathletes and the Greatest Race the World Has Never Seen*. New York: Alfred A. Knopf, 2009.

McKeating, Carl and Rachel Crolla. *Europe's High Points*. Cumbria, UK: Ciccerone, 2009.

Middleton, William D. *Yet There Isn't a Train I Wouldn't Take*. Bloomington: Indiana University Press, 2000.

Morgan Szybist, Richard. *The Lake Atitlan Reference Guide*. Panajachel, Guatemala: Adventuras in Education, USA, 2004.

Muir, John. "Snow-Storm on Mount Shasta." *Harper's New Monthly Magazine*. September, 1877.

Pohl, John, and Charles M. Robinson, III. *Aztecs and Conquistadors*. Oxford, UK: Osprey, 2005.

Porcella, Stephen F., and Cameron M. Burns. *Climbing California's Fourteeners*, rev. ed. Seattle: Mountaineers Books, 2008.

Pratt, Sara E. "Danger in Paradise: The Hidden Hazards of Volcano Geotourism." *Earth*. April 2012.

Restall, Matthew. *Seven Myths of the Spanish Conquest*. New York: Oxford University Press, 2003.

Rolfes, Ellen. "Sweating for Survival: Extreme Runners Race 135 Miles Through Death Valley." *The Rundown* (blog), *PBS Newshour*. July 16, 2013. pbs.org/newshour/rundown/sweating-for-survival-extreme-runners-race-135-miles-through-death-valley/.

Romero, Jordan. *No Summit out of Sight: The True Story of the Youngest Person to Climb the Seven Summits*. With Linda LeBlanc. New York: Simon & Schuster, 2014.

Schiller, Dane. "Texas Climbers Recount Death-defying Fall on Mount Rainier." *Houston Chronicle*. June 22, 2013.

Secor, R. J. *Mexico's Volanoes: A Climbing Guide*, 3rd ed. Seattle: Mountaineers Books, 2001.

Stephens, John L. *Incidents of Travel in Central America, Chaipas and Yucatan.* 2 vols. New York: Dover, 1969.

Terry, Fiona. *Condemned to Repeat? The Paradox of Humanitarian Action.* Ithaca, NY: Cornell University Press, 2002.

Whymper, Edward. *Scrambles Amongst the Alps in the Years 1860–69.* London: John Murray, 1871.

Wood, Michael. *Conquistadors.* Berkeley: University of California Press, 2000.

Yasso, Bart. *My Life on the Run: The Wit, Wisdom and Insights of a Road Racing Icon.* Emmaus, PA: Rodale Books, 2009.

ABOUT THE AUTHOR

GARRY HARRINGTON is a peakbagger, an ultramarathoner, a freelance sports-writer, and a film promoter. His writing has appeared in *The Boston Globe*, *The Kansas City Star*, among other publications. A New Hampshire native, Garry lives wherever his adventures take him.

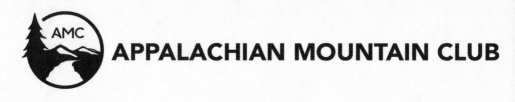

APPALACHIAN MOUNTAIN CLUB

At AMC, connecting you to the freedom and exhilaration of the outdoors is our calling. We help people of all ages and abilities to explore and develop a deep appreciation of the natural world.

AMC helps you get outdoors on your own, with family and friends, and through activities close to home and beyond. With chapters from Maine to Washington, D.C., including groups in Boston, New York City, and Philadelphia, you can enjoy activities like hiking, paddling, cycling, and skiing, and learn new outdoor skills. We offer advice, guidebooks, maps, and unique lodges and huts to inspire your next outing. You will also have the opportunity to support conservation advocacy and research, youth programming, and caring for 1,800 miles of trails.

We invite you to join us in the outdoors.

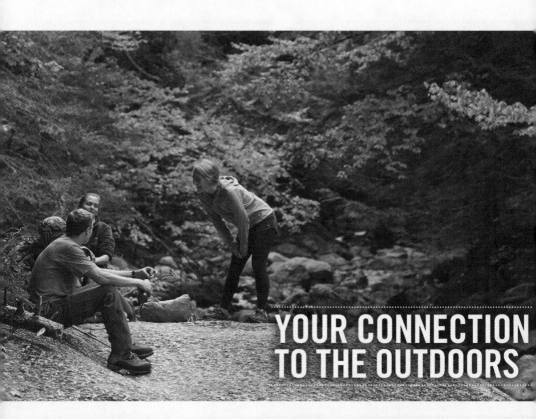

YOUR CONNECTION TO THE OUTDOORS

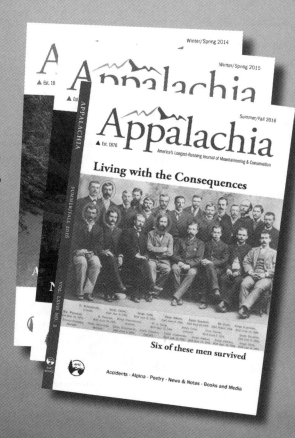

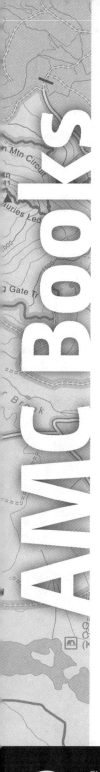
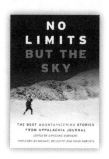
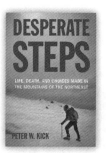
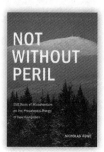
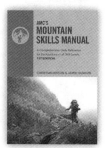

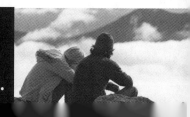